D0761496

SUCCESSFUL COGNITIVE AND EMOTIONAL AGING

SUCCESSFUL COGNITIVE AND EMOTIONAL AGING

Edited by

Colin A. Depp, Ph.D.

Dilip V. Jeste, M.D.

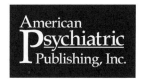

Washington, DC
London, England

If you would like to buy between 25 and 99 copies of this or any other APPI title, you are eligible for a 20% discount; please contact APPI Customer Service at appi@psych.org or 800-368-5777. If you wish to buy 100 or more copies of the same title, please e-mail us at bulksales@psych.org for a price quote.

Copyright © 2010 American Psychiatric Publishing, Inc.
ALL RIGHTS RESERVED

Manufactured in the United States of America on acid-free paper
13   12   11   10   09   5   4   3   2   1
First Edition

Typeset in Adobe's Berkley and Franklin Gothic

American Psychiatric Publishing, Inc.
1000 Wilson Boulevard
Arlington, VA 22209-3901
www.appi.org

Library of Congress Cataloging-in-Publication Data
Successful cognitive and emotional aging / edited by Colin A. Depp, Dilip V. Jeste. — 1st ed.
 p. ; cm.
 Includes bibliographical references and index.
 ISBN 978-1-58562-351-8 (alk. paper)
 1. Cognition in old age. 2. Emotions in old age. I. Depp, Colin A. II. Jeste, Dilip V. [DNLM: 1. Aged. 2. Cognition—physiology. 3. Aging—physiology. 4. Aging—psychology. 5. Cognition Disorders—prevention and control. 6. Emotions—physiology. WT 145 S942 2010]
 BF724.85.C64S83 2010
 155.67—dc22

                2009015493

British Library Cataloguing in Publication Data
A CIP record is available from the British Library.

To my wife Krista, parents Bonnie and Steven,
and grandparents Jane and Wallace
C.A.D.

To Kiran, Nischal, Neelum,
Shafali, Richard, and Sonali
D.V.J.

Contents

PART I Behavioral and Psychosocial Aspects

PART II Biological Aspects

PART III Prevention and Intervention Strategies

Contributors

Monika Ardelt, Ph.D.
Associate Professor, Department of Sociology and Criminology & Law, University of Florida, Gainesville, Florida

Sherry A. Beaudreau, Ph.D.
Clinical Assistant Professor, Department of Psychiatry and Behavioral Sciences, Stanford University School of Medicine, Palo Alto, California; Associate Director, MIRECC (Mental Illness Research, Education and Clinical Centers) Fellowship Program, Palo Alto VA Healthcare System, Palo Alto, California; Sierra-Pacific Mental Illness Research and Education Center, Palo Alto, California

Dan G. Blazer, M.D., Ph.D.
J.P. Gibbons Professor of Psychiatry and Behavioral Sciences, Duke University School of Medicine, Durham, North Carolina

Adam M. Brickman, Ph.D.
Assistant Professor of Neuropsychology, Cognitive Neuroscience Division, Taub Institute for Research on Alzheimer's Disease and the Aging Brain, Department of Neurology, College of Physicians and Surgeons, Columbia University, New York, New York

Ashley Cain, B.S.
Staff Research Associate, Department of Psychiatry, University of California, San Diego, School of Medicine

Susan Turk Charles, Ph.D.
Associate Professor, Department of Psychology and Social Behavior, University of California, Irvine

Sara J. Czaja, Ph.D.
Co-Director, Center on Aging; Professor, Department of Psychiatry and Behavioral Sciences, University of Miami Miller School of Medicine, Miami, Florida

Sharron E. Dawes, Ph.D.
Postdoctoral Fellow, Department of Psychiatry, University of California, San Diego, School of Medicine

Colin A. Depp, Ph.D.
Assistant Professor, Department of Psychiatry, University of California, San Diego, School of Medicine, La Jolla, California

Lisa T. Eyler, Ph.D.
Assistant Professor, Department of Psychiatry, University of California, San Diego, School of Medicine; Clinical Research Psychologist, VA San Diego Healthcare System, San Diego, California

Danny R. George, A.B.D., M.Sc.
Doctoral Candidate in Medical Anthropology, Institute of Social and Cultural Anthropology, University of Oxford, United Kingdom

Mina Hah, M.D.
Postdoctoral Fellow, National MIRECC (Mental Illness Research, Education and Clinical Centers) Fellowship Program, Palo Alto, California; Sierra-Pacific Mental Illness Research and Education Center and Department of Psychiatry and Behavioral Sciences, Stanford University School of Medicine, Palo Alto, California

Hugh C. Hendrie, M.B., Ch.B., D.Sc.
Professor, Department of Psychiatry, Indiana University School of Medicine, and Research Scientist, Indiana University Center for Aging Research, Regenstrief Institute, Inc., Indiana University School of Medicine, Indianapolis, Indiana

Briana N. Horwitz
Student, Department of Social Ecology Administration, University of California, Irvine

Jeffrey T. Hubbard, B.A.
Doctoral Student, University of Strasbourg, Strasbourg, France

Dilip V. Jeste, M.D.
Estelle and Edgar Levi Chair in Aging, Distinguished Professor of Psychiatry and Neurosciences, and Director, Sam and Rose Stein Institute for Research on Aging, University of California, San Diego, School of Medicine, La Jolla, California

Jacqueline Kerr, Ph.D.
Postdoctoral Employee, Department of Family and Preventive Medicine, University of California, San Diego, School of Medicine

Sanja Kovacevic, Ph.D.
Postdoctoral Scholar, Department of Psychiatry, University of California, San Diego, School of Medicine, San Diego, California

Avinoam Luzon, B.S.
Research Assistant, Department of Psychiatry and Behavioral Sciences, Stanford University School of Medicine, Palo Alto, California

Jennifer Margrett, Ph.D.
Assistant Professor, Department of Human Development and Family Studies, Iowa State University, Ames, Iowa

Peter Martin, Ph.D.
Professor, Department of Human Development and Family Studies, and Director, Gerontology Program, Iowa State University, Ames, Iowa

John Martin-Joy, M.D.
Visiting Clinical Instructor, Harvard Medical School and Brigham and Women's Hospital, Boston, Massachusetts; Research Associate, Study of Adult Development

Mark P. Mattson, Ph.D.
Chief, Laboratory of Neurosciences, National Institute on Aging Intramural Research Program, Baltimore, Maryland

Keith G. Meador, M.D., Th.M., M.P.H.
Professor of Psychiatry and Behavioral Sciences, Duke University School of Medicine, and Co-Director, Center for Spirituality, Theology, and Health, Duke University, Durham, North Carolina

Thomas Meeks, M.D.
Assistant Professor of Psychiatry, University of California, San Diego, La Jolla, California

Hunhui Oh, M.S.W., C.G.
Graduate Student, Department of Sociology and Criminology & Law, University of Florida, Gainesville, Florida

Ruth O'Hara, Ph.D.
Associate Professor, Department of Psychiatry and Behavioral Sciences, Stanford University School of Medicine, Palo Alto, California; Associate Director, Sierra-Pacific Mental Illness Research and Education Center, Palo Alto, California

Raymond L. Ownby, M.D., Ph.D., M.B.A.
Professor and Chair, Department of Psychiatry, Nova Southeastern University College of Medicine, Fort Lauderdale, Florida

Barton W. Palmer, Ph.D.
Professor, Department of Psychiatry, University of California, San Diego, School of Medicine

Kevin Patrick, M.D., M.S.
Professor, Department of Family and Preventive Medicine, University of California, San Diego, School of Medicine

Leonard W. Poon, Ph.D.
Distinguished Research Professor, Department of Health Policy and Management, and Director, Institute of Gerontology and Georgia Education Center, University of Georgia College of Public Health, Athens, Georgia

Christianna Purnell, B.A.
Research Coordinator, Indiana University Center for Aging Research, Regenstrief Institute, Inc., Indiana University School of Medicine, Indianapolis, Indiana

Brinda K. Rana, Ph.D.
Assistant Professor, Department of Psychiatry, University of California, San Diego, School of Medicine

Victoria Risbrough, Ph.D.
Assistant Professor, Department of Psychiatry, University of California, San Diego, School of Medicine; Center of Excellence for Stress and Mental Health, Veterans Affairs Hospital, San Diego, California

Cheryl L. Rock, Ph.D., R.D.
Professor, Department of Family and Preventive Medicine, University of California, San Diego, School of Medicine, Moores UCSD Cancer Center, La Jolla, California

Dori Rosenberg, M.P.H., M.S.
Doctoral Candidate, Joint Doctoral Program in Clinical Psychology, University of California, San Diego, School of Medicine, and San Diego State University

Karen L. Siedlecki, Ph.D.
Postdoctoral Research Fellow, Cognitive Neuroscience Division, Taub Institute for Research on Alzheimer's Disease and the Aging Brain, Department of Neurology, College of Physicians and Surgeons, Columbia University, New York, New York

Gary W. Small, M.D.
Parlow-Solomon Professor on Aging and Director, UCLA Center on Aging, Los Angeles, California

Barbara Sommer, M.D.
Director, Geriatric Psychiatry Program and Associate Professor, Department of Psychiatry and Behavioral Sciences, Stanford University School of Medicine, Stanford, California

Yaakov Stern, Ph.D.
Professor of Clinical Neuropsychology and Division Leader, Cognitive Neuroscience Division of the Gertrude H. Sergievsky Center, Taub Institute for Research on Alzheimer's Disease and the Aging Brain, Department of Neurology, College of Physicians and Surgeons, Columbia University, New York, New York

Ipsit V. Vahia, M.D.
Postdoctoral Fellow, Department of Psychiatry, University of California, San Diego, School of Medicine

George E. Vaillant, M.D.
Professor of Psychiatry, Harvard Medical School and Brigham and Women's Hospital, Boston, Massachusetts; Co-Director, Study of Adult Development

Sandra Weintraub, Ph.D.
Professor of Psychiatry and Behavioral Sciences, Cognitive Neurology and Alzheimer's Disease Center, Northwestern University, Feinberg School of Medicine, Chicago, Illinois

Catherine C. Whitehouse, Ph.D.
Principal, The Intergenerational School, Cleveland, Ohio

Peter J. Whitehouse, M.D., Ph.D.
Professor of Neurology, Case Western Reserve University School of Medicine; Attending Physician, University Hospitals Case Medical Center; Director, Adult Learning, The Intergenerational School, Cleveland, Ohio

Alissa H. Wicklund, Ph.D.
Research Neuropsychologist, Cognitive Neurology and Alzheimer's Disease Center, Northwestern University, Feinberg School of Medicine, Chicago, Illinois

Jared W. Young, Ph.D.
Postdoctoral Employee, Department of Psychiatry, University of California, San Diego, School of Medicine

The following contributors to this book have indicated a financial interest in or other affiliation with a commercial supporter, a manufacturer of a commercial product, a provider of a commercial service, a nongovernmental organization, and/or a government agency, as listed below:

Susan Turk Charles, Ph.D.—*Grant:* National Institute on Aging (NIA AG023845).

John Martin-Joy, M.D.—*Stock:* Family member has stock in three drug companies. The author does not have control over these investments.

The following contributors to this book have no competing interests or conflicts to declare:

Monika Ardelt, Ph.D.
Sherry A. Beaudreau, Ph.D.
Dan G. Blazer, M.D., Ph.D.
Adam M. Brickman, Ph.D.
Ashley Cain, B.S.
Sara J. Czaja, Ph.D.
Sharron E. Dawes, Ph.D.
Colin A. Depp, Ph.D.
Lisa T. Eyler, Ph.D.
Danny R. George, A.B.D., M.Sc.
Mina Hah, M.D.
Hugh C. Hendrie, M.B., Ch.B., D.Sc.
Briana N. Horwitz
Jeffrey T. Hubbard, B.A.
Dilip V. Jeste, M.D.
Jacqueline Kerr, Ph.D.
Sanja Kovacevic, Ph.D.
Avinoam Luzon, B.S.
Jennifer Margrett, Ph.D.
Peter Martin, Ph.D.
Mark P. Mattson, Ph.D.
Keith G. Meador, M.D., Th.M., M.P.H.
Thomas Meeks, M.D.
Hunhui Oh, M.S.W., C.G.
Ruth O'Hara, Ph.D.
Raymond L. Ownby, M.D., Ph.D., M.B.A.
Barton W. Palmer, Ph.D.
Kevin Patrick, M.D., M.S.
Leonard W. Poon, Ph.D.
Christianna Purnell, B.A.

Brinda K. Rana, Ph.D.
Victoria Risbrough, Ph.D.
Cheryl L. Rock, Ph.D., R.D.
Dori Rosenberg, M.P.H., M.S.
Karen L. Siedlecki, Ph.D.
Barbara Sommer, M.D.
Yaakov Stern, Ph.D.
Ipsit V. Vahia, M.D.
George E. Vaillant, M.D.
Sandra Weintraub, Ph.D.
Catherine C. Whitehouse, Ph.D.
Peter J. Whitehouse, M.D., Ph.D.
Alissa H. Wicklund, Ph.D.
Jared W. Young, Ph.D.

Foreword

Gary W. Small, M.D.

Remarkable advances in medical technology have increased life expectancy. The average woman today can anticipate living to age 81 and the average man to 75 years. Recent estimates indicate that the number of older adults in the United States will nearly double by 2030. We are living longer but, unfortunately, not necessarily better. While many older adults remain independent and healthy well beyond age 65, more than three-quarters of them suffer from at least one chronic medical condition, such as Alzheimer disease, Parkinson disease, arthritis, heart disease, hypertension, and diabetes. The management and accompanying costs of these illnesses exceed $200 billion annually, challenging an already burdened Medicare program. As the nation's 80 million baby boomers turn 65 and grow older, our nation faces an impending social, financial, and health care crisis.

Despite greater recognition of the needs of our older population and attempts to overcome widespread ageism, society continues to emphasize youth as the ideal. The media have focused their marketing strategies on youthful looks and attitudes to attract consumers to their products; however, recently, we are witnessing a shift in tactics. Instead of pursuing youthful demographics, there is an emphasis on "psychographics"—marketing focused toward the age group that consumers actually *perceive* themselves as being in. Today's 78 million baby boomers tend to consider themselves mentally and physically younger than their actual physical age. Many will confess they still have the attitude of a 20-year-old and feel nowhere near their chronological age.

Most of us protest against the idea of aging in the way our parents did and vow to fight against the process as long as possible. While consumers continue to search for safe, convenient, medically sound ways to live longer and remain healthy and fulfilled throughout that long life, scientists are pushing forward to understand, define, and promote successful aging. The Mac-Arthur Study of Successful Aging helped gerontologists shift their research emphasis from illness to wellness. Among other important lessons, it taught us that genetics accounts for only about one-third of what determines health as people age. Thus, nongenetic factors—healthy lifestyle strategies and medical advances to prevent and ameliorate age-related illnesses—can have a major influence on how well and how long each person lives.

And these nongenetic factors could potentially result in major benefits to the public's health and well-being. For example, in one study, positive and satisfied middle-aged people were twice as likely to survive over 20 years compared with more negative individuals. Optimists have fewer physical and emotional difficulties, experience less pain, enjoy higher energy levels, and are generally happier and calmer in their lives. Positive thinking has been found to boost the body's immune system so we can better fight infection.

Diabetes afflicts 16 million individuals in the United States, while Alzheimer disease and milder cognitive declines debilitate another 10 million people. Regular physical exercise alone has been shown to have an impact in lowering the risk for these illnesses and possibly preventing them. Several studies have demonstrated the significant cognitive benefits from memory training, which can be sustained for years. Although stimulating our minds has not yet been proven to protect brain health, several studies have demonstrated a significant association between mentally stimulating leisure activities like reading, doing crossword puzzles, or playing board games, and a lower the risk for Alzheimer disease. Recent estimates suggest that if nearly every individual in the United States adopted just one healthy lifestyle habit (e.g., eating fish twice each week or taking a daily brisk walk), the incidence of Alzheimer disease would be lowered substantially and the estimated number of cases would be reduced by one million within the next 5 years. Given that Alzheimer disease alone costs the United States over $100 billion annually, teaching and encouraging successful aging lifestyles could have a considerable financial and social impact

This new science of successful aging spans a range of topics, and in this volume, Professors Depp and Jeste have done a remarkable job in bringing together some of the foremost experts in the field to update the reader. In addition to cognitive and physical approaches, the role of nutrition, spirituality, positive outlook, resilience, and other emotional factors are thoughtfully addressed. Relatively new topics, such as the impact of technology on healthy aging, are included as well. I am optimistic that we will witness major breakthroughs in the biological and medical technologies to further improve quality of life as we age, and chapters on molecular genetics, animal models, and biomarkers are appropriately included. *Successful Cognitive and Emotional Aging* is an important and timely volume that will become a valuable resource for students and researchers in the field who want a broad and scholarly overview of this exciting and rapidly developing field.

Parlow-Solomon Professor on Agin and Director, UCLA Center on Aging

Bibliography

Ball K, Berch DB, Helmers KF, et al: Effects of cognitive training interventions with older adults: a randomized controlled trial. JAMA 288:2271–2281, 2002

Barberger-Gateau P, Letenneur L, Deschamps V, et al : Fish, meat, and risk of dementia: cohort study. Br Med J 395:932–933, 2002

Colcombe SJ, Erickson KI, Raz N, et al: Aerobic fitness reduces brain tissue loss in aging humans. J Gerontol: Med Sci 58A:176–180, 2003

de Lorgeril M, Salen P, Martin J-L, et al: Mediterranean diet, traditional risk factors, and the rate of cardiovascular complications after myocardial infarction: final report of the Lyon Diet Heart Study. Circulation 99:779–785, 1999

Del Ser T, Hachinski V, Merskey H, et al: An autopsy-verified study of the effect of education on degenerative dementia. Brain 122:2309–2319, 1999

Dickey RA, Janick JJ: Lifestyle modifications in the prevention and treatment of hypertension. Public Health Nutr 2:383–390, 1999

Eriksson J, Lindström J, Tuomilehto J: Potential for the prevention of type 2 diabetes. Br Med Bull 60:183–199, 2001

Kahn RL, Rowe JW: Successful Aging. Pantheon, New York, 1998

Knoops KTB, de Groot LCPGM, Kromhout D, et al: Mediterranean diet, lifestyle factors, and 10-year mortality in elderly European men and women. JAMA 292:1433–1439, 2004

Menec VH: The relation between everyday activities and successful aging: a 6-year longitudinal study. J Gerontol Series B: Psychol Sci Soc Sci 58:S74–S82, 2003

Small G, Vorgan G: The Longevity Bible. New York, Hyperion, 2006

Small G, Vorgan G: iBrain: Surviving the Technological Alteration of the Modern Mind. New York, HarperCollins, 2008

Verghese J, Lipton RB, Katz MJ, et al: Leisure activities and the risk of dementia in the elderly. N Engl J Med 348:2508–2516, 2003

1

Phenotypes of Successful Aging

Historical Overview

Colin A. Depp, Ph.D.
Dilip V. Jeste, M.D.

> But it is not enough for a great nation merely to add to
> the years of life. Our object also must be to add new life
> to those years.
>
> *John F. Kennedy (1963)*

> To get back my youth, I would do anything in the world,
> except take exercise, get up early, or be respectable.
>
> *Oscar Wilde (1891)*

Media attention regarding the "graying of the world" and the "age crisis" often overshadows the tremendous positive changes to the human life span and health span that have occurred during the past 100 years. In the United States, the number of Americans age 65 and older has increased from 3 million in 1900 to 35 million today (U.S. Census Bureau 2001). Yet this historical rise will be dwarfed by the rise that will begin in the year 2011 when the oldest of the baby boomers (those born between the years 1946 and 1964) reach age 65—the traditional definition of "old age." The number of people over age 65 will rise to nearly 70 million (20% of the population) by 2030. The fastest-growing segment of the population in the United States is that of individuals over age 85. The 85-year-and-older age group is expected to increase from about 3 million in 2008 to more than 18 million in 2050. To put these changes in historical perspective, the number of adults over age 60 will outnumber children under 14 for the first time in recorded history (White House Conference on Aging 1996), and two-thirds of all the people in the entire history of the world who have reached the age of 65 are alive today.

People now have a better chance of living to 100 than ever before. While there were only about 5,000 centenarians in the United States in 1900, today there are 125,000 people over age 100 (U.S. Census Bureau 2001). By 2050, that number is expected to reach 835,000. In addition to more of us living longer, older people are far healthier now than their predecessors of just a few generations ago. In Fogel's (2005) pioneering studies contrasting Civil War era soldiers with their modern descendants, the average male has gained 4 inches in height and 50 pounds in weight in just over 150 years. Whereas infectious diseases were the most common cause of our demise, now, by far, the most common causes of death in the United States are age related (cardio-vascular disease, cancer, and stroke). Furthermore, the mean age at onset of these age-related chronic illnesses, comparing the Civil War cohort with current data, is about 10 years later. These remarkable changes to the age distribution of our species, and the increasing prominence of age-related diseases as determinants of mortality, have made aging the number one public health issue faced by the developed world (Cutler and Mattson 2006).

Along with our need to understand and treat pathological aging (e.g., identifying early prodromes of Alzheimer disease), a complementary body of scientific literature has emerged to define what differentiates "successful" from normal aging. It is an understatement to say that little consensus exists as to what that the definition of *successful aging* is or should be—indeed, there is even disagreement on the descriptor to be used (e.g., *successful aging, robust aging, healthy aging, optimal aging, productive aging*). For a variety of reasons, we argue that definitions, and the concept of healthy aging, will increasingly center on the brain and cognitive and emotional health. In this chapter, we review the historical precedent to today's definitions of successful aging, survey the breadth of definitions of successful aging, and present a rationale for why cognitive and emotional health may become more central to these definitions and to interventions tied to aging. We close this chapter with an overview of the contents of this book.

Historical Definitions of Successful Aging

Although the term *successful aging* might not have appeared in ancient texts, human cultures have long and often unsuccessfully grappled with why we age and what to do about it. A sampling of these early conceptualizations reveals the roots of modern thinking about aging (Birren and Schroots 2001).

Aristotle (384–322 B.C.) was not particularly kind to older adults, describing them as follows:

> They have lived many years; they have often been taken in, and often made mistakes; and life on the whole is bad business. The result is that they are sure about nothing and *underdo* everything. They "think," but they never "know"; and because of their hesitation they always add a "possibly" or a "perhaps," putting everything this way and nothing positively. They are cynical; that is, they tend to put the worst construction on everything. Furthermore, their experience makes them distrustful and therefore suspicious of evil....They are small-minded, because they have been humbled by life....They are not generous, because money is one of the things that they must have....They are cowardly, and are always anticipating danger....They are too fond of themselves....They are not shy, but shameless rather....They lack confidence in the future...They live by memory rather than hope. (Aristotle *Rhetoric* 2:12–14; quoted in Birren and Schroots 2001, pp. 7–8)

The explanation for aging at the time corresponded with the humoral theory of health, in which balance of bodily humors dictated the absence or presence of disease. Aging was interpreted by Aristotle and later by Galen as a primary process involving drying and cooling of the body. Thus, to Aristotle, the model of aging corresponded to deterioration and was a disease unto itself—counteracting this deterioration was all that one could hope to accomplish.

A more positive view of aging came from Cicero (106–43 BC), who, in his fascinating essay on aging titled *De Senectute* (Cicero 2001), systematically provided counterpoints to the assumptions that aging was an inevitable "disease." Among his arguments, Cicero noted that aging persons could transition to advisory roles if they could no longer pursue active work. He asked: "Are there then no old men's employments to be after all conducted by the intellect, even when bodies are weak?" (para. 14).

Cicero further noted that the diminution of pleasures in life, and the related decrease in consumptive desires (e.g., libido), might lead to the pursuit of more virtue. Furthermore, he suggested that memory impairment might be a cause of not using the mind rather than a primary process, suggesting a behavioral component to the rate of decline:

But, it is said, memory dwindles. No doubt, unless you keep it in practice, or if you happen to be somewhat dull by nature....Old men retain their intellects well enough, if only they keep their minds active and fully employed. (Cicero 2001, para. 16)

Cicero added that memory is less impaired for things that truly matter—"*Nor, in point of fact, have I ever heard of any old man forgetting where he had hidden his money*" (para. 16). Cicero's model of aging, in contrast to Aristotle's, provided some hope that healthy aging could be attained, framed in terms of adaptation to physiological changes.

Long before Aristotle or Cicero, Chinese texts provided proscriptions for attaining the goal of longevity. The concept of *yang sheng*, translated as "cultivating life," invokes a number of practices that were thought to lengthen the life span, including regular exercise (e.g., *qi gong*), balancing exertion with rest, and coordinating daily life with the rhythms of nature. Chinese approaches to healthy aging provide a stark contrast with Aristotle's in their reverence for the pursuit of longevity. The role of preventive behaviors in lengthening life is seen in these texts. The themes of deterioration, adaptation, and prevention persist today, as we still grapple with the question of why we age and what we can do about it.

In the early twentieth century, during the emergence of the fields of psychology and psychiatry, the emphasis placed on late-life development varied (Jeste 1997). Some authors such as Freud placed much, if not all, of the action of personality development in childhood and young adulthood, whereas other authors extended their models of development into late life. Most psychiatrists today would not agree with Freud's assertion in 1924 that near or above the age of 50, the "elasticity of mental processes is lacking and, therefore, older individuals are no longer educable." Erik Erikson extended his concept of the stages of development to the end of life, and he depicted positive outcomes in the last stage in terms of reconciliation of the past, contrasted with despair. Jung wrote about the concept of wisdom that could be attained in older age through introspection. Each of these theories was largely based on observations that, although astute, did not derive from systematic scientific observation.

Successful Aging: Emergence as a Research Focus

The first concerted efforts to define healthy aging corresponded with the birth of gerontology as a distinct discipline. In the first issue of *The Gerontologist* in 1961, editor Robert Havighurst called for more research on the determinants of successful aging. Drawing from the Kansas City Studies of Adult Life, Havighurst defined successful aging as "getting a maximum of satisfaction out of life" (Havighurst 1961). His contemporaries Cumming and Henry (1961) developed the *disengagement theory,* one of the first empirically based gerontological theories; disengagement was depicted as the withdrawal from social contacts and from productivity as a natural and functional process in aging. Later theorists (Lemon et al. 1972; Ryff 1982; Atchley 1989) challenged whether disengagement was desirable, instead depicting healthy aging as the maintenance of preferred activities of middle age (the *continuity theory*) and engagement in meaningful activities (the *activity theory*).

Although authors disagreed on the concept of successful aging, it was agreed that longevity in and of itself was not the ideal phenotype with which to measure healthy aging. In 1980, Fries authored a pivotal paper on the concept of *compression of morbidity* (Fries 1980), essentially arguing that medical advances might yield two scenarios, one in which the life span is lengthened but so, too, is the duration of time spent disabled (*extension of morbidity*), and another in which a delay in the onset of disability is emphasized (compression of morbidity). Thus, the time spent free of disability, or the *health span,* was proposed as a better marker for public health policies in relation to aging than longevity, and it was argued that efforts to address aging should target the compression of morbidity at least as much as the expansion of longevity.

Although they helped push the field of successful aging forward, what the above theories often lacked was integration with the biology of aging. In a landmark paper in the journal *Science,* Rowe and Kahn (1987) posited that successful aging is on the upper end of a continuum that extends from pathology to normal aging to successful aging, and that, to a fault, much of the body of research on aging was dedicated to distinguishing pathological from normal aging. On the basis of this article, a model of successful aging was proposed, with three components:

1. Freedom from disability and disease
2. High cognitive and physical functioning
3. Social engagement (in terms of both social and productive activities)

This definition was operationalized and studied extensively by the MacArthur Research Network on Successful Aging in a cohort study that followed a sample of more than 1,000 older adults who met these criteria (Rowe and Kahn 1999).

Another model of successful aging was the *Selection, Optimization, and Compensation* model, proposed by the German psychologist Baltes and colleagues (Baltes 1997). On the basis of longitudinal investigations, the Berlin Aging Study, Baltes conceptualized successful adaptation to aging in developmental terms. Several interlocking components were involved:

1. Selective optimization, or restriction of the range of activities to a smaller set and an increase in practice of selected activities
2. Compensation, or alteration of behavioral patterns to attain similar performance

A tennis player who has experienced decreased speed and power, for example, may work to emphasize and perfect a specific shot, and may work to enhance accuracy in placement to compensate for losses in power. Together, these models propelled the study of successful aging into a broader biopsychosocial context.

Larger Quantitative Studies

A number of quantitative studies have attempted to operationalize various sets of criteria in an effort to identify the characteristics of the subgroup of persons who were successfully aging. Phelan and Larson (2002) conducted extensive reviews of this body of literature, as did we (Depp and Jeste 2006). In our 2006 attempt at a comprehensive review, among peer-reviewed English-language studies with samples of more than 100 older (>60 years of age) adults each, we found a total of 28 reports that had an operational definition of successful aging. These 28 studies had remarkable diversity in the definitions employed; in fact, there were 29 different definitions (one study had two), and each varied in terms of components, measures, and cutoffs on those measures. What most studies agreed on was that physical functioning/ freedom from disability was a component of successful aging. However, no other component appeared in more than half of the definitions (Figure 1–1).

Because of the wide variation in the definitions used, the prevalence of successful aging among these studies varied from 1% to 94%. When one teases apart which components of these definitions led to exclusion of the most older individuals, those definitions that did not exclude individuals on the basis of chronic diseases and/or physical disabilities were associated with a higher proportion of people who were categorized as having aged successfully. This is consistent with findings from The Cache County Memory Study (Østbye et al. 2006), which examined indicators of cognitive and emotional health separately from indicators of physical health. That study found that a majority of older adults sampled were cognitively intact, were satisfied with life, and had adequate social networks. Physical functioning and disability appeared as both the primary domain measured in defining

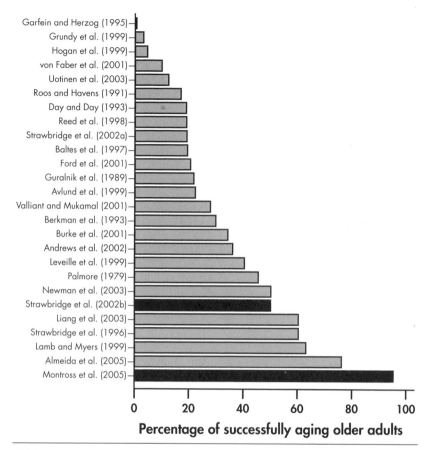

FIGURE 1–1. Reported proportion of persons who were aging successfully, by study.

Note. Among peer-reviewed English-language studies with samples of more than
100 older adults (>60 years of age) each. The two deeply shaded bars represent self-
rated successful aging. Other bars represent researcher-defined successful aging. Of
the 28 studies, 2 used continuous definitions, so these studies were not included in
this figure. See Depp and Jeste 2006 for study citations.
Source. Reprinted from Depp CA, Jeste DV: "Definitions and Predictors of Successful Aging: A Comprehensive Review of Larger Quantitative Studies." *American Journal of Geriatric Psychiatry* 14:6–20, 2006. Used with permission.

successful aging and the primary limiting factor in excluding people from
meeting criteria for successful aging. Of course, the lack of agreement on
definitions used limits the capacity of the field to yield consistent findings
on the contributors to successful aging. It also highlights how difficult it is
to characterize a positive attribute, such as successful aging.

Qualitative Studies

In their review of the literature on successful aging, Phelan and Larson (2002) concluded that the definitions of successful aging too often fail to capture the perspective of older adults themselves about what constitutes successful aging. A small body of literature has used qualitative methods, including personal interviews, surveys, and focus groups, to obtain definitions of successful aging (Reichstadt et al. 2007; von Faber et al. 2001). Among the striking discrepancies from the qualitative data described above, most older adults believe they are aging well, in contrast to the more restrictive attempts of researchers in defining successfully aging adults (Montross et al. 2006; Reichstadt et al. 2007; von Faber et al. 2001). (The age-related divergence in subjective estimations of health from objective measures was described by Baltes [1997].) In addition, when asked what constitutes a definition of successful aging, older adults appear to emphasize psychological factors, such as having a positive outlook, being adaptable, and being happy, over being free of chronic disabilities and diseases (Reichstadt et al. 2007). This contrast corresponds to the paradox in gerontology in which known contributors to depression (e.g., disability, disease) increase in incidence with age, whereas the frequency of depressive symptoms and negative affect appears to decrease. Finally, these qualitative studies highlight the importance of cultural context in defining successful aging—for example, Western ideals of independence and youth likely make for a different conception of successful aging than Eastern ideals of familial piety. In one study, "independence" was ranked as less salient to successful aging among Japanese older adults asked to define successful aging than among seniors in the United States (Phelan et al. 2004).

Intermediate Phenotypes and Biomarkers of Aging

Parallel to studies examining successful aging, there have been increasing numbers of empirical efforts to develop indices of biological age, or *aging biomarkers*. According to Karasik et al. (2005), these biomarkers would track the rate of biological aging, defined by their ability to predict functioning and/or mortality better than chronological age does. These biomarkers would, in their ideal form, be indicators of basic processes, not disease effects, and, ideally, would be translatable across species. One could thus define successful biological aging as being biologically younger than what would be predicted by one's chronological age. A repeatable biomarker of aging would be a potential outcome of interventions to enhance basic processes in aging.

As with the definitions of successful aging, there is no single "panel" of biomarkers that represents biological age to date. Considerable research is currently being conducted to identify the most sensitive and specific combinations of biomarkers to create indices. Much excitement has surrounded research on the *telomere,* the region of the chromosome that protects a cell from fusing with other cells. The telomere shortens with successful cell replications, and thus can provide an indicator of the number of replications a cell has undergone—seen as a marker for cellular aging. Landmark studies have also shown that environmental stress can accelerate the shortening of the telomere, and theoretically accelerate aging (Epel et al. 2004). Other aging-related biomarkers combine multiple markers of basic physiological data to form indices of oxidative stress, or *allostatic load* (see Chapter 10, "Stress, Resilience, and the Aging Brain"). Similar approaches to cognitive functioning have been used. Although these indices of biological age may not be as tangible to the public as is well-being or disability, assays likely offer promise in their ability to provide reliable biologically based mechanisms of the aging process.

What Can Be Said About Definitions of Successful Aging?

Although successful aging remains a somewhat elusive construct, one can conclude a few things about its definition:

1. Longevity is not necessarily the ideal phenotype; certainly extending longevity is a less ideal goal than maximizing the number of well years, howsoever defined.
2. No single dimension or attribute used to measure successful aging appears to be satisfactory; therefore, nearly all attempts have combined multiple indicators to form composite indices of successful aging.
3. The prevalence of successful aging depends on what is being assessed and who is being asked, because objective definitions are often centered on the absence of physical illnesses and disability and, as a result, typically exclude most elderly people from being considered to have aged successfully. In contrast, most elderly people believe they are aging well, as their definitions emphasize adaptations to physical changes.

   The discrepancy between researcher-defined and layperson-defined concepts of successful aging is an important issue, and one that harks back to the debate among ancient Greek philosophers. Much depends on whether optimal aging is seen as the avoidance or deceleration of deterioration, as Aristotle might have seen it, or whether it represents adaptation to deterioration, as portrayed by Cicero.

4. Many of the quantitative studies of successful aging have derived data from studies that were aimed at monitoring physical disease progression (e.g., cardiovascular disease). Therefore, measurements in some arenas (e.g., cognitive functioning) may not have been adequately sensitive to differentiate supranormal from normal performance, and, more importantly, some constructs such as resilience or positive attitudes were unmeasured.

Importance of Cognitive and Emotional Aging

There are several reasons why the concept of successful aging may increasingly hinge on cognitive and emotional phenotypes. By *cognitive aging*, we are referring not only to traditional neuropsychological domains such as memory and executive function, but also to broader constructs such as cognitive schemas and wisdom. In terms of *emotional aging*, we are referring to constructs that extend beyond the absence of depression or anxiety, to include optimism, personal mastery, and other cognitive-emotional constructs. From our review of quantitative studies of successful aging, it seems clear that cognitive and emotional domains have been less well studied than physical attributes. Many of the studies we reviewed used measures designed to rule out dementia or depression and that lack sensitivity in distinguishing between normal and successful aging. The same can be said for freedom from depression, which does not portray the great variability in well-being among those who are not depressed. Therefore, cognitive and emotional aging represent a new frontier in terms of systematic approaches to defining successful aging.

We anticipate that brain health, and the modulation and delay of degenerative brain diseases, may become more relevant to functioning with aging. Fogel (2005) and others have shown that the onset of chronic medical illnesses, such as cardiovascular disease, has been pushed to later in the life span, with a dividend of research on treatments for these diseases. In contrast, current treatments for brain illnesses, such as Alzheimer disease, appear to slow, but not reverse, the effects of the disease process. Signs of the increasing prominence of brain illnesses are already apparent: as of 2008, Alzheimer disease was the sixth leading cause of death in the United States, supplanting diabetes (Alzheimer's Association 2009). Therefore, brain health may become more of a rate-limiting factor in extending the health span, as the care for cardiovascular and other chronic illnesses improves.

As Cutler and Mattson (2006) point out, even if any one of the major chronic illnesses were eliminated, the total gain in years of life would be less than 10 years on average. Most older individuals will have chronic illnesses of aging, at least for now. In a study of centenarians, very few had avoided chronic illnesses; most had survived with some chronic illness (Perls et al. 2002). It may therefore be unreasonable to depict successful aging as involving freedom from deterioration due to disease or disability; rather, the adaptation to those diseases and disabilities may define success.

Behavioral adaptation is mediated by the brain. Much of the burden of chronic diseases and disabilities experienced by older people involves substantial behavioral components. Diet, exercise, and cognitive stimulation all need to start with motivation for lifestyle change. Furthermore, if positive health behaviors are our best strategy toward promoting successful aging, then emotional distress and depression can be seen as primary obstacles to healthy lifestyles. Social engagement, nutrition, stress resistance, and physical activity are all negatively impacted by depression across the life span. Conversely, social and physical activity interventions appear to have antidepressant effects as well as perhaps cognitive-enhancing properties in older people.

Our review suggests that older adults themselves tend to cite cognitive and emotional constructs as being more central to successful aging (e.g., having a positive attitude, being socially engaged) than physical aspects. The views of older people on the topic of successful aging are important, because any public health intervention must first take into account the desired goals of the target population. On the subject of intervention, an impressive body of translational research and a handful of large-scale clinical trials have dispelled notions about the inflexibility of the aging brain (see Chapter 17, "Cognitive Interventions." for review). Thus, physical activity, cognitive training, and other interventions lead to improvements in cognitive functioning and even brain structure. Furthermore, depression treatments work about as well in older people as they do in younger people (Centers for Disease Control and Prevention 2007). However, older adults are most at risk for sedentary lifestyles, and they are least likely to get treatment for depression (2007). Therefore, the opportunities to enhance the health of an aging global population through targeting cognitive and emotional interventions are both immense and challenging. We expect (and hope) that mental health researchers and practitioners will play an increasing role in developing and implementing interventions directed toward successful aging.

Overview of This Book

In this text, our aim is to provide an overview of the state of science in the biological, psychological, and social aspects of cognitive and emotional health. We have divided the book into three parts: 1) behavioral and psychosocial aspects, 2) biological aspects, and 3) prevention and intervention strategies.

In the first part, the view of cognitive and emotional health from the U.S. National Institutes of Health is described by Hendrie and colleagues (Chapter 2, "Defining and Assessing Cognitive and Emotional Health in Later Life"). Then, in Chapters 3 ("Cognitive Aging") and 4 ("Positive Emotions and Health"), the fundamentals of cognitive, emotional, and personality aging are reviewed. Next, two domains that have long captured the interest of gerontologists—spirituality and wisdom—are described (Chapters 5, "The Role of Spirituality in Healthy Aging," and 6, "Wisdom"). In the last chapter (Chapter 7, "Cognition and Emotion in Centenarians"), the status of the above constructs in the oldest of the old, the centenarians, is discussed.

The second part covers cognitive and emotional aging from the basic sciences perspective. The revolutionary capacity to understand the brain with neuroimaging is discussed, in Chapter 8 ("Neuroimaging of Successful Cognitive and Emotional Aging"), in relationship to aging and healthy aging. The concept of cognitive and brain reserve is described in depth by Brickman et al. (Chapter 9, "Cognitive and Brain Reserve"). The fascinating processes involved in cellular aging, as they relate to environmental influences of stress and dietary intake, are discussed in Chapters 10 ("Stress, Resilience, and the Aging Brain) and 11 ("Influence of Dietary Factors on Brain Aging and the Pathogenesis of Alzheimer Disease"). The last two chapters show how the array of techniques used in genetics/genomics (Chapter 12, "Molecular Genetic Building Blocks of Successful Cognitive and Emotional Aging") and animal models (Chapter 13, "Animal Models of Successful Cognitive Aging") can accelerate hypothesis testing in understanding cognitive aging and lead to potential interventions.

In the third, and final, part, we cover what may be most of interest to readers: interventions to enhance cognitive and emotional aging. The status of the current evidence base for physical activity (Chapter 14, "Creating Environments to Encourage Physical Activity"), dietary recommendations (Chapter 15, "Diet, Nutritional Factors, and the Aging Brain"), and pharmacotherapy (Chapter 16, "Pharmacological Approaches to Successful Cognitive and Emotional Aging") is reviewed. The evidence for traditional and nontraditional approaches to cognitive stimulation and interventions (Chapter 17, "Cognitive Interventions") is summarized. The "digital divide" and the potential uses of technology in enhancing adaptation to aging (Chapter 18, "Aging, Cognition, and Technology") are discussed. Finally, two long-standing efforts in the field of aging and mental health are described—one, a 70-year longitudinal study that reveals some of the coping strategies that seem to bring about well-being in older age (Chapter 19, "Recognizing and Promoting Resilience"); the other, an innovative intergenerational program that shows the potent impact of meaningful activity on both older adults and the community (Chapter 20, "Gaining Wisdom Through Multiage Learning").

In the epilogue, which draws from all the chapters in this book, we attempt to consolidate the empirical base and provide a user-friendly collection of strategies for enhancing cognitive and emotional aging. It is our sincere hope that, with much left to know, this book will convince its readers that there is a rapidly developing and scientifically sound basis for optimism about cognitive and emotional aging.

References

Alzheimer's Association: 2009 Alzheimer's Disease Facts and Figures. Chicago, IL, Alzheimer's Association, 2009 [Alzheimer's & Dementia 5(3)]

Atchley RC: A continuity theory of normal aging. Gerontologist 29:183–190, 1989

Baltes PB: On the incomplete architecture of human ontogeny. Am Psychol 52:366–380, 1997

Birren JE, Schroots JJF: The history of geropsychology, in Handbook of the Psychology of Aging, 5th Edition. Edited by Birren JE, Schaie KW. San Diego, Academic Press, 2001, pp 3–28

Centers for Disease Control and Prevention and The Merck Company Foundation: The State of Aging and Health in America 2007. Whitehouse Station, NJ, The Merck Company Foundation, 2007

Cicero MT: On old age, in The Harvard Classics, Vol 11. New York, PF Collier, 2001, pp 1909–1914

Cumming E, Henry WE: Growing Old: The Process of Disengagement. New York, Basic Books, 1961

Cutler RG, Mattson MP: The adversities of aging. Ageing Res Rev 5:221–238, 2006

Depp CA, Jeste DV: Definitions and predictors of successful aging: a comprehensive review of larger quantitative studies. Am J Geriatr Psychiatry 14:6–20, 2006

Epel ES, Blackburn EH, Lin J, et al: Accelerated telomere shortening in response to life stress. Proc Natl Acad Sci USA 101:17312–17315, 2004

Fogel RW: Changes in the physiology of aging during the twentieth century. NBER Working Paper No W11233. Cambridge, MA, National Bureau of Economic Research, March 2005. Available at: http://ssrn.com/abstract=693094. Accessed June 17, 2009.

Fries JF: Aging, natural death, and the compression of morbidity. N Engl J Med 303:130–135, 1980

Havighurst R: Successful aging. Gerontologist 1:4–7, 1961

Jeste D: Psychiatry of old age is coming of age. Am J Psychiatry 154:1356–1358, 1997

Karasik D, Demissie S, Cupples LA, et al: Disentangling the genetic determinants of human aging: biological age as an alternative to the use of survival measures. J Gerontol A Biol Sci Med Sci 60:574–587, 2005

Kennedy JF: Special message to Congress on the needs of the nation's senior citizens, February 21, 1963. Public Papers of the Presidents of the United States: John F Kennedy, 1963, p 189

Lemon BW, Bengtson VL, Petersen JA: An exploration of the activity theory of aging: activity types and life expectation among in-movers to a retirement community. J Gerontol 27:511–523, 1972

Østbye T, Krause KM, Norton MC, et al: Ten dimensions of health and their relationships with overall self-reported health and survival in a predominately religiously active elderly population: the Cache County memory study. J Am Geriatr Soc 54:199–209, 2006

Perls T, Levenson R, Regan M, et al: What does it take to live to 100? Mech Ageing Dev 123:231–242, 2002

Phelan EA, Larson EB: "Successful aging"—where next? J Am Geriatr Soc 50:1306–1308, 2002

Phelan EA, Anderson LA, LaCroix AZ, et al: Older adults' views of "successful aging"—how do they compare with researchers' definitions? J Am Geriatr Soc 52:211–216, 2004

Reichstadt J, Depp CA, Palinkas LA, et al: Building blocks of successful aging: a focus group study of older adults' perceived contributors to successful aging. Am J Geriatr Psychiatry 15:194–201, 2007

Rowe JW, Kahn RL: Human aging: usual and successful. Science 237:143–149, 1987

Rowe JW, Kahn RL: Successful Aging. New York, Dell, 1999

Ryff CD: Successful aging: a developmental approach. Gerontologist 22:209–214, 1982

U.S. Census Bureau: Age: 2000. Census 2000 Brief, October 2001. Available at: http://www.census.gov/prod/2001pubs/c2kbr01-12.pdf. Accessed April 15, 2009.

White House Conference on Aging: The Road to an Aging Policy for the 21st Century: Final Report of the 1995 White House Conference on Aging. Washington, DC, U.S. Department of Health and Human Services, 1996

Wilde O: The Picture of Dorian Gray. London, Ward, Lock, 1891

PART I

Behavioral and Psychosocial Aspects

2

Defining and Assessing Cognitive and Emotional Health in Later Life

Hugh C. Hendrie, M.B., Ch.B., D.Sc.
Christianna Purnell, B.A.
Alissa H. Wicklund, Ph.D.
Sandra Weintraub, Ph.D.

The demographic revolution of the last century has led to greatly increased numbers and proportions of adults living past the age of 65 years. In particular, the oldest-old age category (85 years and older), in the United States as well as in the rest of the world, has created new challenges for society at large and especially for its health services.

The research community and the medical disciplines have responded to this challenge by increasing the emphasis on diseases of the elderly and by developing specialties such as geriatrics and geriatric psychiatry. In the field of geriatric psychiatry, for example, there have now been major initiatives on the management of late-life depression (Lebowitz et al. 1997) and dementia (American Psychiatric Association 2007). Community groups such as the Alzheimer's Association and the American Association of Retired Persons (AARP) have led successful campaigns to increase funding for research on diseases such as Alzheimer disease. Recently, these organizations have recognized the need not only to study the diseases of the elderly but also to try to preserve patients' functioning, including cognitive functioning. Thus, the Alzheimer's Association ("Maintain Your Brain"; http://www.alz.org) and AARP ("Staying Sharp"; http://www.aarp.org) have launched educational campaigns.

This change of focus from disease to health has also been seen in the programs at major government research institutes. In 2001, three institutes of the U.S. National Institutes of Health (NIH)—the National Institute on Aging, the National Institute of Mental Health, and the National Institute of Neurological Disorders and Stroke—launched a new trans-NIH initiative, Cognitive and Emotional Health Project (CEHP): The Healthy Brain. This initiative seeks to identify the demographic, social, and biological determinants of cognitive and emotional health in the older adult. A description of the activities of this project is included on its Web site (http://trans.nih.gov/cehp). The Centers for Disease Control and Prevention, together with the Alzheimer's Association, has also recently published a report, "The Healthy Brain Initiative: A National Public Health Road Map to Maintaining Cognitive Health" (Centers for Disease Control and Prevention and the Alzheimer's Association 2007) (http://www.alz.org/national/documents/report_healthy braininitiative.pdf).

In this chapter we discuss the rationale for measuring cognitive and emotional health and defining cognitive and emotional health and the subdomains of cognition and emotion; provide examples of cognitive and emotional subdomain use in the clinical and epidemiological literature; recommend instruments to measure cognitive and emotional health for use in clinical and research settings; and speculate on future directions for the field. We end with a brief description of a major NIH initiative to develop a comprehensive "toolbox" of measurements of cognition, emotion, and motor and sensory function, applicable throughout the life span, for use in clinical and epidemiological settings.

Why Measure Cognitive and Emotional Health?

There is clearly great public interest in maintaining cognitive and emotional health, probably reflecting the major concern of the elderly, loss of independence. In the foreword to *Successful Aging* (Rowe and Kahn 1998), a report on the MacArthur Foundation study (the MacArthur Research Network on Successful Aging Community Study), the authors define a "new gerontology" in which the emphasis is not only on disease prevention but also on improving or maintaining older Americans' (ages 70–79) physical and mental abilities, including consideration of cognitive and emotional health. This approach parallels a greater interest among government and public health agencies in monitoring states of well-being and quality of life, particularly health-related quality of life, in national and international surveys. The NIH-sponsored CEHP report (Hendrie et al. 2006) recommended that the research community pursue the study of brain health maintenance as vigorously as it does the quest to understand brain disease. Furthermore, it suggested that a focus on optimal cognitive and emotional health and the prevention of cognitive decline and emotional distress may identify a different set or combination of risk factors, and, thus, different prevention strategies for healthy elderly subjects (age 65 and older), than would a focus on single disease outcomes. For example, of the few studies of healthy brain aging, the aforementioned MacArthur Research Network community study of successful aging (Rowe et al. 1998) suggested that a combination of lifestyle and health behaviors is more likely to be predictive of high functioning over time than any single factor alone.

Syndromes such as major depression and dementia often develop slowly and are preceded by symptoms of cognitive decline and emotional distress. Monitoring cognition and emotion over time might provide the clinician with an early indication of incipient disease and thus an opportunity for early intervention (Unverzagt et al. 2001). Finally, measurements of psychological well-being and cognitive function are both good predictors of health-related outcomes such as mortality and institutionalization, as we discuss later in the chapter (see section "Measuring Cognition").

Defining Emotional and Cognitive Health

Emotional Health

There is as yet no widely accepted definition of what constitutes emotional health in the elderly. The report from the National Institute on Aging–sponsored Healthy Brain Workshop (http://trans.nih.gov/cehp/NINDSSummary.pdf) concluded that emotional health is not just the absence of psychiatric illness or even the absence of negative affect, which in certain circumstances (such as grief) can be constructive. Rather, it should be defined more comprehensively, and positively, and include constructs such as emotional regulation and emotional intelligence. (*Emotional regulation* refers to the ability to control emotion, whereas *emotional intelligence* refers to the ability to use and identify emotions constructively.) Most studies of emotional health in the elderly have emphasized the importance of coping and adaptation. In the Berlin Aging Study, Baltes and Baltes (1990) suggested adapting to the realities of aging, with its accompanying reduction in physical capacity, by a process of selection, optimization, and compensation. Blazer (2002) has characterized this process of accepting the limits of aging yet at the same time compensating for these limits by recognizing other potentials for happiness and productivity, a process he calls *self-efficacy*. The processes and determinants involved in the maintenance of emotional health in aging are discussed by Charles and Horwitz in Chapter 4 ("Positive Emotions and Health: What We Know About Aging") of this handbook.

Cognitive Health

Cognitive health with aging, as noted above, is a relatively recent concept in medicine and psychology and lacks a firm definition. Unlike indices of physical health, such as blood pressure, for which there are absolute standards across all individuals, the parameters of cognitive health are not easily defined. This is true in part because there are large interindividual differences in baseline levels of cognitive ability. Moreover, virtually every longitudinal and cross-sectional study of cognitive aging has shown that mean scores decline over time but that standard deviations around the mean, a measure of dispersion, increase. This implies increased cognitive heterogeneity with age, so some individuals seem able to maintain cognitive functioning at a level consistent with younger cohorts, whereas others show a more malignant course. Ardila (2007) analyzed data from 2,450 American adults divided into 13 age groups and 4 education levels. Mean subscale scores declined with age, but the dispersion of scores around the mean increased in magnitude. This dispersion was more apparent on measures of attention, executive functioning, and some nonverbal abilities, with more homogeneous patterns of performance on tests of visuospatial abilities and a person's general fund of knowledge. In another study of cognitive test performance in 1,100 physician volunteers, among the 151 subjects over age 75, the 20 who obtained the highest total score on a computerized test performed within the average range for the youngest cohort, ages 28–34 (Weintraub et al. 1994). The youngest cohort included house officers at a major university medical center, implying that aging can be compatible with a very high level of cognitive functioning.

The concept of "normal aging" needs to be revisited, because it oversimplifies the complex nature of cognitive aging. Interindividual differences in trajectories of cognitive function over time are compounded by interindividual differences in baseline peak levels of ability. Thus, for an 85-year-old with an earlier peak level of cognitive function at the 98th percentile, test scores in the average range for age constitute a decline. Conversely, for an 85-year-old whose peak cognitive level was below the average range, a score below average for age may represent stable functioning.

Many factors influence cognitive health. High educational attainment, high socioeconomic status, physical activity, and an emotionally supportive environment all positively influence healthy cognitive aging. In contrast, hypertension, diabetes, stroke, and depression and anxiety, all of which may increase with age, are negative influences (Hendrie et al. 2006). As suggested above, some individuals are better able to withstand age-associated changes in the brain than others. One explanation for the lack of cognitive decline in some individuals has been referred to as *cognitive reserve*, a factor believed to represent the protective nature of education and high socioeconomic status, as discussed by Brickman et al. in this handbook (see Chapter 9, "Cognitive and Brain Reserve").

All of these factors imply that any definition of cognitive health with aging must be flexible enough to encompass individual differences in cognitive ability at an earlier, peak point in life, and individual differences in customary activities of daily living, personal hobbies, and patterns of social engagement.

Measuring Emotion

Emotion consists of a number of interacting domains with fluid boundaries. It includes positive and negative affect and a very large domain of stress and coping, which itself consists of several subdomains (see National Institutes of Health 2009). The subdomains include self-efficacy, hardiness, resilience, emotional regulation, and social relationships. It often incorporates other concepts such as well-being and quality of life, which involve consideration of emotion in its social and environmental context. Coping and social relationships are the subjects of other chapters in this handbook, so our review focuses on positive and negative affect, well-being, and quality of life, particularly health-related quality of life.

Positive and Negative Affect

The relationship between positive and negative affect can best be characterized as orthogonal rather than bipolar. High levels of positive affect can coexist with high levels of negative affect or vice versa, and their effects on health-related outcomes are relatively independent. Measurements of emotion should therefore include both domains:

- Positive affect has been described as "feelings that reflect a level of pleasurable engagement with the environment such as happiness, joy, excitement, enthusiasm, and contentment" (Pressman and Cohen 2005, p. 925).

- Negative affect comprises unpleasant feelings and emotions such as sadness, anger, and fear, which can range in severity from daily mood fluctuations to the unbearable emotions experienced by sufferers of the major mental disorders.

Both positive and negative affect have a relatively enduring, stable personality component, a person's *traits,* as well as more transient feelings that occur situationally, a *state.* The set point for trait affect is likely to be established early in life as a result of genetic and early-life experiences and can account for up to half of the levels of affect at any given moment (Huppert et al. 2005; Sheldon and Lyubomirsky 2006).

The scales most familiar to psychiatrists, such as the Geriatric Depression Scale (Yesavage 1982–1983), the Center for Epidemiologic Studies Depression Scale (Radloff 1977), and the Hopkins Anxiety Scale (Derogatis 1974), can also be used to monitor subsyndromal negative affect, although they are relatively insensitive to recording daily fluctuations of mood. More specific scales to separate trait and state components and measure daily fluctuations have been used in older populations; these include the State-Trait Anxiety Inventory (Spielberger 1983) and the Worries Scale (Kubzansky et al. 1997).

Relationship of Positive and Negative Affect to Positive Health Outcomes

Pressman and Cohen (2005), in their comprehensive review of the effects of positive affect on health indices, found a consistent association between studies measuring positive affect and lower mortality rates in community-residing adults but, interestingly, not for nursing home residents. They also reported good evidence for positive affect being associated with less risk of illness and injury and generally better health indices in adult populations, including older adults. There was also considerable evidence linking positive affect with fewer reported symptoms and less pain. Another study reported that measurements of hope were significantly inversely associated with a diagnosis of hypertension in older adults (ages 55–69) (Richman et al. 2005).

The negative effect of late-life depression on health is well known. It is associated with diminished health-related quality of life and increased risk for death from suicide or medical illness (Unutzer et al. 2002). Depressed older patients (age 60 and older) are more frequent users of general medical services and have poor adherence to medical treatments (Unutzer et al. 2002).

Anxiety disorder in older adults (age 65 and older) has been associated with increased disability and diminished well-being. Persons with chronically high levels of anxiety tend to be higher utilizers of medical care and have higher rates of emergency room visits, have impaired functional status, and engage in fewer physical activities (Brenes et al. 2005).

Chronic anger and hostility may represent an important risk factor for coronary heart disease (Miller et al. 1996) as well as mortality in general (Smith and Christensen 1992). They may also be associated with risky lifestyle behaviors such as smoking and excessive alcohol consumption (Miller et al. 1996).

Well-Being

Measurements of well-being are now a major part of most government-sponsored surveillance programs both in the United States and in Europe. Measurements of well-being—for example, the General Well-Being Schedule (Dupuy 1984)—frequently consist of components of both positive and negative affect together with consideration of motivational and other factors.

Health-Related Quality of Life

Quality of life measurements, particularly health-related quality of life, are widely used in health surveys. *Health-related quality of life* is a broad concept and refers to an individual's perception of his or her physical and mental health and state of well-being. It is extensively used in population surveys by national and international organizations such as the Centers for Disease Control and Prevention and the World Health Organization. Physicians use health-related quality of life measures to assess the effects of both chronic illnesses and their treatments in patients in order to better understand how these interfere with patients' everyday lives. Instruments commonly used include the Short Form–36 Health Survey (Ware 1993) and the WHOQOL-100 (World Health Organization 1995).

Emotional Vitality

Occasionally researchers combine instruments or items from instruments from different subdomains to create new concepts. A particularly intriguing example of this is *emotional vitality*, which was described by Penninx et al. (2000). They combined questions about mastery and happiness from the Women's Health Initiative questionnaire with a subset of anxiety items from the Hopkins Symptom Checklist–90 (Derogatis et al. 1974) and the Geriatric Depression Scale to create this concept. High levels of emotional vitality (good positive affect, low scores for anxiety and depression) were associated with a lower risk for subsequent new disability and mortality in older disabled women (age 65 and older).

A comprehensive compilation of measurements of cognition and emotion that have been used in older populations can be found at the Cognitive and Emotional Health Project: The Healthy Brain (http://trans.nih.gov/cehp/ HBPcog1.htm and http://trans.nih.gov/CEHP/HBPemot-findings.htm).

Measuring Cognition

In the last quarter of the 20th century, cognitive measurement in aging was dominated by the division of mental processes into two categories, influenced by the types of mental abilities measured on intelligence tests such as the Wechsler scale and the Stanford-Binet Intelligence Scale. *Crystallized intelligence* refers to acquired knowledge related to one's cultural experience and ways of reasoning about social and moral issues, whereas *fluid intelligence* refers to mental operations independent of context and content, such as problem-solving skills and inductive reasoning. A large body of research has shown that aging has a greater impact on fluid than crystallized mental abilities.

More recently, the era of neuropsychology and cognitive neuroscience has supported a classification of cognitive subdomains by their behavioral constructs and also by the brain networks that mediate them. The Cognitive and Emotional Health Project: The Healthy Brain (http://trans.nih.gov/CEHP/) recommended domains of cognitive functioning that should be targeted to assess cognitive health (Hendrie et. al. 2006). Some of the major domains of cognition that have been well studied from a psychological and biological perspective are attention, working memory, episodic memory, language, executive functions, and social cognition. Speed of mental processing is not technically a separate domain, but cuts across all domains. It is included below because of the overwhelming evidence for general and specific changes in aging on processing speed and their impact on cognitive performance. More descriptive information and references to all tests mentioned can be found in *A Compendium of Neuropsychological Tests* (Strauss et al. 2006) and a chapter of *Principles of Behavioral and Cognitive Neurology* ("Neuropsychological Assessment of Mental State"; Weintraub 2000).

Cognition can be measured for clinical purposes or, in basic and epidemiological research, to examine causative, risk, and correlated factors. In the clinical realm, there is increasing awareness about the impact of aging on episodic, or retentive, memory because of the implications for the onset of Alzheimer disease. A decline in memory clearly poses serious limitations on one's ability to maintain autonomy. Aside from the clinical value of memory loss, however, other cognitive functions are important for the maintenance of independence and skill in complex daily living activities. For example, driving, a major symbol of autonomy in developed countries, relies on attention and executive functions, such as rapid decision making. Managing finances requires calculation ability and judgment, and the maintenance of relationships relies on social cognition. Thus, the focus on cognition may differ depending on the purpose of the measurement.

In addition to interindividual variability in baseline performance discussed above, intraindividual differences must be considered when measuring cognitive health (Salthouse 2000). For example, an individual's test scores on the same measure may vary from one time to another. In addition, an individual may perform in the superior range on one measure and the average range on another. Some studies have shown that measures of intraindividual variability at one point in time may be predictive of the future maintenance of cognitive health (MacDonald et al. 2003; Strauss et al. 2007). Intraindividual variability may be exacerbated by health conditions, such as arthritis, that can contribute to decrements in the speed of information processing that accompany the aging process (Salthouse 2000). Common physical conditions of the elderly, such as arthritis, can influence performance on cognitive tests. Finally, sporadic physiological factors that can affect central nervous system function, such as dehydration, metabolic conditions, and medication use, also add to the variability of cognitive test performance. All of these factors combine to make cognitive measurement in the elderly challenging.

Attention

Attention, a complex construct that refers to the allocation of the brain's limited information-processing capacities to deal with an abundance of environmental stimulation, is the foundation for all other types of mental processes (Weintraub 2000). There are several different forms of attention, including sustained, selective, and divided. *Sustained attention* is closely linked to the level of wakefulness or the maintenance of an alert state. *Selective attention* serves to direct sensory and thought processes to a particular stimulus or sector of the environment, including one's own internal thoughts, so that action can be taken. *Divided attention* is the ability to attend to more than one stimulus, spatial sector, or modality simultaneously. The human brain has a limited capacity for processing information. As a result, attention serves to identify and extract stimuli from the environment and focus on what is essential for achieving a goal at any point in time.

- Sustained attention, also called *vigilance,* is closely linked to the level of wakefulness and can be influenced by medical conditions that alter arousal and alertness. It is commonly measured by continuous performance-type tasks in which the subject must monitor a series of signals and react to the target signal (e.g., the letter *A* in a random string of letters presented over a 10-minute interval). The skills of radar and sonar operators rely on this form of attention.

- Selective attention is easiest to conceptualize in the visual modality, where it serves to identify significant stimuli from the mass of environmental stimuli. Aging narrows the window of visual attention (Greenwood and Parasuraman 2004), also referred to as the *useful field of view* (Ball et al. 1993). As a result, despite having adequate primary vision, older individuals may be slower to react to stimuli that suddenly appear in regions of the visual field where attention is not specifically focused. Visual perimetry testing is usually not sufficient to assess visual attention, and tasks such as those that assess the useful field of view and experimental tests of covert attention (Greenwood and Parasuraman 2004) may be more revealing. Changes in the useful field of view, quantified by a computerized test that varies the level of distraction in the visual field and measures its impact on target detection (Ball et al. 1988), have been of value in predicting driving safety in the elderly (Ball et al. 1993).
- Divided attention operates when two tasks or sources of stimuli must be processed; some consider this aspect of attention to also involve executive functions. *Multitasking* is a vernacular term for this form of attention, a real-life example of which is driving while speaking on a cell phone or while using an in-vehicle display. Older individuals have difficulty dividing their attention, which may put them at increased risk for accidents. The dichotic listening technique, in which two different stimuli are presented simultaneously, one to each ear, is a classic example of a method for testing divided attention. The subject must be able to store information from one ear while reporting information from the other.

Working Memory

Working memory refers to a limited-capacity storage buffer that becomes overloaded when the amount of information exceeds capacity. Classical studies have shown the human limit to be, on average, seven bits of discrete information (Miller 1956). Working memory is composed of several components that serve to 1) process information across a series of tasks and modalities (auditory, visual, spatial), 2) hold the information in a short-term buffer, 3) manipulate the information, and 4) hold the products in the same short-term buffer (Baddeley 2003). This concept replaces the traditional construct of "short-term memory" as a passive storage buffer, to signify the notion of an active computational workspace.

The Digit Span test, a simple measure of working memory in the auditory modality, measures the longest sequence of random numbers an individual can repeat in forward and backward sequence. A normal forward digit span is approximately seven digits, and the backward span, under normal circumstances, does not differ from the forward by more than two digits.

Working memory is integral to other cognitive processes such as learning a list of words, recalling a series of verbal instructions or directions, and performing complex sequences of tasks, in which information must be held online for later recall or manipulation. The ability to call for telephone information, hear the phone number, and immediately dial it depends on working memory.

Executive Functioning

Executive functioning is defined as the capacity to plan, organize, and monitor the execution of behaviors that are strategically directed in a goal-oriented manner. The precise definition of executive functioning is controversial, but executive functioning is generally agreed to consist of several distinctive processes, including planning, cognitive flexibility, problem solving, response inhibition, fluency, and self-monitoring. Many of these functions rely on the integrity of disparate regions in the frontal lobes and are difficult to measure in the laboratory or clinical setting because they are most operative in situations of uncertainty or situations in which several possible alternatives exist. The National Institute of Neurological Disorders and Stroke's EXAMINER project (Executive Abilities: Methods and Instruments for Neurobehavioral Evaluation and Research) is a large-scale project that has defined key constructs in this multidimensional domain and has recommended measurements (http://examiner.ucsf.edu/Related_Literature/literature_search.htm).

The ability to shift among different trains of thought, different actions, and different sources of outside stimulation is well suited for testing in an office or laboratory. Tests of shifting usually require the establishment of a response set and the ability to then alter the response once it is no longer successful. The Wisconsin Card Sorting Test rewards the subject for sorting a stack of cards based on three possible attributes: color, shape, and number. The initial sorting category, color, is rewarded by positive feedback from the examiner. Then, without warning, the response contingency is shifted by the examiner, requiring the subject to adapt accordingly and sort by one of the other attributes, that is, either shape or number. Errors on this test consist of *perseveration,* the persistence of the incorrect response despite negative feedback, and *impersistence,* or failing to maintain the relevant strategy despite positive feedback.

Another component of executive functioning, response inhibition, is required whenever an ordinarily automatic response tendency must be inhibited because of the exigencies of the context. An example of automatic behavior is stepping on the brake pedal when a traffic light turns red. However, this response may need to be overridden if the driver notices a truck in the rearview mirror that is not slowing down. A simple test of this function is the Stroop Color-Word Interference Test. In the first of three conditions, the subject reads rows of the words *red, blue,* and *green,* presented in random sequence. In the second, the subject is asked to name the colors (red, blue, or green) in rows of colored swatches. In the interference condition, the subject is presented with the words for the colors but each is printed in an opposing color (e.g., *red* is printed in blue, *green* is printed in red, etc.). The task is not to read the word, the more automatic of the responses, but instead to suppress that response and name the color of the ink. Response time normally slows in the interference condition, but in individuals with deficits in this function response time slows excessively, and there may also be errors of commission (i.e., naming the word instead of the color).

Episodic Memory

There are many types of memory but only *episodic memory* is discussed here. The ability to consciously register, consolidate, store, and retrieve information related to an experience is the essence of this type of memory. It is well known that this form of memory is dependent on the integrity of the hippocampus and entorhinal cortex, structures deep in the mesial temporal lobe. Episodic memory can be easily tested by training an individual to learn a list of words, a story, or a geometric design, then testing recall of the information after time has elapsed (typically 20–30 minutes). Examples of such tests are the word list from the Consortium to Establish a Registry for Alzheimer's Disease (CERAD) battery (Morris et al. 1989), the Rey Auditory Verbal Learning Test (Strauss et al. 2006), and the story and design recall tests from the Wechsler Memory Scale–III (Wechsler 1998). An impairment of this type of memory is *amnesia,* a core sign in early Alzheimer disease because the earliest pathological changes in this disorder destroy neurons in the hippocampus and entorhinal cortex.

Language

Language functions, which are mediated by the left cerebral hemisphere, service communication through speaking, understanding, reading, and writing (Mesulam 1998). Language processes can be divided into two main components: syntactic and lexical-semantic. The former includes word sequence and modifications of words to alter meaning, such as the affix *-ed* to convert a verb to the past tense in English. The latter includes the store of words in a language and their meanings, similar to a dictionary. Although there are many ways to measure language, literacy is one component that is relatively easy to assess and that is also very relevant to cognitive health, especially in a population where there is cultural and ethnic diversity and, therefore, highly variable levels of this skill. Literacy can be measured by the ability to read single words and also to comprehend paragraph-length material, both of which can be measured on the reading subtests of the Wide Range Achievement Test–4 (Wilkinson and Robertson 2006). Reading single words aloud correlates strongly with IQ, but also is heavily influenced by past educational exposure, which has an impact on performance on standard cognitive tests in minority populations (Manly et al. 2004; Mehta et al. 2004).

The ability to read has broad implications for many functional skills, including financial management, recreation, employment, and safety. One very practical application of literacy, namely *health literacy,* may have more direct application to health outcomes. Health literacy can be broadly defined as the ability to comprehend health information in printed and oral form (Baker 2006), and it has been shown to influence mortality in elderly individuals (Baker et al. 2008).

Processing Speed

Processing speed is defined as either the amount of time it takes to process a set amount of information, or, conversely, the amount of information that can be processed within a certain unit of time. It is a measure that reflects mental efficiency. Processing speed is central for many cognitive functions and domains, and it is very sensitive to change and/or disease. It is well established that the speed at which information is processed slows with increasing age (Salthouse 2000). This can be tested with relatively simple measures such as comparing pairs to stimuli (e.g., digit strings) to determine whether they are the same or different (i.e., the *identical pairs test;* Cornblatt et al. 1988). In addition, simple or choice reaction time tests can be used. A Sternberg-type task provides a method for assessing mental processing speed by measuring the amount of time it takes to scan internal memory stores while searching sets of information of increasing size. For example, if one is given a set of four numbers to keep in mind and then asked to determine whether each number in a subsequent series of single digits is a member of the set, reaction time is longer than if the original set size is three numbers or two numbers. The increase in response time is not due to slowing of motor speed, since motor speed is constant across all set sizes, but rather represents a true slowing of mental processing time.

Social Cognition

Social cognition is the subdomain that is the most recent to be studied experimentally in adults. The capacity for sympathy and empathy, both of which require perspective taking, is a simple construct of this complex subdomain. The *theory of mind* currently dominates thinking about social cognition, asserting that humans are able to imagine that they and others have minds that guide behavior and that other minds and perspectives can be different from their own (Gallagher and Frith 2003). Tasks that measure this function typically consist of presenting a vignette where one must attempt to determine what the actors are thinking and how this might alter their behavior. Studies have shown that performance of these tasks may actually *improve* with aging, perhaps representing the construct of "wisdom" (Happe et al. 1998; Saltzman et al. 2000).

Relationship of Cognition to Positive Health Outcomes

None of the cognitive domains outlined in the previous subsections are mutually exclusive. For example, it is easy to see how working memory, attention, and processing speed can influence the ability to learn new information. In aging, the confluence of a decline in any one or more of the abilities may result in a change in information-processing capacity. Furthermore, cognitive performance may be affected even in healthy older individuals as resources shift to accommodate for deficits in hearing and vision and decreased processing speed that occur in normal aging (Wingfield et al. 2005).

An increasing number of studies have looked at health and other risk factors for cognitive decline in the elderly. However, relatively few studies have measured the converse, namely the impact of cognitive health on general health outcomes. Several studies have shown that poor cognition, usually in the form of "mild cognitive impairment" or dementia, is associated with negative health outcomes, including increased mortality (Bosworth et al. 1999; Hunderfund et al. 2006; Jagger et al. 2007; Lee et al. 2006) and morbidity (Weiler et al. 1991). Links have been made between specific types of cognitive deficits, such as decreased attention, and the impairment of specific activities, such as driving, as described above. There is a need for more research on the impact of cognitive decline that does not meet criteria for mild cognitive impairment or dementia but that can arise from a variety of causes, including medically induced alterations of mental state (also referred to as *delirium*) and the cognitive consequences of stroke and traumatic brain injury.

Future Directions:
The NIH Toolbox Project

In the CEHP report (Hendrie et al. 2006) it was noted that although many large-cohort epidemiological studies have included some information on cognition and emotion, they tended to evaluate only limited aspects of these domains and there was little commonality among the studies on the instruments used. This made comparisons between studies and combining data from studies difficult, thus limiting the useful information on cognitive and emotional health that could be derived from these large and expensive projects. The CEHP report therefore recommended that a multidimensional but brief instrument be developed to measure cognition and emotion, which could be included in such large studies. In partial response to this proposal and also to other perceived needs of the neuroscience research community, the NIH Toolbox was conceived.

The NIH Toolbox is a 5-year project with the goal of creating brief, comprehensive assessment tools to measure outcomes in longitudinal epidemiological and intervention studies across the life span in the areas of cognition, emotion, motor functioning, and sensation. State-of-the-art computerized assessment techniques will be employed to create an instrument that is psychometrically robust, relatively brief, and readily available to clinicians and researchers. Computerized testing has many advantages, including standardized administration, advanced testing formats, and easy centralization of data. Computer-adaptive testing is a method for administering tests that adapt to the test taker's ability level (i.e., tailored testing). Questions are successively selected to maximize precision of ability estimation based on responses to prior questions. Most often, fewer items are needed to arrive at equally accurate trait estimates (Revicki and Cella 1997), a benefit for testing older individuals, in whom fatigue could interfere with more lengthy assessment measures.

The NIH Toolbox (National Institutes of Health 2009) will examine many aspects of cognition, including the following:

- Attention (visual attention, using a "flanker-type" task [Fan et al. 2002]) in the presence of spatially congruent and incongruent cues
- Working memory (complex span and continuous updating tasks)
- Processing speed (letter/pattern comparison tasks)
- Executive functioning (dimensional change card-sorting and flanker tasks)
- Language (auditory-picture vocabulary comprehension)
- Episodic memory (imitation-based assessment of memory)

Once available, this instrument will allow cross-study comparisons. Tests are intended to target indices of health rather than signs of disease. Eventually, it will be important to introduce instruments that can be used in a wide variety of settings that provide services and programs for older individuals, and to help physicians monitor cognitive health, incorporating such monitoring into mainstream primary care.

Conclusion

With the continuing demographic changes and possible advent of new prevention and early treatment interventions, interest in studying and measuring cognitive and emotional health in the elderly is only likely to increase. There are currently available a number of instruments measuring the various domains and subdomains of cognition and emotion that have demonstrated good predictive validity for health outcomes. There is, however, no available well-recognized test battery that incorporates measurements of cognition and emotion. When completed in 2011, the NIH Toolbox instrument will represent a unique, state-of-the-art resource for measuring cognition and emotion in such epidemiological and clinical settings.

KEY POINTS

- Preserving function, including cognitive and emotional health, in the elderly is now a major public health goal. Measurements of these domains should be capable of measuring health as well as illness.

- Emotional health should be defined comprehensively. It should not be limited to the absence of psychiatric illness or negative affect but should also include consideration of positive affect.

- A definition of cognitive health in aging must be flexible enough to encompass individual differences in cognitive ability at an earlier, peak point in life and individual differences in customary activities of daily living, personal hobbies, and patterns of social engagement.

- Measurements of emotion should incorporate a number of interacting domains, including positive and negative affect and stress and coping. Both positive and negative affect influence health outcomes, but in different directions.

- Major domains of cognitive function include attention, working memory, executive functioning, episodic memory, language, and social cognition. Poor cognitive function is associated with negative health outcomes.

- The ongoing NIH Toolbox project has the goal of creating brief, comprehensive assessment tools to measure cognition, emotion, motor functioning, and sensation. When completed in 2011, the Toolbox instrument will represent a unique, state-of-the-art resource for measuring cognition and emotion that will be applicable to older populations.

References

American Psychiatric Association Work Group on Alzheimer's Disease and Other Dementias, Rabins PV, Blacker D, et al: American Psychiatric Association practice guideline for the treatment of patients with Alzheimer's disease and other dementias: second edition. Am J Psychiatry 164:5–56, 2007

Ardila A: Normal aging increases cognitive heterogeneity: analysis of dispersion in WAIS-III scores across age. Arch Clin Neuropsychol 22:1003–1011, 2007

Baddeley A: Working memory: looking back and looking forward. Nature Reviews Neuroscience 4(10):829–839, 2003

Baker DW: The meaning and the measure of health literacy. J Gen Intern Med 21:878–883, 2006

Baker DW, Wolf MS, Feinglass J, et al: Health literacy, cognitive abilities, and mortality among elderly persons. J Gen Intern Med 23:723–726, 2008

Ball KK, Beard BL, Roenker DL, et al: Age and visual search: expanding the useful field of view. Journal of the Optical Society of America A: Optics, Image Science, and Vision 5:2210–2219, 1988

Ball K, Owsley C, Sloane ME, et al: Visual attention problems as a predictor of vehicle crashes in older drivers. Invest Ophthalmol Vis Sci 34:3110–3123, 1993

Baltes PB, Baltes MM (eds): Successful Aging: Perspectives From the Behavioral Sciences. New York, Cambridge University Press, 1990

Blazer DG: Self-efficacy and depression in late life: a primary prevention proposal. Aging Ment Health 6:315–324, 2002

Bosworth HB, Schaie KW, Willis SL: Cognitive and sociodemographic risk factors for mortality in the Seattle Longitudinal Study. J Gerontol B Psychol Sci Soc Sci 54:P273–P282, 1999

Brenes GA, Guralnik JM, Williamson J, et al: Correlates of anxiety symptoms in physically disabled older women. Am J Geriatr Psychiatry 13:15–22, 2005

Centers for Disease Control and Prevention and the Alzheimer's Association: The Healthy Brain Initiative: A National Public Health Road Map to Maintaining Cognitive Health. Chicago, IL, Alzheimer's Association, 2007. Available at: http://www.alz.org/national/documents/report_healthybraininitiative.pdf. Accessed April 14, 2009.

Cognitive and Emotional Health: The Healthy Brain Workshop. Available at: http://trans.nih.gob/cehp/NINDSSummary.pdf. Accessed April 14, 2009.

Cornblatt BA, Risch NJ, Faris G, et al: The Continuous Performance Test, Identical Pairs Version (CPT-IP), I: new findings about sustained attention in normal families. Psychiatry Res 26:223–238, 1988

Derogatis LR, Lipman RS, Rickels K, et al: The Hopkins Symptom Checklist (HSCL): a self-report symptom inventory. Behav Sci 191:1–15., 1974

Dupuy HJ: The Psychological General Well-Being (PGWB) Index, in Assessment of Quality of Life in Clinical Trials of Cardiovascular Therapies. Edited by Wenger NK. Darien, CT, Le Jacq Publishing, 1984, pp 170–183

Fan J, McCandliss BD, Sommer T, et al: Testing the Efficiency and independence of attentional networks. J Cogn Neurosci 14:340–347, 2002

Gallagher HL, Frith CD: Functional imaging of "theory of mind." Trends Cogn Sci 7:77–83, 2003

Greenwood PM, Parasuraman R: The scaling of spatial attention in visual search and its modification in healthy aging. Percept Psychophys 66:3–22, 2004

Happe FG, Winner E, Brownell H: The getting of wisdom: theory of mind in old age. Dev Psychol 34:358–362, 1998

Hendrie HC, Albert MS, Butters MA, et al: The NIH Cognitive and Emotional Health Project: report of the Critical Evaluation Study Committee. Alzheimers Dement 2:12–32, 2006

Hunderfund AL, Roberts RO, Slusser TC, et al: Mortality in amnestic mild cognitive impairment: a prospective community study. Neurology 67:1764–1768, 2006

Huppert F, Baylis N, Keverne B (eds): The Science of Well-Being. New York, Oxford University Press, 2005

Jagger C, Matthews R, Matthews F, et al: The burden of diseases on disability-free life expectancy in later life. J Gerontol A Biol Sci Med Sci 62:408–414, 2007

Kubzansky LD, Kawachi I, Spiro A 3rd, et al: Is worrying bad for your heart? A prospective study of worry and coronary heart disease in the Normative Aging Study. Circulation 95:818–824, 1997

Lebowitz BD, Pearson JL, Schneider LS, et al: Diagnosis and treatment of depression in late life: consensus statement update. JAMA 278:1186–1190, 1997

Lee HB, Kasper JD, Shore AD, et al: Level of cognitive impairment predicts mortality in high-risk community samples: the memory and medical care study. J Neuropsychiatry Clin Neurosci 18:543–546, 2006

MacDonald SW, Hultsch DF, Dixon RA: Performance variability is related to change in cognition: evidence from the Victoria Longitudinal Study. Psychol Aging 18:510–523, 2003

Manly JJ, Byrd DA, Touradji P, et al: Acculturation, reading level, and neuropsychological test performance among African American elders. Appl Neuropsychol 11:37–46, 2004

Mehta KM, Simonsick EM, Rooks R, et al: Black and white differences in cognitive function test scores: what explains the difference? J Am Geriatr Soc 52:2120–2127, 2004

Mesulam M-M: Apahsias and other focal cerebral disorders, in Harrison's Principles of Internal Medicine, 14th Ed. Edited by Fauci A, Braun E, Isselbacher K, et al. New York, McGraw-Hill, 1998, pp 134–142

Miller GA: The magical number seven, plus or minus two. Psychol Review 63(2):81–97, 1956

Miller TQ, Smith TW, Turner CW, et al: A meta-analytic review of research on hostility and physical health. Psychol Bull 119:322–348, 1996

Morris JC, Heyman A, Mohs RC, et al: The Consortium to Establish a Registry for Alzheimer's Disease (CERAD): part I: clinical and neuropsychological assessment of Alzheimer's disease. Neurology 39:1159–1165, 1989

National Institutes of Health: Emotion. NIH Toolbox: Assessment of Neurological and Behavioral Function. Available at: http://www.nihtoolbox.org/WebPart%20Pages/Emotion.aspx. Accessed April 14, 2009.

Penninx BW, Guralnik JM, Bandeen-Roche K, et al: The protective effect of emotional vitality on adverse health outcomes in disabled older women. J Am Geriatr Soc 48:1359–1366, 2000

Pressman SD, Cohen S: Does positive affect influence health? Psychol Bull 131:925–971, 2005

Radloff LS: The CES-D Scale: a self-report depression scale for research in the general population. Applied Psychological Measurement 13:385-401, 1977

Revicki DA, Cella DF: Health status assessment for the twenty-first century: item response theory, item banking and computer adaptive testing. Quality of Life Research 6:595600, 1997

Richman LS, Kubzansky L, Maselko J, et al: Positive emotion and health: going beyond the negative. Health Psychol 24:422–429, 2005

Rowe JW, Kahn RL: Successful Aging. New York, Pantheon, 1998

Royall DR, Lauterbach EC, Cummings JL, et al: Executive control function: a review of its promise and challenges for clinical research. J Neuropsychiatry Clin Neurosci 14:377–405, 2002

Salthouse TA: Aging and measures of processing speed. Biol Psychol 54:35–54, 2000

Saltzman J, Strauss E, Hunter M, et al: Theory of mind and executive functions in normal human aging and Parkinson's disease. J Int Neuropsychol Soc 6:781–788, 2000

Sheldon KM, Lyubomirsky S: Achieving sustainable gains in happiness: change your actions, not your circumstances. J Happiness Stud 7:55–86, 2006

Smith TW, Christensen AJ: Hostility, health and social contexts, in Hostility, Coping, and Health. Edited by Friedman HS. Washington, DC, American Psychological Association, 1992, pp 33–48

Spielberger CD: Manual for the State-Trait Anxiety Inventory (Form Y). Palo Alto, CA, Consulting Psychologists Press, 1983

Strauss E, Sherman EMS, Spreen O: A Compendium of Neuropsychological Tests: Administration, Norms, and Commentary, 3rd Edition. New York, Oxford University Press, 2006

Strauss E, Bielak AA, Bunce D, et al: Within-person variability in response speed as an indicator of cognitive impairment in older adults. Neuropsychol Dev Cogn B Aging Neuropsychol Cogn 14:608–630, 2007

Unutzer J, Katon W, Callahan CM, et al: Collaborative care management of late-life depression in the primary care setting: a randomized controlled trial. JAMA 288:2836–2845, 2002

Unverzagt FW, Gao S, Baiyewu O, et al: Prevalence of cognitive impairment: data from the Indianapolis Study of Health and Aging. Neurology 57:1655–1662, 2001

Ware JE: SF-36 Health Survey: Manual and Interpretation Guide. Boston, MA, The Health Institute, New England Medical Center, 1993

Wechsler D: Wechsler Memory Scale–III. San Antonio, TX, Psychological Corporation, 1998

Weiler PG, Lubben JE, Chi I: Cognitive impairment and hospital use. Am J Public Health 81:1153–1157, 1991

Weintraub S: Neuropsychological assessment of mental state, in Principles of Behavioral and Cognitive Neurology. Edited by Mesulam MM. New York, Oxford University Press, 2000, pp 121–173

Weintraub S, Powell D, Whitla D: Successful cognitive aging: individual differences among physicians on a computerized test of mental state. J Geriatr Psychiatry 28:15–34, 1994

Wilkinson GS, Robertson GJ: Wide Range Achievement Test 4 (WRAT4). Lutz, FL, Psychological Assessment Resources, 2006

Wingfield A, Tun PA, McCoy SL: Hearing loss in older adulthood: what it is and how it interacts with cognitive performance. Curr Dir Psychol Sci 14:144–148, 2005

World Health Organization: Field Trial, WHOQOL-100. Geneva, World Health Organization, February 1995. Available at: http://www.who.int/mental_health/who_qol_field_trial_1995.pdf. Accessed April 2, 2009.

Yesavage JA, Brink TL, Rose TL, et al: Development and validation of a geriatric depression screening scale: a preliminary report. J Psychiatr Res 17:37–49, 1982–1983

Recommended Readings and Web Sites

Cognitive and Emotional Health: The Healthy Brain Workshop. Available at: http://trans.nih.gob/cehp/NINDSSummary.pdf. Accessed April 14, 2009.

Hendrie HC, Albert MS, Butters MA, et al: The NIH Cognitive and Emotional Health Project: report of the Critical Evaluation Study Committee. Alzheimers Dement 2:12–32, 2006

National Institutes of Health: Emotion. NIH Toolbox: Assessment of Neurological and Behavioral Function. Available at: http://www.nihtoolbox.org/WebPart%20Pages/Emotion.aspx. Accessed April 14, 2009.

Weintraub S: Neuropsychological assessment of mental state, in Principles of Behavioral and Cognitive Neurology. Edited by Mesulam MM. New York, Oxford University Press, 2000

3

Cognitive Aging

From Basic Skills to Scripts and Schemata

Barton W. Palmer, Ph.D.
Sharron E. Dawes, Ph.D.

What happens to cognitive abilities as people reach and move through "older age"? Through much of the history of Western civilization, the assumed answer was that aging is virtually synonymous with cognitive as well as physical decline (Berchtold and Cotman 1998). That bleak view is still reflected in contemporary language. The term *senile,* deriving from the Latin stem *sen-* ("pertaining to old age"), originally had no inherent connotations of pathology. In contemporary use, however, the term tends to be restricted to descriptions of age-related disease states, and in colloquial English it is often used as a virtual synonym for *dementia.*

Fortunately, the traditionally pessimistic view of normal cognitive aging began to change in the latter third of the twentieth century. Accumulating empirical data established that severe cognitive deterioration in the elderly, previously categorized under the nebulous label of *senile dementia,* is in fact attributable to specific neuropathological conditions such as Alzheimer disease (Katzman and Bick 2000). A by-product of the improved understanding of specific forms of senile dementia was that it helped diminish the assumption that dementia is an inevitable result of aging (Jeste and Palmer 2003); this change in view also fostered increased interest and empirical attention to nonpathological/"normal" cognitive aging, as well as to superior or particularly successful cognitive aging.

A fundamental question in successful aging research is, apart from prevention of dementia, what is it that distinguishes those who maintain high levels of functioning throughout the later years of life? Are *successful cognitive agers* people who have escaped the modal, albeit subtle, age-related cognitive declines? Are they persons who functioned at such high levels in earlier life that even with normal degrees of decline, they retain sufficient residual levels so that no functional impairments are evident? Or are successful cognitive agers those who have found some means of compensating for the functional effects of normal cognitive declines? To understand the degree to which each of these possibilities may play a role in successful cognitive aging, it is helpful to consider how aging normally (in the absence of specific neuropathological conditions) affects cognitive functioning. Because normal aging does not affect all cognitive abilities to the same degree (Christensen 2001), it is also helpful to consider the meaning of common labels for various cognitive constructs, and how those constructs are typically operationalized in research or applied settings. (Except where otherwise indicated by a more specific citation, wherever specific tests are named below, further details and original citations are available in Lezak et al. 2004 and/or Strauss et al. 2006.)

Our goal in this chapter is to provide an overview of the differential effects of normal aging on specific cognitive abilities, as well as to describe some of the prototypical methods commonly used to operationalize/measure the key cognitive constructs. Following that overview, in our Conclusion section, we discuss the potential relevance of normal age-related changes in cognition to the concept of "successful cognitive aging." Key in the latter discussion is a description of the notion of accumulated knowledge structures, such as scripts and schema, and the potential value in considering such structures as a means of further elucidating the nature of, and fostering the occurrence of, successful cognitive aging.

Specific Cognitive Domains: Measurement and Effects of Aging

Despite remarkable advances in cognitive neuroscience over the past few decades, including detailed understanding of the neurobiology of some specific cognitive processes (e.g., initial consolidation of new memories), questions remain regarding the natural categorization of cognitive abilities (as well as other mental processes such as emotions and temperament). For instance:

- How many types of cognition are there?
- How much homogeneity is appropriate among abilities with a single label (e.g., How many forms of *attention* are there? How many forms of *executive functions* exist?)?

- Should all abilities within a given category be more closely related to one another than to cognitive abilities in other categories? If so, how should *relatedness* be defined (e.g., in terms of the degree of statistical covariation, in terms of common neurobiological underpinnings, and/or in terms of the effects on independent/everyday functioning)?
- Do the groupings have equal ontological and/or heuristic status across different age, cultural, and/or neurodiagnostic groups?

We do not pretend to have the definitive answers to these questions, but we note the questions here to acknowledge that there is no clear consensus on any one finite set of cognitive categories or labels. Nevertheless, the eight categories discussed in the following subsections are among those frequently used among contemporary neuropsychologists to describe differences in various cognitive dimensions.

Crystallized Knowledge

One of the common distinctions made when describing human cognitive abilities is the difference between those emphasizing acquired knowledge, such as word meanings and general facts, and those that require more active "online" problem solving, abstraction, and information-processing resources. The most widely known form of this distinction is provided in the various forms of Cattell's and Horn's theory of *crystallized* versus *fluid* intelligence (e.g., Cattell 1943; Horn and Blankson 2005). Although the theory evolved and was expanded with additional cognitive constructs after Cattell's original formulation in 1943, the notion of crystallized ability remains important in the context of the present chapter because it is the one dimension for which the empirical evidence most consistently suggests that normal aging has little deleterious influence (in fact, accumulated experience with aging may have a positive influence on crystallized abilities throughout much of the adult life span) (Christensen 2001; Ryan et al. 2000). Therefore, in the context of successful aging, the crystallized abilities represent a common strength that older adults may use to compensate for the functional effects of declines experienced in other cognitive dimensions.

Prototypical examples of tests emphasizing crystallized abilities include the Information and Vocabulary subtests from the Wechsler intelligence scales (in any of their various incarnations). The Information subtest requires examinees to answer a series of questions about general facts of the type typically learned in school or through acculturation (e.g., "Who was the first president of the United States?"), whereas on the Vocabulary subtest the examinee is asked to provide dictionary-level definitions for a series of words of increasing difficulty. Another commonly used type of task in this category is word reading, such as the American National Adult Reading Test, in which examinees are asked to read and pronounce a series of words, most of which do not follow standard rules of English pronunciation (and therefore require prior exposure/knowledge for accurate pronunciation).

As is true of other crystallized abilities, cross-sectional and longitudinal data indicate that performance on vocabulary tests tends to remain stable, and may even improve during much of the adult life span (Bowles and Salthouse 2008; Ryan et al. 2000). Because performance on measures of crystallized knowledge also tends to be resilient to many forms of brain injury, such tests are sometimes described as *hold tests* and are frequently used by clinical neuropsychologists to estimate patients' levels of premorbid cognitive functioning.

Processing Speed

Slowed processing speed may be viewed as the very hallmark of cognitive aging. Indeed, some influential theorists and researchers suggest that many, albeit not all, of the normal age-related changes in other cognitive dimensions likely reflect inefficiency due to slowed information processing (Birren and Fisher 1995; Salthouse 1996). *Processing speed* is appropriately conceptualized as the speed of thinking, although when the construct is operationalized, the measures frequently include a psychomotor component—that is, the speed with which thought and action are integrated. Another overlapping construct is that of *reaction time,* which also slows with age. Regardless of which of these formulations is used, a gradual slowing of mental processing speed occurs throughout much of mid and later adulthood (Christensen 2001; Ryan et al. 2000; Salthouse 1996). Indeed, as summarized by Christensen (2001), "cognitive speed drops by approximately 20% at age 40 and by 40%–60% at age 80 [years]" (p. 769). It does not appear that such slowing can be attributed merely to sensory or motor effects, but rather it appears to reflect a genuine slowing of mental processing within the central nervous system (Birren and Fisher 1995).

Two prototypical measures of processing or psychomotor speed are the Trail Making Test and the Digit Symbol task (also known as the Coding task). The Trail Making Test consists of two parts: In part A, the examinee's task is to use a pencil to rapidly connect a series of circled numbers in ascending order. In part B, the examinee must alternate between circled numbers and circled letters; part B is thus sometimes viewed as a measure of mental flexibility and thereby grouped among the tests of executive functioning. Both part A and part B are highly affected by normal aging; in one large normative study of neuropsychiatrically healthy persons (i.e., persons with no reported history of neurological or neuropsychiatric conditions that might deleteriously affect cognitive functioning) ages 20–80 years, 30%–

34% of the variance in scores (time to completion) among healthy individuals was predicted by current age (Heaton et al. 1991).

The Digit Symbol task dates back at least to the early 1900s (reviewed in Boake 2002), but together with the Trail Making Test it remains among the most widely used measures of processing or psychomotor speed. The examinee is presented with a sheet containing a key in which each of the numbers from 1 to 9 is paired with a graphic symbol, and a larger matrix of numbers in random order with empty boxes below each number. The examinee's task is to rapidly fill in the symbol paired with each number within the empty boxes. This simple test can be administered very quickly. (The form in the Wechsler Adult Intelligence Scale, 4th Edition, and that in all of the prior editions of the Wechsler scale, can be administered in less than 5 minutes, including instruction time.) It has consistently proven to be among the most reliable psychometric measures and is particularly sensitive to virtually all forms of neurocognitive impairment (Dickinson et al. 2007). Approximately 28%–38% of the variance in Digit Symbol task scores among healthy normal adults is accounted for by current age (Heaton et al. 1991).

Attention

Attention is a broad term that may refer to any one function or a combination of more specific functions, such as distinguishing between relevant and irrelevant stimuli or information, keeping mentally "on track," and waiting and efficiently responding to a specific targeted stimulus or event that occurs over time. The term *basic attention* is sometimes applied to transient working memory, such as when briefly rehearsing and holding an unfamiliar telephone number actively in one's mind to facilitate immediate accurate dialing (Baddeley 2007). However, the concept of *working memory* is also closely related to that of *executive functioning,* both of which are discussed in separate sections below.

The construct of *selective attention* is itself a heterogeneous one that may refer to an early stage of precognitive filtering as well as to later, effortful selective attention; older adults may have evidence of declines in both forms of selective attention (de Fockert 2005; Gaeta et al. 2003). Oltmanns and Neal (1975) designed an interesting task to measure a person's ability to selectively attend to relevant stimuli. The examinee listens to an audiotape of a woman saying a series of digit strings; the task is to remember the numbers and, after each string is spoken, to write down the digits in the presented sequence. During distractibility trials, the recoding includes a man's voice presenting additional numbers between each digit spoken by the woman. The examinee's task is to ignore the man's voice and to selectively attend to and recall only the numbers spoken by the woman. To our knowledge this particular task has not yet been used in published, large-scale longitudinal studies of normal aging. However, we mention it in the present context because it is easy to administer and score, is generally well tolerated by examinees, and has been shown to be sensitive to the selective attention deficits associated with some neuropsychiatric conditions such as schizophrenia (Oltmanns and Neale 1975).

Letter or number cancellation tests are another commonly used type of task used to measure attention deficits. For instance, on the Digit Vigilance Test, examinees are required to search for and cross out every instance of a specific number on a sheet containing a large matrix of numbers. Performance on this task is measured in terms of both speed and accuracy. In a normative study of healthy adults ages 20–80 years, age accounted for 24% of the variance in time for completion, and for 15% of the variance in number of errors (Heaton et al. 1991), thereby suggesting that older adults are not simply sacrificing speed for accuracy but in fact also tend to make more errors.

Continuous Performance Tests (CPTs) are a different but also widely used form of tasks used to measure attention or vigilance. The CPTs are not a single test but rather a method or family of tests having similar underlying procedures and response demands. The examinee is rapidly presented with a large series of trials (usually on a computer screen); the task is to watch for an identified target and make a response when that target appears. The target may be a simple standard value (e.g., "Press a button every time you see the letter *H*"); it may involve vigilance to a specific sequence over successive trials (e.g., "Press a button every time you see the letter *Y* followed by the letter *H*"); or it may involve a specified relationship among the stimuli (e.g., "Press a button every time you see two numbers of identical value in two successive trials"). The CPT method was originally developed to detect brain injury (Beck et al. 1956), but performance on CPTs is also clearly affected by normal aging (Mani et al. 2005).

Receptive and Expressive Language

Receptive and expressive areas of language involve the ability to listen or otherwise receive external language communications (vocalized, signed, and/or written) and the ability to speak, write, or otherwise communicate effectively using appropriate vocabulary and grammar.

An example of a simple receptive language task is the Token Test, in which examinees are presented with a set of plastic tokens that vary in size, color, and shape. The examinee is then given a series of commands of increasing complexity. For instance, an early item may be simply "Touch a red square," whereas a later item may be in the form "Using a blue circle, touch a square that is not red, but first touch a green triangle." This simple task can be very helpful in discerning the level of complexity in spoken language sentence structure that an individual is capable of comprehending. There are also myriad tests for assessing reading comprehension in which examinees are given a short passage to read and then asked questions about the content of those passages. Although receptive communication can be affected by some age-related changes in sensory perception (hearing or vision loss), basic auditory and reading comprehension in and of themselves are not strongly affected by normal aging.

One of the most common complaints among older adults is that of word-finding difficulties, or what is known as the "tip of the tongue" experience. Tip of the tongue experiences (anomia) do in fact appear to increase with normal aging (Brown and Nix 1996). However, as anomia can also be an early sign of some cortical dementias, it can be particularly helpful to assess word-finding abilities using standardized measures (i.e., measures that permit comparison of an individual's performance with the performance of similarly aged healthy persons). The most widely used test of that sort for applied use in clinical settings is the Boston Naming Test, in which the examinee is presented with a series of line drawings depicting nameable objects. For example, simple items early in the test might include very common objects such as a cow or a spoon. If the examinee is unable to spontaneously name the pictured object, he or she may be given a phonemic cue wherein the examiner tells the examinee the first phoneme in the target word. Instances in which an examinee cannot spontaneously generate the name for an item but can do so with a phonemic cue are of particular interest, because these are the items for which it is most clear that the examinee actually knows the word but is having difficulty with retrieval. Approximately 18% of the variance in performance on the Boston Naming Test is accounted for by current age (Heaton et al. 1991); thus, word-finding ability is not unaffected by normal aging, but the influence of age on this ability is less than that on some other domains such as processing speed.

Visuospatial and Constructional Skills

Visuospatial and constructional skills allow one to recognize objects and their location or orientation in three-dimensional space, identify the shape of objects, and coordinate motor movements with the visual-spatial information (such as the hand-eye coordination involved in drawing). A prototypical example of a visuospatial-constructional task is the Block Design subtest from the Wechsler intelligence scales. Examinees are given a set of dual-colored blocks (white and red), which they must arrange to match pictured designs of increasing complexity. Cross-sectional studies suggest that Block Design performance begins to decline gradually after about age 30

(Rönnlund and Nilsson 2006; Ryan et al. 2000), but the results of longitudinal research suggest that some of the differences in Block Design performance are due to cohort effects, and that notable within-person deterioration does not emerge until age 60 or later (Rönnlund and Nilsson 2006). (The issue of cohort effects, which is in fact an interpretive limitation across much of the cognitive aging literature, is considered in more detail in the section "Cognitive Effects of Normal Aging: Caveats" below).

The Block Design task, like many tests used to evaluate this domain, has both a visuospatial component and constructional (psychomotor integration) demands. There are a few visuospatial tasks that do not involve motor skills, such as the Hooper Visual Organization Test (VOT). The VOT uses pictured objects similar to those on the Boston Naming Test, except that on the VOT the pictures have been cut into pieces and arranged in random order. The examinee must mentally rotate and rearrange the pieces in order to discern and then state the pictured object. Cross-sectional data suggest the VOT is highly sensitive to age, with a negative correlation of approximately $r=-0.42$ to -0.50 (Tamkin and Jacobsen 1984). However, to our knowledge the effects of normal aging on this test have not been evaluated in large-scale, published, longitudinal studies of healthy aging, so the within-person effects of normal aging on this task need further documentation.

Memory

As is true of the terms *attention* and *executive functioning,* the term *memory* is a broad one that may refer to any of a number of loosely related cognitive processes. It is important to distinguish between declarative and nondeclarative memory. *Declarative memory* refers to specifically nameable/consciously retrievable memory traces (i.e., things one can "declare") and may itself be divided into episodic memory (memories tied to specific episodes in time, such as "Where did I park my car when I came to work today?" or "What were the words on the list I just read to you?") and semantic memory. *Semantic memory* refers to declarable facts that are not tied to a specific learning episode and is grossly synonymous with the construct of crystallized knowledge, discussed earlier. Adding further confusion, one may also speak of *prospective memory*— memory for intentions, such as paying the electric bill—and *working memory.* Prospective memory is generally viewed as a form of executive functioning, and working memory is considered below (see subsection "Working Memory").

Nondeclarative memory can be conceptualized as the products of experience that cannot necessarily be consciously verbalized. Common examples include motor or procedural memory (e.g., how to use the clutch to shift gears in a manual transmission car), as well as implicit memories, such as those resulting from priming or classical conditioning.

Episodic declarative memory tends to be the form of memory most affected by normal aging. Indeed, reports of failing episodic declarative memory are among the most ubiquitous cognitive concerns expressed by older adults (Jonker et al. 2000). The heightened concern about such deficits may in part reflect the fact that certain types of failure of episodic declarative memory are among the hallmarks of Alzheimer disease and related cortical dementias. Some of the most common tests of learning and memory are those in which examinees are asked to memorize short lists of words (generally over several aurally presented learning trials) (e.g., the Auditory Verbal Learning Test [see Boake 2000]), short stories or paragraphs (e.g., the Story Memory Test [see Heaton et al. 1991]), and/or geometric designs/figures (e.g., the Figure Memory Test [see Heaton et al. 1991]). Many of these tests include several learning trials (to help discern how much examinees may benefit from repeated exposure) and delayed recall (to determine how much information initially recalled has been stored and retained), as well as cued recall and/or recognition formats (to distinguish deficits in efficient retrieval from those reflecting genuine deficits in storage) (Lezak et al. 2004; Strauss et al. 2006).

Together with the age-related decline in processing speed, age-related deficits in episodic memory test performance are among the most consistently documented in the empirical literature (Christensen 2001). Craik (2008) summarized some of the key aspects of memory loss in older adults, noting that difficulties are most common in

> situations requiring large amounts of self-initiated processing…[i.e., those involving] cognitive operations that are neither habitual nor well supported by the environmental context…[but rather must be] initiated and performed in a conscious, effortful manner….Older people are also penalized when the information sought from memory is highly specific in nature….Older people are relatively unimpaired when retrieving general information about a topic, but do less well when specifics are required. (p. 343)

Assessment of memory with tests that provide multiple learning trials, as well as tests with cued or recognition formats, suggests that normal aging—in contrast to the pattern seen with cortical dementia—does not affect retention per se, but rather affects encoding and efficient retrieval (Price et al. 2004). Such findings of differential impairment of specific memory functions have obvious implications for compensating for other declines to maintain independent functioning.

Working Memory

Working memory may be conceptualized as the "mental workbench" wherein auditory or visual information is temporarily held (via active, effortful, resource-demanding processes such as rehearsal) for brief storage and manipulation (Baddeley 2007; Jarrold and Towse 2006). The most commonly cited model of working memory was initially proposed by Baddeley and Hitch in the early 1970s, but it has been expanded and elaborated by Baddeley over the subsequent decades to incorporate additional empirical findings (Baddeley 2007 provides a comprehensive overview). The most basic form of the model includes two resource-limited storage systems (the *phonological* or *articulatory loop* and the *visuospatial sketchpad*), which process verbal or visual/spatial information, respectively, and a *central executive,* which coordinates and updates allocation of processing resources to the two storage systems.

Two widely used measures of auditory working memory are the Digit Span and Letter-Number Sequencing subtests from the Wechsler scales. The Digit Span test has appeared on virtually every form of the Wechsler intelligence and memory scales since publication of the Bellevue Intelligence Examination in 1939, but its origins go back at least to the 1880s (for review, see Boake 2002). It remains among the most widely used psychometric procedures to this day. The procedures are extremely simple: On the first portion (forward span), the examiner reads aloud a series of digit (number) sequences of increasing length, and the examinee's task is to repeat the numbers in the presented sequence. The second portion (backward span) is virtually identical to the first, except that the examinee is required to report the number sequences in reverse order. Thus, the latter portion requires examinees not only to hold the information in working memory but also to actively manipulate that information for appropriate response. The latter form is sometimes said to require *executive working memory*, which is also emphasized on the Letter-Number Sequencing task.

The Letter-Number Sequencing task is similar to the Digit Span task except that the sequences presented involve intermixed letters and numbers. The examinee's task is to repeat the numbers in ascending order and then the letters in terms of their standard order in the English alphabet. There has also been a spatial version of the Digit Span task on some versions of the Wechsler Memory Scale.

Working memory tasks are highly influenced by age (Bopp and Verhaeghen 2005), but the effects may differ by the difficulty of the specific task. For instance, examining the standardization sample data for the third edition of the Wechsler Adult Intelligence Scale, Ryan et al. (2000) found that age decrements (relative to younger subjects) on the Letter-Number Sequencing task began to emerge in the 45- to 54-year age group, and those decrements gradually increased in older age cohorts. However, performance on the Digit Span test remained relatively unchanged through the 70- to 74-year age group. These findings may indicate that passive working memory (as emphasized in the forward span portion of the Digit Span task) is relatively resilient to the effects of aging, whereas executive working memory may be more prone to aging's effects. Longitudinal studies that focus on passive and executive forms of auditory and visual working memory would be helpful to tease out these possibilities and any neurobiological underpinnings.

Executive Functioning

Executive functioning is a label that is widely used but difficult to precisely define. It clearly refers to a range of specific processes. After reviewing several published definitions of this construct, Palmer and Heaton (2000) concluded that executive functions are those that provide

> an adaptive balance of maintenance and shifting of cognitive or behavioral responses to environmental demands, permitting longer-term goal-directed behavior rather than reflexive automated action.... Abilities underlying such activities may include: search of knowledge, abstraction and planning, evaluation/decision-making skills, initiation, self-monitoring, mental flexibility and [response inhibition]. (p. 53)

It must be acknowledged that even the preceding definition speaks more to the purpose of executive skills than to their fundamental nature. Nonetheless, that summary statement appears to capture the gist of what is generally being referred to with this term.

As is to be expected given the nebulous nature of the construct of executive functions, many different tests have been used to measure executive functioning. Some of the most commonly used are the Wisconsin Card Sorting Test (WCST), the Stroop Test, Letter and Category Fluency tasks, and part B of the Trail Making Test (the latter was described earlier in the subsection "Processing Speed"). Detailed descriptions of these and many other executive function measures are available in the review by Palmer and Heaton (2000), as well as in standard neuropsychological textbooks (e.g., Lezak et al. 2004; Strauss et al. 2006). To convey a hint of the diversity of skills incorporated under this construct, we limit our description here to the WCST and the Stroop Test.

On the WCST, the examinee is presented with four stimuli with designs that vary (between cards, not on the same card) in terms of the number of elements, the shape of those elements, and the color of those elements. The examinee is given a deck of response cards, which also vary along these dimensions (but may not match any one of the stimulus cards across all three dimensions), and he or she must serially match each response card to one of the stimulus cards. After each attempted match, the examinee is informed as to whether his or her response was correct or incorrect. To effectively perform this task, the examinee must generate (abstract) a viable hypothesis about the underlying sorting rule, test that hypothesis, and incorporate feedback to maintain or alter his or her strategy.

Innumerable studies of aging have included the WCST (Rhodes 2004). In fact, one of the first two studies to employ the WCST was a 1946 master's thesis by Morrow (1946), in which she found profound age effects on test results. The magnitude of age-related findings in Morrow's study was likely confounded by the procedures employed for recruiting elderly participants, all of whom were "residents of county homes for the aged" (Morrow 1946, p. 5). However, results of a meta-analysis of more recent and methodologically stronger studies still indicated robust deleterious effects on WCST performance with normal aging (Rhodes 2004).

Another widely used measure of executive functions is the Stroop Test. As is true of the CPT method (reviewed earlier in the subsection "Attention"), the term *Stroop Test* actually refers not to a single test but rather to a common method. In particular, the traditional Stroop paradigm is based on the long-known fact that among literate adults, word reading is more automatic (or perhaps more quickly processed) than is color naming. The *Stroop effect* derives its name from John Ridley Stroop, who published an influential paper on the phenomenon in 1935, but the roots of this task date back at least to the 1880s (for review, see MacLeod 1991). Examinees are presented with a series of word names that are printed in ink of a color discordant with the content of the word. (For instance, the word *green* may be printed in red ink.) The examinee's task is to ignore the meaning of each word and instead rapidly identify and state the color of the ink in which each is printed. Performance on the Stroop Test is deleteriously affected by age, although the degree to which the age-related decrement can be accounted for simply by slowed processing speed remains a point of controversy (Verhaeghen and Cerella 2002).

Cognitive Effects of Normal Aging: Caveats

Before considering the implications that the patterns of age-related decline in the cognitive domains described above have for successful aging, we offer two interpretive caveats that apply across the cognitive dimensions that have been considered.

One clear caveat in interpreting empirical findings on the effects of normal aging is that much of the published research rests on cross-sectional comparisons. Yet there are clear interpretive problems with cross-sectional age comparisons. Specifically, the presence of age-cohort effects on cognitive test results has been unequivocally established, in that newer cohorts tend to have better test performance. (For example, the average performance for 65-year-olds in 2009 on any particular cognitive test will tend to be higher than that shown by the average 65-year-old tested 50 years ago.)

The presence of cognitive cohort effects is a fascinating and not fully explained phenomenon in itself. A wealth of data collected within many different cultures and countries suggests that there has been (and continues to be) an incremental rise in average cognitive test performance over at least the past 100 years. This rise is known as the *Flynn effect,* named after James R. Flynn, who first brought it to widespread attention (although Flynn does not use that term for the phenomenon; Flynn 1998). At present, there remains no clear consensus on the cause and nature of the Flynn effect. For instance, is it merely improvement in test-taking ability, or does it reflect a genuine improvement in the cognitive functions being assessed by our measures? If the latter, what accounts for such a rise?

Answers about the cause of the Flynn effect await resolution, but for our present purposes it is sufficient to note that cohort effects cloud interpretation of cross-sectional studies of aging. Indeed, some researchers suggest that the degree of age-associated cognitive decline prior to age 60 or 65 is substantially less when cohort effects are taken into account (Schaie 2005).

A second caveat in interpreting findings on the effects of normal aging on cognition is that the studies cited above emphasized mean or average changes with aging. Mean or average changes may not accurately communicate the pattern of change at the level of individuals. Indeed, there is considerable interindividual variability in test performance, and this degree of variability clearly increases with advanced age (Ardila 2007; Christensen 2001). As discussed elsewhere in this book, a host of candidate factors, including genetic, social, lifestyle, and health factors, have been and continue to be actively investigated to understand why some individuals experience greater decline, whereas others retain relatively stable and unimpaired cognitive functions.

Despite the above caveats, the empirical literature nonetheless appears strong enough to support at least two conclusions in regard to the cognitive effects of normal aging:

1. Crystallized knowledge is not only spared by normal aging (at least through much of the adult life span) but may even improve with accumulated experience.
2. Aging has a deleterious effect on processing speed.

There also appears to be little controversy that advanced age is associated with decreased memory, particularly in regard to free recall on tests of episodic declarative memory. In contrast, healthy elderly adults appear to benefit from cued or recognition memory formats, suggesting that age-related memory deficits do not represent storage difficulties per se, but rather deficits in efficient encoding and/or retrieval processes. Deficits in other cognitive dimensions are also apparent, but the degrees to which each may reflect a primary impairment or the result of reduced processing resources and speed remain points of contention. In our concluding remarks, we consider the potential implications of these patterns in reference to successful aging.

Conclusion

As noted in the introductory comments, it is possible that individuals who achieve successful cognitive aging have escaped manifestation of the common age-related cognitive impairments, either because of a relative absence of decline or because of high premorbid cognitive reserve capacity. However, another possibility is that some successful cognitive agers have learned to compensate for declines in some cognitive abilities. For instance, Salthouse (1991) considered various domains of human expertise. In speculating on what, beyond a mere lack of proficiency, represent common performance barriers for nonexperts across domains, he suggested several related to accumulated knowledge, such as "not knowing what to expect...not knowing what to do and when to do it...lack of knowledge of interrelations among variables...[and] not knowing what information is relevant" (p. 294).

Accumulated knowledge is the one area of cognitive functioning that appears relatively unaffected (and even improved) by aging. Is it possible that older adults can use accumulated knowledge as expert agers in compensating for decrements in processing speed, working memory, and/or declines in other cognitive dimensions? One set of theories of knowledge representation and application that is potentially relevant to this possibility is those regarding *schemata*, and particularly the subtype commonly referred to as *scripts* (Schank and Abelson 1977). The concept of schemata has ancient origins, but in contemporary cognitive psychology and neuroscience it is generally traced to the early twentieth-century work of Bartlett (1932). Although Bartlett emphasized the role of schemata in memory, as a more general contemporary construct it can be loosely conceptualized as referring to mental structures or organized bundles of knowledge and expectations that guide, foster, and shape efficient perception, comprehension, memory, and response behaviors in regard to a specific type of object, event, or situation (Schank 1980). The term *scripts* refers to a subtype of schematic knowledge/ expectancy structures, specifically referring to those involving prototypical, sequenced actions or events (Schank and Abelson 1977).

The potential functional value of scripted or other schematic knowledge in compensating for age-related declines in basic cognitive functions seems self-evident. Decreased processing speed or other basic cognitive processing components such as working memory may result in a bottleneck for many nonautomated cognitive tasks; reducing the needs for conscious (nonautomated) cognitive resources during perception, information processing, and/or response selection, generation, or implementation should facilitate more efficient performance in routine situations (Norman and Shallice 1980) . On the other hand, to the degree that processing speed and other cognitive abilities affected by normal aging may also be required in the activation, selection, implementation, and adaptation of a particular script to the unique aspects and demands of a particular instance, it is possible that some aspects of schema- and/or script-guided behavior could be adversely affected by normal aging. To our knowledge, the potential value of scripted knowledge as a model of successful aging, or as a means to foster its development, has not been systematically evaluated, but this is clearly an avenue warranting empirical attention.

The easiest way to foster successful aging may be to help individuals develop and rely on relevant knowledge structures. That is, it may be easier for some persons to learn successful compensatory strategies than it is to increase premorbid cognitive reserve capacity. Clearly, a multipronged approach to understanding the nature of successful cognitive aging, and to fostering its occurrence in others, is appropriate. Consideration of the modal and individual cognitive strengths and limitations among older adults may be a key component in efforts to foster successful aging through compensatory mechanisms.

KEY POINTS

- As one ages, there is usually a decline in processing speed and certain aspects of memory (particularly free recall).

- Crystallized abilities (vocabulary, general knowledge) tend to remain stable or even increase.

- A broad number of domains can be tested with standardized tests (e.g., crystallized intelligence, processing speed, attention, receptive and expressive language, visuospatial and constructional abilities, memory, working memory, and executive functioning).

- Difficulties with interpreting available data in regard to the degree of cognitive change in nonpathological ("normal") aging include limited longitudinal data, the presence of cohort effects in cross-sectional comparisons of age groups, and descriptions based on mean performances with lack of attention to the degree of variability between the individuals.

▪ Successful cognitive aging may be a result of an individual's cognitive reserve capacity or effective use of compensation strategies.

▪ Scripts and schemata may promote maintenance of cognitive performance in aging, but this possibility has not yet received comprehensive research attention.

References

Ardila A: Normal aging increases cognitive heterogeneity: analysis of dispersion in WAIS-III scores across age. Arch Clin Neuropsychol 22:1003–1011, 2007

Baddeley A: Working Memory, Thought, and Action. New York, Oxford University Press, 2007

Bartlett FC: Remembering: A Study in Experimental and Social Psychology. Cambridge, UK, Cambridge University Press, 1932

Beck LH, Bransome ED Jr, Mirsky AF, et al: A continuous performance test of brain damage. J Consult Psychol 20:343–350, 1956

Berchtold NC, Cotman CW: Evolution in the conceptualization of dementia and Alzheimer's disease: Greco-Roman period to the 1960s. Neurobiol Aging 19:173–189, 1998

Birren JE, Fisher LM: Aging and speed of behavior: possible consequences for psychological functioning. Annu Rev Psychol 46:329–353, 1995

Boake C: Édouard Claparède and the Auditory Verbal Learning Test. J Clin Exp Neuropsychol 22:286–292, 2000

Boake C: From the Binet-Simon to the Wechsler-Bellevue: tracing the history of intelligence testing. J Clin Exp Neuropsychol 24:383–405, 2002

Bopp KL, Verhaeghen P: Aging and verbal memory span: a meta-analysis. J Gerontol B Psychol Sci Soc Sci 60:P223–P233, 2005

Bowles RP, Salthouse TA: Vocabulary test format and differential relations to age. Psychol Aging 23:366–376, 2008

Brown AS, Nix LA: Age-related changes in the tip-of-the-tongue experience. Am J Psychol 109:79–91, 1996

Cattell RB: The measurement of adult intelligence. Psychol Bull 40:153–193, 1943

Christensen H: What cognitive changes can be expected with normal ageing? Aust NZJ Psychiatry 35:768–775, 2001

Craik FIM: Memory changes in normal and pathological aging. Can J Psychiatry 53:343–345, 2008

de Fockert JW: Keeping priorities: the role of working memory and selective attention in cognitive aging. Sci Aging Knowledge Environ Nov 2(44):pe34, 2005

Dickinson D, Ramsey ME, Gold JM: Overlooking the obvious: a meta-analytic comparison of digit symbol coding tasks and other cognitive measures in schizophrenia. Arch Gen Psychiatry 64:532–542, 2007

Flynn JR: IQ gains over time: toward finding the causes, in The Rising Curve: Long-Term Gains in IQ and Related Measures. Edited by Neisser U. Washington, DC, American Psychological Association, 1998, pp 25–66

Gaeta H, Friedman D, Ritter W: Auditory selective attention in young and elderly adults: the selection of single versus conjoint features. Psychophysiology 40:389–406, 2003

Heaton RK, Grant I, Matthews CG: Comprehensive Norms for an Expanded Halstead-Reitan Battery: Demographic Corrections, Research Findings, and Clinical Applications. Odessa, FL, Psychological Assessment Resources, 1991

Horn JL, Blankson N: Foundations for better understanding of cognitive abilities, in Contemporary Intellectual Assessment: Theories, Tests, and Issues. Edited by Flanagan DP, Harrison PL. New York, Guilford, 2005, pp 41–68

Jarrold C, Towse JN: Individual differences in working memory. Neuroscience 139:39–50, 2006

Jeste DV, Palmer BW: The changing view of Alzheimer disease. Trends in Evidence-Based Neuropsychiatry 5:32–35, 2003

Jonker C, Geerlings MI, Schmand B: Are memory complaints predictive for dementia? A review of clinical and population-based studies. Int J Geriatr Psychiatry 15:983–991, 2000

Katzman R, Bick KL: The rediscovery of Alzheimer disease during the 1960s and 1970s, in Concepts of Alzheimer Disease: Biological, Clinical, and Cultural Perspectives. Edited by Whitehouse PJ, Maurer K, Ballenger JF. Baltimore, MD, Johns Hopkins University Press, 2000, pp 104–114

Lezak MD, Howieson DB, Loring DW, et al: Neuropsychological Assessment, 4th Edition. Oxford, UK, Oxford University Press, 2004

MacLeod CM: Half a century of research on the Stroop effect: an integrative review. Psychol Bull 109:163–203, 1991

Mani TM, Bedwell JS, Miller LS: Age-related decrements in performance on a brief continuous performance test. Arch Clin Neuropsychol 20:575–586, 2005

Morrow MA: Performance on the Hunt test with differential vocabulary scoring compared with performance on a card sorting test. Master's thesis, Madison, University of Wisconsin, 1946

Norman DA, Shallice T: Attention to Action: Willed and Automatic Control of Behavior (Report No 8006). La Jolla, CA, Center for Human Information Processing, University of California, San Diego, 1980

Oltmanns TF, Neale JM: Schizophrenic performance when distractors are present: attentional deficit or differential task difficulty? J Abnorm Psychol 84:205–209, 1975

Palmer BW, Heaton R: Executive dysfunction in schizophrenia, in Cognition in Schizophrenia: Impairments, Importance and Treatment Strategies. Edited by Sharma T, Harvey P. New York, Oxford University Press, 2000, pp 52–72

Price L, Said K, Haaland KY: Age-associated memory impairment of logical memory and visual reproduction. J Clin Exp Neuropsychol 26:531–538, 2004

Rhodes MG: Age-related differences in performance on the Wisconsin Card Sorting Test: a meta-analytic review. Psychol Aging 19:482–494, 2004

Rönnlund M, Nilsson LG: Adult life-span patterns in WAIS-R Block Design performance: cross-sectional versus longitudinal age gradients and relation to demographic factors. Intelligence 34:63–78, 2006

Ryan JJ, Sattler JM, Lopez SJ: Age effects on Wechsler Adult Intelligence Scale–III subtests. Arch Clin Neuropsychol 15:311–317, 2000

Salthouse TA: Expertise as the circumvention of human processing limitations, in Toward a General Theory of Expertise: Prospects and Limits. Edited by Anders Ericsson K, Smith J. New York, Cambridge University Press, 1991, pp 286–300

Salthouse TA: The processing-speed theory of adult age differences in cognition. Psychol Rev 103:403–428, 1996

Schaie KW: What can we learn from longitudinal studies of adult development? Res Hum Dev 2:133–158, 2005

Schank RC: What's a schema anyway? Contemporary Psychology: APA Review of Books 25:814–816, 1980

Schank RC, Abelson RP: Scripts, Plans, Goals and Understanding: An Inquiry Into Human Knowledge Structures. Hillsdale, NJ, Erlbaum, 1977

Strauss E, Sherman EMS, Spreen O: A Compendium of Neuropsychological Tests: Administration, Norms, and Commentary, 3rd Edition. New York, Oxford University Press, 2006

Tamkin AS, Jacobsen R: Age-related norms for the Hooper Visual Organization Test. J Clin Psychol 40:1459–1463, 1984

Verhaeghen P, Cerella J: Aging, executive control, and attention: a review of meta-analyses. Neurosci Biobehav Rev 26:849–857, 2002

Recommended Readings and Web Sites

Jeste DV, Palmer BW: The changing view of Alzheimer disease. Trends in Evidence-Based Neuropsychiatry 5:32–35, 2003

Longitudinal Studies on Aging: http://oregonstate.edu/~hofers/LLDR/longitudinal_aging_studies.htm. Accessed April 24, 2009.

Salthouse TA: The processing-speed theory of adult age differences in cognition. Psychol Rev 103:403–428, 1996

Schank RC: What's a schema anyway? Contemporary Psychology: APA Review of Books 25:814–816, 1980

4 Positive Emotions and Health

What We Know About Aging

Susan Turk Charles, Ph.D.
Briana N. Horwitz

What happens to people when they age? Are they happier? Grumpier? Do people become lonelier or more content? Most people hold beliefs about aging. Although some mention increasing wisdom or benevolence, these descriptions are generally in the minority. Instead, we commonly hear a person describe his or her uncle's behavior as typical of how people become more difficult with age, or mention how older people are always complaining about their health problems.

People readily volunteer their opinions about how emotional well-being and personalities change with aging, but these opinions do not always correspond with research findings. Accurate expectations of aging are critical for healthy functioning: overly positive portraits often underestimate challenges that many people face in late life and can leave them ill prepared in planning for the future. At the other extreme, overly negative expectations lead to self-fulfilling prophecies, in which people experience lower cognitive functioning and affective well-being partially in response to their own expectations.

In this chapter, we provide an overview of the literature regarding emotion and aging. First, we discuss patterns of personality and emotional well-being in adulthood. We review findings suggesting that personality remains relatively stable in adulthood but that the few changes that do occur show age-related improvements. Similarly, we discuss age-related changes in the experience of both positive and negative emotions. We then present the socioemotional selectivity theory to explain age differences in well-being, and we show how the changes in emotional processing influence social and cognitive functioning. Next, we mention three specific life circumstances that threaten psychosocial and physical well-being and that occur with greater frequency in old age. Finally, we provide practical advice for older adults when they are faced with difficult situations in their own lives.

Patterns of Personality and Emotional Well-Being Across the Adult Life Span

Newborns exhibit different temperaments at birth: some are easy to soothe and others are easily upset; some are active and others are calm. These temperaments are hypothesized to unfold across childhood and adulthood into personality traits (McCrae et al. 2000). In young adulthood, people form a fairly stable self-identity and fairly consistent patterns of emotional and behavioral responses. Life events can lead to changes in personality traits, such as positive work experiences that predict greater conscientiousness and more emotional stability. Despite these influences, rank-ordering of personality traits among groups of individuals is often fairly stable. For example, the person who was voted as most outgoing at the 10-year high school reunion will most likely be the most extraverted person attending the fiftieth high school reunion.

As a group, however, mean levels of personality traits change with age, and they change for the better. Neuroticism—the tendency to become easily upset or depressed (Eysenck 1963)—decreases slightly with age. Conscientiousness and social dominance (assertiveness) increase slightly in young adulthood and throughout middle age (Roberts and Mroczek 2008). Agreeableness, the tendency to be cooperative and compassionate rather than suspicious and antagonistic, also increases with age. If we extend the example of the high school reunion above, the attendees of the 10-year high school reunion are likely more sensation-seeking and more easily upset if a disaster strikes than the 50-year-reunion attendees in the next room. Thus, the term *grumpy old men* once used for a Hollywood movie title is not supported in research. The tendency to make health complaints is also inaccurate; older men and women actually report fewer minor aches and pains than do young and middle-age adults, even though they have greater numbers of chronic health conditions (Almeida and Horn 2004).

Emotional Experience and Aging

Personality is tied strongly to emotional experiences. Extraversion is related to the experience of positive emotions (positive affect), and neuroticism is associated with the experience of negative emotions (negative affect). The decrease in neuroticism, then, would suggest decreases in the experience of negative affect. Indeed, research findings are consistent with this view. In a longitudinal study examining reported negative affect across as much as 23 years, negative affect decreased with age among groups of younger adults (aging from 19 years to their mid-thirties), middle-aged adults (who aged from their mid-thirties to their late fifties), and older adults (aging from 63 years to their mid-eighties) (Charles et al. 2001). Across all age groups, the people reporting the highest levels of negative affect were the youngest adults in the group. In other cross-sectional studies, negative affect is similarly highest among people in young adulthood (Charles and Carstensen 2007); however, the age-related decreases in negative affect are often observed in people only up to their mid-sixties. People in their seventies and eighties report slightly higher negative affect than people in their sixties, although they never report the levels observed in younger adults (Carstensen et al. 2000).

In studies of people in the last decades of life, spanning from septuagenarians to centenarians, findings are more mixed. In a large German community sample, negative affect decreased with age only after functional health problems were controlled for (Kunzmann et al. 2000). In another study examining depressive symptoms among older adults across 6 years, people experienced higher levels of symptoms over time even after controlling for the effects of poor health (Davey et al. 2004).

The experiences of positive and negative emotions are not strongly tied together. People can experience both positive and negative emotions simultaneously, so changes in negative affect poorly predict changes in positive affect. Positive affect follows a different trajectory with age than negative affect, remaining markedly stable across 23 years in one study as people aged from youth to middle adulthood and from middle to older adulthood (Charles et al. 2001). Among samples of adults ranging from people in their seventies to those over 100, positive affect increased with older age after the effects of functional health problems were controlled for (Kunzmann et al. 2000).

Socioemotional Selectivity Theory

The overall picture of emotion and aging, as assessed by both personality characteristics and reported emotional experiences, is one characterized by decreases in negative experiences and stability if not increases in emotional stability and positive emotional experiences. One interpretation of these findings concerning general decreases in negative affect is that over the years, older adults have accumulated necessary skills at regulating their emotions and have honed these skills through continual practice. Older adults have become sophisticated in applying cognitive-behavioral strategies (such as reappraising stressful events to make themselves less upset, or disengaging from a negative situation) to regulate their emotions in response to stressors in their lives. Older adults appear to better understand what bothers them, and they learn to avoid these situations or to ignore or cope with what they cannot avoid. Additionally, older adults may realize that their time left is growing shorter, and they choose activities that make them feel content and happy in order to fully appreciate the time remaining in their lives (Carstensen et al. 1999).

Socioemotional selectivity theory describes how time left in life is related to the ways in which people structure their lives and the emotions they experience (Carstensen et al. 1999). According to this theory, all people have an awareness of how much time is left in their lives, and this temporal horizon structures people's goals. When time is perceived as expansive, people select goals that focus on gaining knowledge for a long and unknown future. Although people enjoy positive experiences, they often choose situations that provide them with the opportunity to gain information even if these situations threaten their affective well-being. For example, people may choose to work with a difficult, disrespectful boss if working for this person is necessary to building a successful career. When the future extends seemingly forever, temporary discomfort for a potential long-term payoff in information is often worth the risk. Even younger adults who are not carefully planning their future activities realize that they have a long life ahead of them.

As time left in life grows shorter, however, people are much more invested in the present than in the future. As a result, people have more emotion-focused rather than information-focused goals. According to socioemotional selectivity theory, as future horizons narrow, maintaining well-being is more important than the potential for gaining new information. In young adulthood, the time perspective is expansive. As people get older, they are more aware that their future is not endless. Their decisions bear more on how they relate to their current well-being and not to an unknown future.

Social Processes Influencing Well-Being in Aging

Age differences in the motivations of older and younger adults are probably best exemplified in their different patterns of social interactions. Older adults interact with fewer social partners than younger adults, a reliable finding documented in multiple gerontological studies (for review, see Charles and Carstensen 2007). Social processes are strongly related to physical health; people who have strong social networks report better physical health at every age and live longer than their same-age peers with weaker social ties (Charles and Mavandadi 2003). Social support is also strongly related to mental health. Friends serve as companions and sources of positive experiences in general as well as provide support during difficult times. Because social support is so strongly tied to mental and physical health, people have viewed age-related decreases in social partners as an age-related deficit (Carstensen et al. 1998). Because older people report interacting with fewer social partners, they have been viewed as lonely and isolated and in need of interventions to boost their social activity.

This assumption, however, was not supported by further research. Older adults had fewer social partners than younger adults, but they were not reporting greater loneliness than their younger counterparts (for review, see Charles and Carstensen 2007). Additionally, they did not report lower levels of well-being than younger adults, even though they had a smaller social network. Why, with a smaller social network, were older adults reporting similar if not higher levels of well-being than younger adults? This paradox was explained by additional research informed by socioemotional selectivity theory. Older adults did have fewer social partners than younger adults, but these smaller social networks comprised a greater proportion of close social contacts. However, older and younger adults did not vary in their total number of very close social partners—those people without whom life would never be quite the same. The levels of well-being found in older adults were instead explained by their having fewer peripheral social partners, those people defined as casual friends and acquaintances. These peripheral social partners are arguably necessary and beneficial when the future is expansive and people are building social networks for future possibilities, including dating to find a future mate or interacting with others for future business or social contacts. For people with foreshortened futures, however, these peripheral partners are arguably less important.

Other research has found that older adults actively cull fewer emotionally close social partners from their social networks and that their social networks are strongly dominated by emotionally meaningful social partners (Lang and Carstensen 1994). Older adults report high levels of satisfaction with their social partners, reporting even greater positive affect when interacting with family members than do younger adults (Charles and Piazza 2007). In contrast, younger adults report higher rates of social interactions with new friends, even though these new friends do not offer the same level of emotionally meaningful engagement that established social partners do (Carstensen et al. 1998).

Cognitive Processes Influencing Well-Being in Aging

Emotional and informational goals influence not only social interactions but also how people appraise the environment around them, make decisions, and remember the events in their lives. The cognitive evaluations and decision-making processes of younger adults reflect the priority they place on knowledge and information. The motivations of older adults lie in emotion-related processes. Their cognitive evaluations and decision-making processes focus on emotion-related outcomes. Motivations to maintain and even enhance levels of well-being translate into active cognitive and behavioral strategies to regulate emotions. For example, older adults focus their attention away from negative stimuli and toward positive stimuli (Mather and Carstensen 2003). They also appraise situations in their lives less negatively (Charles and Almeida 2007) and choose strategies of disengaging from situations that continue the experience of negative emotions. When confronted with a social conflict, older adults are more likely to walk away from tense interpersonal interactions, choosing coping strategies such as preserving harmony in social interactions over active confrontations with close family members; in contrast, younger adults often choose more active confrontational approaches when handling interpersonal conflicts (Lefkowitz and Fingerman 2003).

Older adults also report more positive memories than younger adults. Memories represent active reconstructions of past events that are influenced by current motivations. Goals related to optimizing emotional experience lead to more positive appraisals and more positive memories. In a study examining memory of positive, neutral, and negative pictures, younger adults remembered the negative pictures best; older adults showed no such bias (Charles et al. 2003). Age differences in the focus on and retention of negative and positive aspects of the environment have been used to explain why older adults often report higher levels of well-being than younger adults, although older adults may not attend to negative aspects of a situation when making decisions in their lives (Charles and Carstensen 2007).

Socioemotional Processes and Health

Older adults place great importance on maintaining well-being, a position that provides additional benefits for physical and cognitive functioning. Folk theories have long promoted the idea that positive emotions are good for health, whereas negative emotions (or stress) are detrimental to physical well-being. Accumulating empirical studies offer both explanations and support for these early intuitions. Positive emotions provide immediate physical health benefits, including their role in promoting healthy habits in diet and exercise that improve cardiovascular functioning (Lefcourt et al.

1997). Positive emotions (e.g., joy, interest, and contentment) are thought to broaden creative thoughts and promote active behaviors. In doing so, positive emotions loosen the hold that negative emotions have on an individual's mind and body by undoing narrowed thoughts and actions that are activated by negative emotions (Fredrickson and Losada 2005). As a result, people can focus their psychological resources on adaptive ways of preserving health, including creative health behaviors. One implication here is that therapies targeted at increasing positive emotions, such as relaxation exercises or cognitive-behavioral therapy, may also influence physical health.

Researchers have also started to examine how stress may impair physical and cognitive functioning. The glucocorticoid cascade hypothesis describes how psychosocial stress directly affects physiological and cognitive functioning (Sapolsky 1996) (see also Chapter 10, "Stress, Resilience and the Aging Brain"). When people experience distress, the physiological system releases cortisol, a hormone that is activated in response to psychosocial stressors, into the bloodstream. Cortisol plays a role in multiple physiological processes, including the release of glucose and the inhibition of insulin so the body has energy available for rapid response to a stressor. Although enabling individuals to be adaptive by mobilizing the body for quick responses, high levels of cortisol over prolonged periods of time lead to adverse physical outcomes, including impaired glucose metabolism and decreased immune system functioning. As a result, cortisol has been hypothesized to be one reason why high levels of chronic stress, such as those resulting from living with an anxiety disorder or living in a stressful environment, are related to higher rates of chronic illness (Sapolsky et al. 1986). These physiological processes also include reductions in the volume of the hippocampus, the area of the brain vital for learning and memory. Animal studies have documented that chronic stress elevates cortisol levels and that these high levels of cortisol are related to impairments in new learning and memory (Sapolsky 1996).

Life Circumstances That Threaten Well-Being

The research reviewed thus far offers a fairly optimistic portrayal of old age. Personality is fairly stable across the adult life span, but the small changes that are noted all indicate age-related increases in functioning: with age, people become more emotionally stable (less neurotic), more agreeable, and more conscientious. Concerning reports of emotional experience, negative affect decreases and positive affect remains fairly stable. Results thus indicate overall higher levels of well-being for older than younger adults. And, when controlling for functional health problems, researchers have found that positive affect levels are higher and negative affect levels are often lower among people in their nineties than among people in their seventies (Kunzmann et al. 2000). Social support also suggests age-related advantages. The smaller social networks of older adults are more selective than those of younger adults because older adults actively shape their social networks to include only emotionally meaningful network members.

These findings represent good news for people who are older adults or who work with older adults. However, certain situations arise in old age that produce challenges to a person's well-being. These situations make engaging in cognitive-behavioral strategies of emotional regulation difficult and often place strain on social support networks. Older adults who face these circumstances must recognize the situation's impact on their abilities to regulate their emotions to maintain well-being. These situations include loss of social belonging, the experience of chronic stressors, and neurological dysregulation.

Loss of Social Belonging

Across the life span, people have a small group of people who provide a sense of attachment, or belonging. The *convoy model of social relationships* describes the importance of this relatively small collection, or convoy, of people who constitute the closest, most meaningful social relationships in a person's life (Antonucci et al. 2004). Members of the convoy are generally long-term friends and family members who provide people with feelings of belonging and strong security. With this secure base, people are free to explore their worlds, knowing that they can always turn to these sources of comfort in times of distress.

People are social animals who need to feel this sense of belonging (Baumeister and Leary 1995). With this convoy, people have a sense of belonging and are integrated into a social group. Without this support, people at every age are at risk for depression. Most older adults report high levels of satisfaction with their social support network (for review, see Charles and Carstensen 2007), but the death of close friends and family members can place older adults at risk as they lose these very important social network members. One study suggests that social integration, described as feeling of belonging within a community, is a protective factor against suicide among older adults (Cutright et al. 2006).

Although loss of social belonging can occur with the loss of any meaningful relationship, such loss has been studied most often in the context of marriage. Spousal bereavement is linked to high levels of emotional distress for both men and women, although men are at higher risk for psychological distress in response to the death of a spouse than are women (Stroebe et al. 2000). One reason for this difference may be that women have stronger social bonds outside of the marriage than do men. Men are more likely to report their wives as their closest social partner, whereas women are more likely to report having a best friend outside of the marital bond (Antonucci and Akiyama 1987).

Constant, Unrelenting Stressors

Constant and unrelenting stressors include any negative situations that are so constant that they do not allow for time and recovery from bombarding interruptions and responsibilities. Unfortunately, some types of unremitting stressors increase in prevalence as people age. Living with chronic disabilities or chronic pain is associated with distress. People who have severe disabilities report lower levels of well-being years after the onset of the condition (Lucas 2007). Taking care of a spouse with dementia is another common source of stress.

Caregiving for a spouse with dementia poses a risk to emotional wellbeing in later life. Among individuals caring for community-dwelling people with dementia, 35% are the spouse of the affected person (Langa et al. 2001). The caregiving experience is more adverse than other types of long-term stressors because this task constitutes unrelenting financial and physical demands on the caregiver. Spousal caregiving represents a situation often referred to as "the long good-bye," where the caregiver must slowly lose his or her partner to dementia. The lack of any reprieve is often a reality for caregivers, and research indicates that caregiving takes a toll on emotional wellbeing. Rates of depression and anxiety among caregivers are higher than among their peers without this responsibility (Schulz et al. 1995). Among caregivers, greater feelings of distress and perceived burden are the best predictors of mental and physical health outcomes, including higher rates of major depressive disorder and higher rates of mortality than among noncaregiving peers (Schulz and Beach 1999). Moreover, caregivers with low levels of social support show greater cardiovascular reactivity to psychological stressors compared with noncaregivers and caregivers with higher levels of social support (Uchino et al. 1992).

Neurological Dysregulation

Emotional regulation strategies do not require superior intelligence, but they often require some judgment and forethought (Charles and Piazza, in press). As a result, individuals with cognitive deficits, dementia, or neurological dysregulation have a more difficult time engaging in these strategies. Without the use of cognitive-behavioral strategies, such as structuring the social network or focusing attention to more positive aspects of the environment, people are more susceptible to experiencing distress. This greater susceptibility leaves them more vulnerable to stressful experiences. People of any age have greater problems using cognitive-behavioral regulation strategies in the face of neurological dysregulation, but these conditions increase in prevalence with age. Two such neurological diseases, Parkinson disease and Alzheimer disease, create chronic and often uncontrollable stressors that can make emotion regulation difficult. They also, unfortunately, lead to organic changes that leave people more susceptible to emotional dysregulation.

Anxiety and depression often accompany Parkinson disease, with rates of clinically significant anxiety estimated as high as 40% (Richard et al. 1996). Even though the functional limitations of this disease also create stressors sufficient to cause affective distress, researchers believe that the high comorbidity of Parkinson disease with anxiety and depression has a neurological basis (Cummings 1992). Alzheimer disease is also associated with emotional dysregulation. Rates of depression are high in people with Alzheimer disease, with an estimated 26% having clinical levels of major depression and another 26% meeting criteria for minor depression (Starkstein et al. 2005). The presence of depressive symptoms has led researchers to debate whether depressive symptoms that often precede a dementia diagnosis reflect early neurological changes that are part of the Alzheimer disease pathology.

Even mild cognitive deficits may lead to minor emotional dysregulation. Among cognitively intact adults, older adults direct their attention away from negative information to a greater extent than do younger adults, and age-related declines in memory are more pronounced for negative material than positive material (Charles et al. 2003). Older adults who score low on working memory tasks assessing cognitive control focus less on positive aspects of the environment and more on negative aspects than do their same-age counterparts who score higher on cognitive tests. Although observed differences may reflect lower cognitive functioning as opposed to cognitive deficits, these findings suggest that low cognitive performance is associated with decreases in strategies that help older adults to optimize their positive information and with decreases in positive emotional experiences as a consequence (Mather and Knight 2005).

When Faced With Adversity: What to Do Next?

When researchers describe the factors that relate to successful aging, the list of attributes often includes being in optimal physical and mental health, having a large social network, and having sufficient financial resources to avoid unnecessary stressors. These requirements, however, are not always possible. Nearly everyone who lives into old age experiences loss in life at some point, whether it is the loss of friends or family members to death or the loss of one's health. Despite engaging in good health behaviors, people are diagnosed with physical health problems. After spending years accruing an emotionally meaningful and invaluable social network, people begin to see members of that network die. Despite having a high degree of education and engaging in mentally challenging activities, they can experience cognitive decline. And marrying someone years younger than you cannot guarantee that you will avoid the role of spousal caregiver or widow or widower.

Anyone can face adverse situations. These situations are difficult, and people vary in their needs during difficult times. People differ in both what they experience and how they perceive these events. Some people thrive in adversity, whereas others may not have adequate resources to cope successfully. Experiences themselves differ in their frequency, intensity, and predictability. The complexity of older adults' needs suggests that it is necessary to consider individual needs when designing therapies and interventions. Below we present three recommendations for older adults who are experiencing stress in their lives, although we realize that modifications and adaptations for each recommendation should take into account specific life circumstances for each individual.

Receiving Adequate Social Support

Humans are social animals, and social support predicts health outcomes as strongly as objective health indicators such as smoking history or cholesterol levels (Charles and Mavandadi 2003). Social support should therefore be regarded as a health behavior and be taken as seriously as other medical prescriptions. The need for social support is vitally related to health and well-being and is perhaps even more important when people encounter difficulties in their lives (Cartensen et al. 1999). Although socioemotional selectivity theory posits that older adults are content with smaller social networks, these social networks are vitally important to maintain.

Life circumstances often make social interactions more difficult. For example, health problems may make social engagement difficult because of transportation issues or because a person is experiencing pain. In these events, barriers must be identified (e.g., finding alternative transportation or recognizing certain times of day when pain is less intense) and social interactions should be organized taking into account the potential problems. If travel is not often possible, then alternative means of social contact such as telephone calls or interactions via computer technology should be considered. Older individuals are less familiar with this technology but can learn through tutoring or computer classes, which may benefit cognitive functioning as well (Gunther et al. 2003).

Another situation that makes maintaining social activities difficult is caregiving. Caregivers have little time to focus on healthy behaviors related to proper nutrition and exercise, let alone time to engage in social activities that are not part of their caregiving responsibilities. Caregivers may also feel guilty spending time away from the person for whom they are providing care. Yet social support affects the well-being of all people involved in a stressful situation and helps to offset the negative effects of stressful experiences. Among caregivers, perceived support is related to lower levels of depression and is related to less distress after experiencing stressors in their lives (Atienza et al. 2001). People must make time for social interactions away from their caregiving role, realizing that these experiences are beneficial to their physical and mental well-being and will help them be more effective at home.

Social support is important for older adults' physical and emotional well-being, but it is important to recognize the types of social interventions that will best meet the needs of the individual. Sometimes existing social ties fail to provide sufficient support. Also, the number of meaningful and close social partners may have been reduced by death. In these cases, people may need to turn to new social partners. Although some older adults may benefit from meeting new people, others may instead prefer to see existing friends and family members more often. By rekindling and strengthening existing relationships, older adults can expand their social relationships from within their existing network.

Sometimes family members and friends lack understanding of the situation, or they may be too emotionally involved to help. For example, adjusting to a chronic health problem affects not just the person affected, but his or her spouse and family members as well. Also, older adults dealing with personal health struggles or caregiving responsibilities may not feel comfortable sharing their thoughts with members of their social networks. In that case, one option is seeking peers in a support group who are going through similar experiences; another is talking to a more objective listener and one who is familiar with the situation, a therapist or counselor who is used to working with clients who have similar issues.

Maintaining Control

Researchers state that the motivation to maintain control is an innate drive present in all species (Heckhausen 1999). High levels of perceived control— the feeling that people can actively shape their environment to achieve their goals—are related to better physical and mental well-being. With aging, limitations develop whereby people feel they have less power or fewer resources with which to exert control in their lives. When they are faced with difficult situations such as the loss of social belonging, exposure to chronic stressors, or neurological dysregulation, the need for control is often more difficult to maintain, but is no less important. Because a sense of control is so strongly tied to well-being, finding ways to maintain a sense of control under difficult circumstances is vitally important. Sometimes people in these situations accept care from well-meaning others, yet this help can carry the unintended negative consequence of taking away the control that people need to maintain healthy functioning. For example, a man who has suffered a stroke and has problems using utensils may receive help from his wife. Although his wife has the best intentions in mind, her actions may lead to greater inactivity from her husband. Instead of practicing and regaining his skills, her husband may remain dependent on her help. Research findings indicate that providing help can often, ironically, lead to greater disability for the older care recipient (Baltes et al. 1994).

Family members and health professionals can help an older adult maintain a feeling of control in his or her life by identifying activities that are personally meaningful. After identifying these areas, they can help the person make a plan to actively engage in these activities. Obviously, these strategies must be tailored to a person's interests and abilities. Even someone with low levels of cognitive functioning, for example, can be given simple choices or simple responsibilities over issues in their lives. For example, a person with mild-to-moderate dementia can be asked to choose between two different activities or food options. Higher functioning people are encouraged to identify valued activities in their lives and find ways to continue to participate in them. If necessary, identifying possible compensatory strategies, such as enlisting the help of others or using technological devices, can help someone maintain independence and a sense of control.

Making Time for Positive Experiences

People must structure their lives so that they experience positive emotions every day. Often, self-care is the activity that is forfeited when older adults are faced with stressful, time-demanding experiences, regardless of whether the stressor is a function of caregiving, coping with a chronic illness of their own, or coping with other losses. People struggling with many challenges in their lives are often too overwhelmed to consider taking time out to experience positive emotions. Additionally, people who are already depressed are often reluctant or lack the energy and motivation to engage in positive experiences. People experiencing distress in response to bereavement or another recent loss may feel that experiencing positive emotions is contrary to proper behavior and response to loss. Yet positive emotions are beneficial for physical health not only for the individual but also for those around that individual. For example, the depression experienced by caregivers spills over to affect the emotional well-being of the patient (Beach et al. 2008). Positive experiences can be something as small as reading a magazine or newspaper, calling a friend, taking a walk, or listening to a favorite song. The best atmosphere is one where people experience almost three times more positive than negative experiences (Fredrickson and Losada 2005). When life experiences are stressful, older adults (or, if they cannot, those who support them) need to strive to intersperse these times with positive events.

Conclusion

Aging has been historically viewed as a time of loss, and losses do occur. Friends and family members die, and physical health problems are more likely to occur. Yet despite these difficulties, older adults do not become less agreeable or more negative. Instead, older adults report lower levels of negative affect and report personality traits of greater assertiveness and emotional stability than in early adulthood. Understanding these findings is vitally important for understanding old age. If older adults are more depressed than usual or report dissatisfaction with their social networks, these symptoms should not be dismissed as typical of aging. Physicians and other health care professionals need to recognize new symptoms or problems and intervene early to prevent further problems.

For some older adults, life circumstances have placed them in situations that are difficult to manage. In these cases, older adults need to recognize that maintaining well-being will be particularly challenging. Maintaining strong social networks, maintaining high levels of control over one's situation, and ensuring that every day contains positive experiences are not an exhaustive list of the necessary ingredients for successful coping, but each recommendation has been supported by empirical research as important for both physical and emotional well-being. By maintaining emotional health, older adults can more effectively make decisions, focus on positive aspects of their lives, and optimize their physical well-being.

KEY POINTS

■ Personality remains relatively stable across adulthood for the majority of adults. Slight changes in personality, including slight decreases in neuroticism and increases in conscientiousness, do occur with age.

I Emotional well-being tends to improve into late adulthood. Negative affect decreases with age up to the mid-sixties. Although negative affect increases slightly in people in their seventies and eighties, it never reaches the high levels documented in younger adulthood. Positive affect is slightly higher among older adults than younger adults, after controlling for health problems.

I Two explanations are advanced for why emotions improve with age. First, people develop better emotional regulation skills as a result of having had more life experiences. Second, according to socioemotional selectivity theory, older adults tend to involve themselves in more emotionally meaningful goals and activities than do younger adults, as a result of an awareness that the time left in life is decreasing.

I Circumstances that increase in likelihood with age can lead to decreases in both emotional and physical well-being and include 1) loss of social belonging, 2) constant and unrelenting stressors (e.g., caregiving for a spouse with dementia), and 3) neurological dysregulation.

I Therapies and clinical interventions designed to improve health and well-being in later life may be more beneficial when they improve older adults' social support, help them maintain or increase their levels of personal control, and make time for positive experiences.

References

Almeida DM, Horn MC: Is daily life more stressful during middle adulthood? in How Healthy Are We? A National Study of Well-Being at Midlife. Edited by Brim OG, Ryff CD, Kessler RC. Chicago, IL, University of Chicago Press, 2004, pp 425–451

Antonucci T, Akiyama H: An examination of sex differences in social support among older men and women. Sex Roles 17:737–749, 1987

Antonucci T, Akiyama H, Takahashi K: Attachment and close relationships across the lifespan. Attach Hum Dev 6:353–370, 2004

Atienza AA, Collins R, King AC: The mediating effects of situational control on social support and mood following a stressor. J Gerontol B Psychol Sci Soc Sci 56:129–139, 2001

Baltes MM, Neumann EM, Zank S: Maintenance and rehabilitation of independence in old age: an intervention program for staff. Psychol Aging 9:179–188, 1994

Baumeister RF, Leary MR: The need to belong: desire for interpersonal attachments as a fundamental human motivation. Psychol Bull 117:497–529, 1995

Beach SRH, Kogan SM, Brody GH, et al: Change in caregiver depression as a function of the Strong African American Families Program. J Fam Psychol 22:241–252, 2008

Carstensen LL, Gross JJ, Fung HH: The social context of emotional experience, in Annual Review of Gerontology and Geriatrics, Vol 17: Focus on Emotion and Adult Development. Edited by Schaie KW, Lawton MP. New York, Springer, 1998, pp 325–352

Carstensen LL, Isaacowitz DM, Charles ST: Taking time seriously: a theory of socioemotional selectivity. Am Psychol 54:165–181, 1999

Carstensen LL, Pasupathi M, Mayr U, et al: Emotional experience in everyday life across the adult lifespan. J Pers Soc Psychol 79:644–655, 2000

Charles ST, Almeida DM: Genetic and environmental effects on daily life stressors: more evidence for greater variation in later life. Psychol Aging 22:331–340, 2007

Charles ST, Carstensen LL: Emotion regulation and aging, in Handbook of Emotion Regulation. Edited by Gross J. New York, Guilford, 2007, pp 307–327

Charles ST, Mavandadi S: Relationships and health across the life span, in Growing Together: Personal Relationships Across the Life Span. Edited by Lang F, Fingerman K. New York, Cambridge University Press, 2003, pp 240–267

Charles ST, Piazza JR: Memories of social interactions: age differences in emotional intensity. Psychol Aging 22:300–309, 2007

Charles ST, Piazza JR: Age differences in affective well-being: context matters. Social and Personality Psychology Compass (in press)

Charles ST, Reynolds CA, Gatz M: Age-related differences and change in positive and negative affect over 23 years. J Pers Soc Psychol 30:136–151, 2001

Charles ST, Mather M, Carstensen LL: Aging and emotional memory: the forgettable nature of negative images for older adults. J Exp Psychol 122:310–324, 2003

Cummings JL: Depression and Parkinson's disease: a review. Am J Psychiatry 149:443–454, 1992

Cutright P, Stack S, Fernquist R: The age structures and marital status differences of married and not married male suicide rates: 12 developed countries. Arch Suicide Res 10:365–382, 2006

Davey A, Halverson CF, Zonderman AB, et al: Change in depressive symptoms in the Baltimore Longitudinal Study of Aging. J Gerontol B Psychol Sci Soc Sci 59:270–277, 2004

Eysenck HJ: Biological basis of personality. Nature 199:1031–1034, 1963 [Republished in Neuropsychiatry and Clinical Neuroscience 10:230–231, 1998]

Fredrickson BL, Losada MF: Positive affect and the complex dynamics of human flourishing. Am Psychol 60:678–686, 2005

Gunther VK, Schafer P, Holzner BJ, et al: Long-term improvements in cognitive performance through computer-assisted cognitive training: a pilot study in a residential home for older people. Aging Ment Health 7:200–206, 2003

Heckhausen J: Developmental Regulation in Adulthood: Age-Normative and Sociostructural Constraints as Adaptive Challenges. New York, Cambridge University Press, 1999

Kunzmann U, Little TD, Smith J: Is age-related stability of subjective well-being a paradox? Cross-sectional and longitudinal evidence from the Berlin Aging Study. Psychol Aging 15:511–526, 2000

Lang FR, Carstensen LL: Close emotional relationships in late life: further support for proactive aging in the social domain. Psychol Aging 9:315–324, 1994

Langa KM, Chernew ME, Mohammed U, et al: National estimates of the quantity and cost of informal caregiving for the elderly with dementia. J Gen Intern Med 16:770–778, 2001

Lefcourt HM, Davidson K, Prkachin KM, et al: Humor as a stress moderator in the prediction of blood pressure obtained during five stressful tasks. J Res Pers 31:523–542, 1997

Lefkowitz ES, Fingerman KL: Positive and negative emotional feelings and behaviors in mother-daughter ties in late life. J Fam Psychol 17:607–617, 2003

Lucas RE: Adaptation and the set-point model of subjective well-being: does happiness change after major life events? Current Directions in Psychological Science 16:75–79, 2007

Mather M, Carstensen LL: Aging and attentional biases for emotional faces. Psychol Sci 14:409–415, 2003

Mather M, Knight M: Goal-directed memory: the role of cognitive control in older adults' emotional memory. Psychol Aging 20:554–570, 2005

McCrae RR, Costa PT Jr, Ostendorf F, et al: Nature over nurture: temperament, personality, and lifespan development. J Pers Soc Psychol 78:173–186, 2000

Richard IH, Schiffer RB, Kurlan R: Anxiety and Parkinson's disease. J Neuropsychiatry Clin Neurosci 8:383–392, 1996

Roberts BW, Mroczek D: Personality trait change in adulthood. Curr Dir Psychol Sci 17:31–35, 2008

Sapolsky RM: Why stress is bad for your brain. Science 273:749–750, 1996

Sapolsky RM, Krey LC, McEwen BS: The neuroendocrinology of stress and aging: the glucocorticoid cascade hypothesis. Endocrinol Rev 7:284–301, 1986

Schulz R, Beach SR: Caregiving as a risk factor for mortality: the Caregiver Health Effects Study. JAMA 282:2215–2219, 1999

Schulz R, O'Brien AT, Bookwala J, et al: Psychiatric and physical morbidity effects of dementia caregiving: prevalence, correlates, and causes. Gerontologist 35:771–791, 1995

Starkstein SE, Jorge R, Mizrah R, et al: The construct of minor and major depression in Alzheimer's disease. Am J Psychiatry 162:2086–2093, 2005

Stroebe MS, Stroebe W, Schut H: Grief and loss, in Encyclopedia of Psychology. Edited by Kazdin AE. New York, Oxford University Press, 2000, pp 11–14

Uchino BN, Kiecolt-Glaser JK, Cacioppo JT: Age-related changes in cardiovascular response as a function of a chronic stressor and social support. J Pers Soc Psychol 63:839–846, 1992

Recommended Readings

Carstensen LL, Isaacowitz DM, Charles ST: Taking time seriously: a theory of socioemotional selectivity. Am Psychol 54:165–181, 1999

Charles ST, Carstensen LL: Emotion regulation and aging, in Handbook of Emotion Regulation. Edited by Gross J. New York, Guilford, 2007, pp 307–327

Charles ST, Reynolds CA, Gatz M: Age-related differences and change in positive and negative affect over 23 years. J Pers Soc Psychol 30:136–151, 2001

Heckhausen J: Developmental Regulation in Adulthood: Age-Normative and Sociostructural Constraints as Adaptive Challenges. New York, Cambridge University Press, 1999

5

The Role of Spirituality in Healthy Aging

Dan G. Blazer, M.D., Ph.D.
Keith G. Meador, M.D., Th.M., M.P.H.

Interest in the association between religion/spirituality and health in later life has heightened in recent years (Coleman 2005; Koenig et al. 2001). Although this interest, broadly defined, crosses all age groups, many studies and writings have focused specifically on the elderly. At least two factors may have driven the increased attention toward religion/spirituality and its relationship to health in later life. First, the longtime boundary between the medical profession and the religious or spiritual has been blurred if not erased. Physicians and other health care professionals have been encouraged to explore the beliefs and religious practices of their patients as a means to better relate to their patients and to increase their understanding of the interactions between these beliefs/practices and their patients' health. For example, diet and lifestyle for some religious groups, such as the Seventh-day Adventists, are strongly determined by the traditions of their faith. Working within those traditions to encourage a healthy diet not only facilitates the therapeutic bond; it also can promote better health (as the Seventh-day Adventists almost completely abstain from smoking and tend toward a vegetarian diet).

Second, the explosion of empirical research about the association between health and the individual's deepest spiritual beliefs, religious practices, and membership in faith communities has been weighted toward the elderly. The reasons for the emphasis on the elderly are not entirely clear but some factors do emerge. Many large community surveys of older adults, such as the Established Populations for Epidemiologic Studies of the Elderly, have included items assessing religious beliefs and practices (Cornoni-Huntley et al. 1990; Koenig et al. 1999). In addition, it is possible that investigators who have an interest in the elderly also tend to have more of an interest in religion and spirituality. Regardless, the literature exploring the association between religion/spirituality and health among the elderly has significantly increased during the past 20 years.

Yet another factor has emerged. Given the tendency in years past to consider aging from a perspective of inevitable decline and loss, a new paradigm emerged during the 1990s—the concept of successful aging. The MacArthur Research Network on Successful Aging is but the most prominent of a number of efforts supporting this new paradigm. Changes in diet and exercise, mental stimulation, self-efficacy, and dynamic social network connections have all been demonstrated to enhance physical, mental, and social well-being among the elderly. This view has naturally attracted further elaborations of what it means to age successfully. One such elaboration has been proposed by Crowther and colleagues (2002). "Positive spirituality," according to these authors, is defined by "a developing and internalized personal relation with the sacred or transcendent that is not bound by race, ethnicity, economics, or class and promotes the wellness and welfare of self and others" (p. 613). Such positive spirituality is less authoritarian, less formal and orthodox. It is more intrinsic, oriented toward emotion and behavior and the capacity to engage in positive actions that promote life-enhancing behaviors and beliefs. Although this construct has yet to be demonstrated to be associated with healthy aging, the intuitive appeal of the construct is apparent.

In this chapter we present an exploration of spirituality and healthy aging from three perspectives. First, we explore briefly the data-based studies that have emerged over the past three decades that inform our understanding of the association between religion/spirituality and health among older adults. Second, we reflect on the role of faith communities as they support and at times hinder the health of older adults. Finally, we explore the unique aspects of spirituality among adults entering the later stages of their lives.

Because the vast majority of older adults in North America who are religious adhere to Jewish or Christian tradition (though religious diversity has become much more apparent in Western societies), and because the vast majority of the empirical studies that have explored the association of religion/spirituality and health have been limited to populations from these traditions, most of our discussion in this chapter falls under the canopy of these traditions.

Throughout this discussion, we do not attempt to artificially define and delineate spirituality and religion, for practical and conceptual reasons. Nevertheless, operational definitions of religion and spirituality might at least set parameters for the discussion below. One example is to define religion as an organized system of beliefs, practices, rituals, and symbols designed to facilitate closeness to the sacred or transcendent and to foster understanding of one's relationship and responsibility to others living together in a faith community. Spirituality, in contrast, may be said to encompass religion but to expand the above definition as an understanding of answers to ultimate questions about life, its meaning, and one's relationship to the sacred or transcendent. Spirituality, therefore, may or may not lead to or derive from the development of religious rituals and the formation of faith communities (Koenig et al. 2001). Unfortunately, such definitions leave much to be desired. For example, some religions do not focus on the transcendent, nor do all spiritual experiences attempt to answer ultimate questions.

Empirical Evidence for the Association Between Spirituality and Health Outcomes in Aging

Empirical studies have explored the association between religion/spirituality and health outcomes (both physical and psychological health). We describe some representative studies briefly below. In general, these studies support an association between participation in religious activities (e.g., church attendance) and better health outcomes, even when baseline health is controlled for. In contrast, studies that explore the association between private religious activities and general measures of spirituality (often measured by a generic scale of spirituality) have been equivocal in their results, strongly supporting neither an association nor the lack of an association.

For example, Markides (1983) examined the relationship between religiosity and life satisfaction in a 4-year prospective cohort study involving older Mexican Americans. He found that church attendance assessed in cross-sectional analyses correlated positively with life satisfaction for both Mexican Americans and Anglos. In contrast, self-rated religiosity and private prayer were correlated with greater life satisfaction for Anglos.

Musick (1996) examined the relationship between religious involvement and subjective health. For African Americans, religious devotion, which included private prayer and Bible reading, was significantly related to subjective health 4 years later. Though religious attendance was related to subjective health cross-sectionally, it dropped out as a predictor of longitudinal subjective health when results were controlled for functional disability. In yet another study, an early study in this field, church attendance was not associated with life satisfaction in later life but was associated with life satisfaction at an earlier age (Spreitzer and Snyder 1974).

The association between religious activity and well-being may be influenced by the perceptions of older adults versus the perceptions of those who work with them. For example, Carp (1974) examined the relationship between church attendance and adjustment among older adults when they relocated from their homes to a new living situation. Although church attendance was a strong predictor of adjustment as judged by administrator evaluations, attendance was not one of the primary predictors of happiness when rated by the subjects themselves.

Many studies have emerged that inform us about both religious beliefs and practices in relationship to health outcomes. Progress in science, however, is iterative, and equivocal results often signify the need to explore the subject more thoroughly, employing conflicts from previous findings to construct better-designed studies (Blazer 2007). Despite the numerous articles that have emerged, the empirical study of religion remains an infant science. More sophisticated methods will be developed over time to better explore this subject.

Studies of religion and health, however, may stimulate a strong visceral response, a response that may be negative or positive (Blazer 2007). One reason for such a response is the predetermined views of many who assess the salutary benefits of religious beliefs and practices for health. Strong proponents of the health benefits of religious practices, such as Larry Dossey, boldly assert that a practice such as prayer has unquestionably been proven to be as valid and vital to healing as drugs or surgery, having perhaps distorted the understanding of prayer as embodied within most major world religious traditions (Dossey 1997). At the opposite pole, critics such as Richard Sloan have challenged all religions and the entire health research enterprise, claiming that proven curative powers remain to be demonstrated in practice (and therefore medical practice has been contaminated by unproven "spiritual" approaches to treatment), while failing to note that the most significant findings regarding the association between religion and health have not been made in clinical samples (Sloan 2006). Of course, such extreme views are frequently driven by the long-standing personal beliefs of those who assert their views forcefully with limited evidence or communal deliberation. Investigators with a strong personal faith and belief in the positive health benefits of faith bring to the task a very different orientation (and perhaps even different methods) than investigators who are nonbelievers and express strong claims about the damage and danger of religion. The upsurge of interest in religion/spirituality in the United States in general has been countered with an upsurge in vigorous opposition, such as Richard Dawkins' book *The God Delusion* (Dawkins 2006).

Even among believers, however, concerns have been expressed about the appropriation of religion as a "means to an end," namely health (Shulman and Meador 2003). One's spirituality and religious practices should be an end in themselves. Popular culture's fascination with the health benefits of religion runs against the grain of the world's great religious traditions. A utilitarian view of faith misrepresents and devalues the true meaning of faithfulness in major world faith traditions. Spiritual formation, or simply learning to be religious, does not mean enlisting faith as a vehicle to obtain what one wants, but rather living in a spirit of gratitude and hope. To put this another way, the suffering that may emerge from the inevitable illnesses and loss of function with age may provide an opportunity for growth, perhaps growth through increasing trust and release.

Faith Communities

Spiritual Formation, Attachment, and Healthy Aging

Despite the emergence of a more individualistic approach to spiritual exploration and development (such as a focus on prayer and meditation), Jews and Christians did not exist per se prior to and do not exist apart from the society that is called Israel or the Church, respectively (Shulman and Meador 2003). Yet religious communities take on a special character apart from people's interactions in the workplace or neighborhood, and even within the family. Pollner (1989), in a secondary analysis of data from the National Opinion Research Center General Social Survey, proposes that although the social support literature focuses on the effects of networks composed of "real" or concrete individuals on psychological well-being, persons interact intrapersonally as well with a wide range of others who may or may not actually exist, which is irrelevant to the potential benefits of such interactions. That is, adults identify and form relationships with spiritual or divine beings. Pollner examined the extent to which relationships with "divine others" affect psychological well-being. These relationships had a significant effect on several measures of well-being in controlled studies that included church attendance. These "imaginary social worlds" not only unify one's beliefs; they also enhance actual social attachments.

Caughey (1984), supporting the role of "divine others," suggests that we all create imaginary social worlds (and faith communities are almost always in part imaginary social worlds). Some individuals, for example, construct elaborate and enduring, even though perhaps imagined, relations with televangelists and turn to them for guidance and support. Religious texts and symbolism provide many resources for personifying the divine (such as "my Father"), who can then be engaged interactionally for support, guidance, and solace. The divine other is the most persuasive symbolic "other" in American society. (Additional symbolic "others" might include the government or the military.)

Spirituality and Clinical Indicators of Health

Maselko and colleagues (2007) demonstrated the unique value of the faith community beyond traditional social support. They found that weekly religious attendance was associated with a lower allostatic load among women, but not men. (*Allostatic load* is a physiological construct introduced to measure overall physiological wear and tear on one's body, which in turn may serve as a preclinical marker of pathophysiological processes that precede the onset of disease.) The association could not be explained by traditional measures of social support. The authors suggested that certain rituals and beliefs linked to religious activity (e.g., the deep inner peace that may result from a practice such as meditation or prayer) may shift the physical state from sympathetic to parasympathetic relaxation.

A community of faith may be especially useful for alleviating depression among older people (Blazer 2000). One means by which the religious community can assist depressed persons and help them find a new sense of meaning is by enabling them to tell their story, thus becoming part of the shared story of the community. Vehicles by which storytelling can be accomplished include individual conversations, sharing groups, and even classroom teaching. This storytelling, in turn, helps older people explore who they are. Another means by which the religious community can buffer the pain of depression is by providing a vision for the community that is incorporated by the individual (e.g., a community that endures together). Many religious communities point to a brighter future than current difficulties present. These communities have, through the ages, enabled people of all ages to tolerate individual and group stress. Finally, religious communities can assist depressed older persons by providing a context for understanding the suffering that they may experience either from physical illnesses or from depressive symptoms.

Social Benefits of Spirituality

Faith communities may also provide practical support. This practical support may be especially valuable to the older adult who has little family in the vicinity or whose family is so occupied that they cannot provide the care and support needed. It is not uncommon that members of the faith community know the immediate needs of the older adult better than family members at some distance. In turn, families often rely on members of the faith community to assist them when they are attempting to help the older adult from a distance.

One means by which these communities provide support is through the reinforcement of beneficial rhythms for older adults. If an older adult is isolated, then the weekly (or more frequent) attendance at gatherings of the faith community provides an ongoing and assured opportunity for social support. If the older adult is not able, for physical or economic reasons, to travel to the regular meetings of the community, frequently someone from the faith community provides transportation, and in the process, one-on-one social interaction.

Faith communities also reinforce the natural cycle of work and rest. The practice of the Sabbath (whether a particular day or as a rhythm within life) reinforces that work must be punctuated with rest. In the modern workplace, this necessary rhythm of Sabbath and rest often is disrupted with nonstop, 7-day-a-week activities with one's work. The older adult may feel isolated in her or his inactivity. The Sabbath (as day or practice) is a reminder that one cannot work at a breakneck pace indefinitely. Regular adherence to the Sabbath in turn supports the older person as he or she enters a period when the energy for work declines and work ultimately gives way to retirement, reframing this as a life-giving opportunity rather than a restriction or imposition within the life course.

Finally, faith communities may provide very practical assistance to older adults. One model program is the parish or congregational nurse movement. Nurses jointly trained in pastoral care as well as health assistance and advocacy are employed by faith communities to provide consultation and guidance to members (frequently older adults). In a health care environment where consumers are faced with a dazzling array of choices (choices of the Medicare Part D drug benefit being a prime example) coupled with difficulty accessing primary care (due to the very busy schedules of primary care providers), negotiating the health care system can be daunting to adults of any age, but especially the elderly. The availability of someone working with a faith community, known and trusted by the older adult, can be of great assistance both in meeting medical needs that need not go beyond the encounter with the congregational nurse and as a bridge to the more formal health care environment.

Individual Spirituality

Divine Relations and Healthy Aging

Robert Browning's well-known poem about old age, "Rabbi Ben Ezra, 1864" (Browning 1915, p. 501), is frequently quoted only in part. We are quite familiar with

> Grow old along with me!
> The best is yet to be,
> The last of life, for which the first was made:

Yet the following lines of the poem set the context for the first three lines:

> Our times are in his hand
> Who saith, "A whole I planned,
> Youth shows but half; trust God see all, nor
> Be afraid!

In other words, a central reason for "the best is yet to be" is that "our times are in his hand." Spiritual practices, including those relating to the transcendent "other," may become, as one ages, more individualistic, less visible and measurable, more subjective, and more unifying (Crowther et al. 2002). Although perhaps not well documented, many believe that as one ages within a faith tradition, successful aging is accompanied by a more flexible, loving, and less judgmental orientation formed through years of adaptively negotiating the inevitable frailties and vulnerabilities of life.

The belief that religion/spirituality is essential for successful aging has a long history in the United States. From the Puritans, the perception emerged that old age was insupportable without religion (Cole 1992). St. Paul (II Corinthians 4:16) suggested, "Though outwardly we are wasting away, yet inwardly we are being renewed day by day." This led to the Puritans' belief that piety was exempt from the inevitable decline with growing old and therefore buttressed the individual through the loss of function with age (Cole 1992). Oliver Wendell Holmes believed that old age might be a special time for a closer relationship with God (Holmes 1891, as quoted in Cole 1992, p. 157): "We must not make too much of…exceptional cases of prolonged activity.…The great privilege of old age is getting rid of responsibilities.… Freed from the harness, an old man could enjoy more intimate relations with his Maker."

One means by which spirituality is thought to enhance one's late life is through the life review. William Adams (1871, p. 10) believed that mature age "is a hill from which one may look in opposite directions—backward (recollecting the many windings of one's pathway through the world, reconciling those memories with humility, acceptance and renunciation)—and forward—the weary pilgrim focusing on the many mansions of his Father's house, where a place is prepared for him."

As noted earlier (see subsection "Controversies in the Study of Spirituality and Health"), however, the objective evidence that a rich inner spiritual life is associated with better health and well-being is not strong. One exception to the equivocal findings to date is the data from the Netherlands (Braam et al. 2008). As part of a pilot project among older adults (age 60 years and older) in the Longitudinal Aging Study Amsterdam, a small sample of older church members filled out a questionnaire that included items exploring feelings about God and perceptions of God. Feelings of discontent toward God correlated positively with feelings of hopelessness, depressive symptoms, and feelings of guilt, and also with depressive symptoms assessed 13 years earlier. These findings were limited to Protestant participants. In general, positive feelings toward God—perceptions of God as supporting and accepting—were more prevalent than their negative counterparts. There was a trend in this study (not statistically significant) for perceiving God as supportive being associated with lower levels of hopelessness. More support was found for feelings of discontent toward God being associated with higher levels of hopelessness, more depressive symptoms, and more feelings of guilt. One critique of these findings is that they were cross-sectional and that, therefore, for example, depression could lead to feelings of discontent toward God.

In addition, when one is interpreting these results, it should be remembered that both discontent toward God and depressive symptoms may originate in a shared underlying construct. An emotional interpretation of religiousness is rooted in primary object relations or, more specifically, in attachment relationships. A negative or critical image of God may originate in an insecure attachment relationship. In turn, inconsistencies in earlier relationships could generate insecure attachment capacities, which in turn are related to depression in adulthood.

In the Braam et al. (2008) study, feelings of guilt were associated with negative feelings about God, and with perceiving God as one who punishes. Feelings of guilt, however, were also strongly associated with positive feelings toward God. In other words, some feelings of guilt may be considered as normal phenomena, belonging to a religious view of guilt covered by grace, and may connect with awareness of responsibility rather than being pathological.

In another positive study, Bosworth et al. (2003) assessed 114 older adults (age 65 and older) who completed measures of both public and private religious practices. In this study, religious coping (defined as "how I think about my life as part of a larger spiritual force"; "I work together with God as partners"; and "I look to God for strength, support, and guidance") was related both cross-sectionally and longitudinally to lower scores on the Montgomery-Åsberg Depression Rating Scale. In contrast, public religious practice, but not private religious practice (such as praying, meditating, or watching or listening to religious programming), was related cross-sectionally to lower scores on the Montgomery-Åsberg scale.

Spirituality and Sense of Meaning, Integrity, and Wisdom in Aging

The work of Erik Erikson provides an excellent approach for understanding the potential problem of meaninglessness in later life (Blazer 2000; Erikson 1963). According to Erikson (1963), individuals negotiate through eight epigenetic stages during the life cycle (not simply sequentially, but with certain stages more prominent at certain ages than others). Each of these stages can be described as a tension between a healthy resolution and a pathological resolution. The tension of integrity (an acceptance that one's life fits together through time) versus despair is the unique psychological challenge faced by older adults. Resolution of this conflict leads to wisdom. In a later study, Erikson et al. (1986) found that during the last stage of life, the life cycle "weaves back on itself," leading to integration of hope, will, perseverance, competence, fidelity, warmth, and care. In order to meet and overcome the existential dread of "not being," looming ever closer as one ages, the older person continually integrates previous actions and restraints, choices and rejections, and strengths and weaknesses of the present with the past. Erikson et al. (1986, p. 145) summarizes this as follows: Integration is "the acceptance of one's one and only life cycle and of the people who have become significant to it as something that had to be and that, by necessity, permitted no substitutions."

Whitehead and Whitehead (1982) expanded on Erikson's theory from a spiritual perspective. Integrity is the acceptance of one's one and only life as well as the people who have become significant to it as something that had to be and that, by necessity, permitted no substitutions; that is, affirmation of the given inevitability of one's life course. Such acceptance brings both freedom from one's past and a deeper respect for its power in one's life all the way to the present. This process may begin with forgiveness of one's parents even as one enters late life and the parents have long since been deceased. Forgiveness of one's parents, especially one's father, can have profound spiritual significance for the older adult. Integrity, however, does not eliminate despair. Despair, in fact, may be an appropriate response to one's awareness of the limits of one's life, to the awareness that not all the possibilities of that life have been realized.

Along with integrity, wisdom may emerge (Whitehead and Whitehead 1982). Wisdom may manifest itself as an inclusive understanding, a widening empathy, a broadened appreciation of diversity, and pluralism in both persons and experience. The core of this psychological strength of wisdom is a detached yet active concern with life itself, especially the lives of others. The recognition that death is approaching can liberate one's concern for one's own life. Wisdom born in the struggle for integrity enables the older person to squarely face the human condition. It enables the elderly person to maintain confidence as he or she faces the decline of bodily and mental functions.

Conclusion

Facing inevitable decline with age is perhaps one of the central psychospiritual challenges, especially in a social context that permits little room for anything but optimal performance. Baltes and Baltes (1990) have described a pattern that includes both declines and continuities as "selective optimization with compensation." The older person is an active agent who negotiates not only with the outside world but with her or his own abilities and resources to maintain as much satisfaction as possible given the inevitability of decline. For example, the elder who has gained much comfort through life from reading scripture but can no longer read may compensate by asking someone to read to him or her, or by listening to recorded readings of scripture. In turn, if disability limits the ability to attend religious services, then the elder may optimize the development of his or her inner spiritual life.

The struggle to come to some integrated sense of one's entire life may naturally require an inner search for, or a wish to communicate with, the mysterious, ultimate "other": to many there can be no "I" without an "other" (Buber 1970). With old age, new possibilities emerge for spiritual growth. One moves beyond a merely deductive and notional dimension of the transcendent (e.g., "I believe that God has a plan for the world") to an affirmation that evolves from personal experience (e.g., "I have experienced the transcendent other in my own life") (Whitehead and Whitehead 1982).

Meaning for the older adult leads to questions such as "Of what value am I?" "What does a human life mean?" and "Why must I die?" (Whitehead and Whitehead 1982). In other words, older adults must establish a sense of self-worth that is increasingly less dependent on their productivity or role. Rather, they must reach to a deeper acceptance of their life, and come to terms with the diminution and the losses that come with aging (not simply compensating for them). With most of their lives lying behind them, elders face questions that can produce considerable anxiety, namely anxiety as to what has been significant in their lives. Reputation, accomplishment, duty, influence, affection, and wealth, important sources of self-esteem, may decrease. Paradoxically, these losses may provide an opportunity to recognize the power that these factors held, powers that may not be congruent with one's sense of a mature spiritual self. This in turn may lead to the affirmation by elders that they are more than what they may seem to others or even previously seemed to themselves. This is an acceptance of one's particularity, finiteness, and limitations, and moves beyond simple acquiescence toward appreciation and celebration of one's unique, though limited, self.

KEY POINTS

■ Religion is an organized system of beliefs, practices, rituals, and symbols designed to facilitate closeness to the sacred or transcendent and to foster understanding of one's relationship and responsibility to others living together in a faith community.

▪ Spirituality encompasses religion but expands the above definition as an understanding of answers to ultimate questions about life, its meaning, and one's relationship to the sacred or transcendent.

▪ Empirical studies support an association between participation in religious activities (e.g., church attendance) and better health outcomes, even when controlling for baseline health, among the elderly.

▪ Even among believers, concerns have been expressed about the appropriation of religion as a means to an end, namely health in late life.

▪ A community of faith may be especially helpful for alleviating depression among older people.

References

Adams W: Retrospect and prospect, in Light at Eventide. Edited by Holm J. New York, Harper Brothers, 1871

Baltes PB, Baltes MM (eds): Successful Aging: Perspectives From the Behavioral Sciences. Cambridge, UK, Cambridge University Press, 1990

Blazer D: Spirituality, aging and depression, in Perspectives on Spiritual Well-Being and Aging. Edited by Thorson J. Springfield, IL, Charles C Thomas, 2000, pp 161–169

Blazer D: Religious beliefs, practices and mental health outcomes: what is the research question? Am J Geriatr Psychiatry 15:269–272, 2007

Bosworth H, Park K-S, McQuoid D, et al: The impact of religious practice and religious coping on geriatric depression. Int J Geriatr Psychiatry 18:905–914, 2003

Braam A, Schaap-Jonker H, Mooi B, et al: God image and mood in old age: results from a community-based pilot study in the Netherlands. Mental Health, Religion, and Culture 11:221–237, 2008

Browning R: Rabbi Ben Ezra, in The Works of Browning. New York, Macmillan, 1915, p 501

Buber M: I and Thou. Translated by Kaufman W. New York, Charles Scribner's Sons, 1970

Carp F: Short-term and long-term prediction of adjustment to a new environment. J Gerontol 29:444–453, 1974

Caughey R: Imaginary Social Worlds. Lincoln, University of Nebraska Press, 1984

Cole T: The Journey of Life: A Cultural History of Aging in America. Cambridge, UK, Cambridge University Press, 1992

Coleman P: Spirituality and ageing: the health implications of religious belief and practice. Age Ageing 34:318–319, 2005

Cornoni-Huntley J, Blazer D, Lafferty M (eds): Established Populations for Epidemiologic Studies of the Elderly: Resource Data Book, Vol 2. Bethesda, MD, National Institute on Aging, 1990

Crowther MR, Parker MW, Achenbaum WA, et al: Rowe and Kahn's model of successful aging revisited: positive spirituality—the forgotten factor. Gerontologist 42:613–620, 2002

Dawkins R: The God Delusion. New York, Houghton Mifflin, 2006

Dossey L: Healing Words: The Power of Prayer and the Practice of Medicine. New York, HarperCollins, 1997

Erikson E: Childhood and Society, 2nd Edition. New York, Basic Books, 1963

Erikson EH, Erikson JM, Kivnick HQ: Vital Involvement in Old Age. New York, WW Norton, 1986

Holmes O: Over the Teacups. Boston, MA, Houghton Mifflin, 1891

Koenig HG, Hays JC, Larson DB, et al: Does religious attendance prolong survival? A six-year follow-up study of 3,968 older adults. J Gerontol A Biol Sci Med Sci 54:M370–M376, 1999

Koenig HG, McCullough M, Larson D: Handbook of Religion and Health. New York, Oxford University Press, 2001

Markides K: Aging, religiosity, and adjustment: a longitudinal analysis. J Gerontol 38:621–625, 1983

Maselko J, Kubzansky L, Kawachi I, et al: Religious service attendance and allostatic load among high-functioning elderly. Psychosom Med 69:464–472, 2007

Musick M: Religion and subjective health among black and white elders. J Health Soc Behav 37:221–237, 1996

Pollner M: Divine relations, social relations, and well-being. J Health Soc Behav 30:92–104, 1989

Shulman J, Meador K: Spirituality, Medicine and the Distortion of Christianity. New York, Oxford University Press, 2003

Sloan R: Blind Faith: The Unholy Alliance of Religion and Medicine. New York, St Martin's Press, 2006

Spreitzer E, Snyder E: Correlates of life satisfaction among the aged. J Gerontol 29:454–458, 1974

Whitehead E, Whitehead J: Christian Life Patterns: The Psychological Challenges and Religious Invitations of Adult Life. New York, Image Books, 1982

Recommended Readings

Blazer D: Spirituality, aging and depression, in Perspectives on Spiritual Well-Being and Aging. Edited by Thorson J. Springfield, IL, Charles C Thomas, 2000, pp 161–169

Blazer D: Religious beliefs, practices and mental health outcomes: what is the research question? Am J Geriatr Psychiatry 15:269–272, 2007

Bosworth H, Park K-S, McQuoid D, et al: The impact of religious practice and religious coping on geriatric depression. Int J Geriatr Psychiatry 18:905–914, 2003

Koenig HG, McCullough M, Larson D: Handbook of Religion and Health. New York, Oxford University Press, 2001

6

Wisdom

Definition, Assessment, and Relation to Successful Cognitive and Emotional Aging

Monika Ardelt, Ph.D.
Hunhui Oh, M.S.W., C.G.

> We can all imagine care without wisdom, but not wisdom without care.
>
> *George E. Vaillant*

Most of us wish to live happy and contented lives. Without any concern for life's vicissitudes and the certainty of age-related losses and death, we usually aspire to be happier in the future than in the past and present. However, we cannot escape the fact that our lives are dynamic and unpredictable. Without prior warning we might experience a perplexing life crisis or hardship, which frustrates us because it seems persistent, inexorable, and exhaustive. Yet while suf-

A slightly different version of this chapter was first published in the *Journal of the Korean Gerontological Society* (Vol. 28, No. 3, pp. 619–643) and is reprinted with permission of the Executive Editor.

fering from depression and frustration, we might learn valuable life lessons (Ardelt 2005). Crises and hardships, such as an encounter with a life-threatening situation, might initiate a life-changing transformation and growth in wisdom (Martin and Kleiber 2005). In this chapter we give an overview of the definitions and assessment of wisdom in the contemporary literature and describe its relation to successful cognitive and emotional aging.

Definitions of Wisdom

Before we discuss the various paradigms used to define wisdom, we first need to explore whether wisdom should be considered part of one's personality, such as intelligence or openness to experience, or part of one's possessions, such as knowledge or life experiences. Or to phrase it differently: is wisdom a quality of being or of having?

Personality Versus Possession

In a very general sense, wisdom can be described as 1) having long-term consequences, 2) requiring insight and reflection, and 3) being concerned with the common good (Bluck 2007). Wisdom encompasses a virtuous value that we can cultivate through life experiences. Its development as a lifelong process requires riding on the waves of life. Life experiences per se, however, do not necessarily make people wise. During and after the ride, we need to reflect on where we were heading and with what purpose. An internalizing process of learning from our experiences is thus required. By doing so, we gain insight into our own life and life in general and are transformed in the process (Ardelt 2004).

Bluck (2007) argues that the rarity of wisdom is related to the rarity of current environments in which it is adaptive to trade off personal benefit in favor of the common good. Current societal values emphasize short-term gains, personal achievement, individual wealth, status, and appearance rather than long-term inner gains, such as insight and a reduction in self-centeredness that benefits the individual and society at large. The rarity of wisdom, in brief, is due to idealizing it as a virtue only rather than implementing it in our daily lives (Bluck 2007), and might be explained further by society's emphasis on having rather than being (Fromm 1976). As Moody (1986, p. 142) states, "One can *have* theoretical knowledge without any corresponding transformation of one's personal being. But one cannot 'have' wisdom without *being* wise" (emphasis as in the original). The conflict between possessive inclination and inner consciousness can easily misguide us to put more value on outward properties than inwardly rich assets in our personalities.

In the following sections, we introduce definitions and assessments of wisdom from a Western and Eastern perspective. Definitions of wisdom can be further subdivided into explicit (or expert) wisdom definitions and implicit (or lay) definitions of wisdom. The distinction between *having* wisdom and *being* wise is part of the discussion of whether wisdom should be defined and assessed as general wisdom–related knowledge or personal wisdom.

Western Definitions of Wisdom

Explicit wisdom theories are constructs of the experts in the field. The definitions of wisdom are drawn from theorists, scholars, philosophers, and researchers (Bluck and Glück 2005). Explicit wisdom theories are distinguished from implicit wisdom theories, which are obtained from laypeople. Bluck and Glück (2005, p. 84) aptly compare these two approaches, characterizing the former as more interested in addressing "How wise is this person compared to that one?" and the latter as concerned with "What do people think wisdom is?"

Western Explicit Wisdom Theories

Wisdom has been defined in many different ways in the contemporary Western research literature, and the following can only provide an overview of the most prominent, explicit definitions of wisdom in the West. A more comprehensive review of Western explicit wisdom theories can be found in works by Sternberg (1990b) and Sternberg and Jordan (2005).

One of the most prominent groups of contemporary wisdom researchers is the Berlin Wisdom Group established by Paul Baltes (1939–2006), which has conducted extensive research on general wisdom or, more precisely, wisdom-related knowledge. From a successful human development and aging perspective, Baltes and colleagues (Baltes and Smith 1990) initiated their study on wisdom with three motivations:

1. To study high levels of human performance
2. To identify strengths that emerge in the aging process
3. To study facets of intelligence that reflect strengths in the pragmatics of human functioning

They define wisdom as an expert knowledge system and emphasize the volume of knowledge amassed by an individual and how the individual is able to use and apply this knowledge. Defined as "a truly superior level of knowledge, judgment and advice," wisdom comprises knowledge with extraordinary scope, depth, measure, and balance (Staudinger et al. 2005, p. 195). With that level of knowledge, expertise and mastery in the fundamental pragmatics of life (which includes life planning, life management, and life review) and the meaning and conduct of life are attainable (Baltes and Staudinger 2000). Kekes (1983), however, cautions that wisdom should not be equated with descriptive knowledge. According to Kekes (1983), wisdom entails a deeper interpretative understanding of the meaning of descriptive knowledge. For example, although most people know at a descriptive intellectual level that humans grow old and are mortal, the deeper interpretive meaning of those truths escapes those who fight against the aging process and act as if they can look and be young forever. Similarly, McKee and Barber (1999) define wisdom as perceiving things as they really are by "seeing through illusion." This requires 1) recognizing the illusion of a belief (e.g., "I can look and be young forever"), 2) not being tempted by or vulnerable to the illusion, and 3) an empathetic understanding of those who still believe in the illusion. As Taranto (1989) remarked, the recognition and acceptance of human limitations might be a prerequisite for the development of wisdom.

Another collection of studies approaches the dynamics of wisdom development through either dialectical or more balanced, synchronized reasoning. Birren and Fisher (1990) claim that the balance between emotion and detachment, action and inaction, and knowledge and doubt is a critical attribute in using wisdom to deal with life's vicissitudes. Similar to Arlin's (1990) statement that wisdom is the art of questioning, Meacham (1990) emphasizes struggling with the balance between knowing and doubting as a necessary antecedent for wisdom, and Brugman (2000) defines wisdom as expertise in dealing with the cognitive, emotional, and behavioral aspects of uncertainty.

It is, however, Sternberg who refines the balance theory of wisdom. This theory entails viewing wisdom as the application of intelligence, creativity, and tacit knowledge, mediated by values aimed at achieving a common good by balancing multiple intrapersonal, interpersonal, and extrapersonal interests, to obtain a balance among the adaptation to and shaping of existing environments and the selection of new environments (Sternberg 1998). In contrast to a conventionally intelligent person who considers ambiguity as something to be resolved, and in contrast to a creative person who can tolerate ambiguity but is uncomfortable with it, a wise person is, as Sternberg (1998) claims, comfortable with ambiguity.

Achenbaum and Orwoll (1991) emphasize the transformative and integrative characteristics of wisdom through intrapersonal, interpersonal, and transpersonal experiences in the domains of personality, cognition, and conation, and Levenson et al. (2005) equate wisdom itself with self-transcendence.

Western Implicit Wisdom Theories

Implicit wisdom theories focus on laypeople's conceptions and descriptions of wisdom or wise persons. Implicit wisdom theories seek not to determine how wise people are compared with others, but instead to examine individuals' mental representations of what constitutes wisdom (Sternberg 1985). People carry views of wisdom that they have learned or constructed through their interactions in the world. Such views are the filters through which people view and judge cultures, individuals, and themselves (Bluck and Glück 2005). Hence, implicit wisdom theories might vary between cultures and people with different personal characteristics (Takahashi and Bordia 2000).

In past research, wisdom characteristics have been described and rated by young, middle-aged, and older laypersons from various educational and occupational backgrounds. Through a multidimensional scaling analysis, Clayton and Birren (1980) came to the conclusion that three wisdom dimensions best summarize the wisdom conception of individuals across age groups:

1. A cognitive dimension (being knowledgeable, experienced, intelligent, pragmatic, and observant)
2. A reflective dimension (being introspective and intuitive)
3. An affective dimension (being understanding, empathetic, peaceful, and gentle)

Sternberg (1990a) found that laypersons and professors of art, physics, philosophy, and business tended to describe wisdom as consisting of one's reasoning ability, sagacity, ability to learn from ideas and the environment, judgment, expeditious use of information, and perspicacity. In research by Holliday and Chandler (1986), a factor analysis of wisdom descriptors resulted in five factors, labeled exceptional understanding, judgment and communication skills, general competencies, interpersonal skills, and social unobtrusiveness. Similarly, Brown (2004) found that recent college graduates tended to depict wisdom as an integration of self-knowledge, understanding of others, judgment, life knowledge, life skills, and willingness to learn. In short, most laypersons characterize wisdom as a combination of cognitive ability, insight, reflective attitude, concern for others, and real-world skills (Bluck and Glück 2005).

Descriptions of laypeople's own wisdom experiences parallel their definitions of wisdom in others. Individuals tend to report that their own wise behavior or growth in wisdom encompasses guidance, compassion, empathy, support for others, knowledge, experience, moral principles, self-determination and assertion, and/or balance and flexibility (Glück et al. 2005).

Eastern Definitions of Wisdom

Although Western and Eastern definitions of wisdom overlap considerably, the emphasis on the various components of wisdom varies, with Western approaches stressing the importance of the cognitive/reflective elements and

Eastern approaches giving equal weight to the cognitive/reflective and emotional/compassionate aspects of wisdom (Takahashi and Overton 2005). Interestingly, the differences between Western and Eastern approaches are less pronounced in implicit wisdom theories than in explicit wisdom theories.

Eastern Explicit Wisdom Theories

Most of the modern conceptions of Eastern explicit wisdom theories are based on the ancient wisdom teachings of the East (Takahashi 2000). One of the oldest and most distinguished wisdom texts of the East, holding 108 discourses by various Eastern saints and sages, is the Upanishads of ancient India (written between 800 and 500 B.C.E.). The Upanishads give advice on how to live a good and meaningful life, and try to explain the unintelligible, nonsensory aspects of this world that require an intuitive rather than an intellectual understanding (Birren and Svensson 2005). Wisdom is considered an internal human asset, that is potentially available to every human being who has gained access to this intuitive understanding. Another highly important wisdom book of the East is the Bhagavad Gita, which gives an overview of Hindu philosophy and was likely written between 500 and 200 B.C.E. (Zaehner 1969). In the Bhagavad Gita, wisdom is depicted as knowledge of life, emotional regulation, control over desires, decisiveness, love of God, duty and work, self-contentedness, yoga (integration of personality), compassion/sacrifice, and insight/humility (Jeste and Vahia 2008).

The teachings of the Buddha, a title given to Siddhartha Gautama (c. 563–483 B.C.E.) after he attained the state of enlightenment, are an important source of ancient Eastern wisdom and have gained greater prominence in recent years in the West through the popularity of mindfulness practices (e.g., Holland 2006). The Buddha emphasized the importance of mindful self-observation, which he considered a prerequisite for growth in equanimity, insight (self-insight), compassion, and wisdom (Ñanamoli 2001).

In ancient China, the philosopher and sage Lao-tzu (c. 604–531 B.C.E.) also stressed the importance of self-observation and self-knowledge for the development of intuition, compassion, and wisdom, whereas the philosopher, political servant, and educator Confucius (c. 551–479 B.C.E.) dismissed the role of intuition in favor of learning and reflection on the material that has been learned (Riegel 2006). Nevertheless, Confucius recognized compassion and personal morality as essential components for the acquisition of wisdom as well (Birren and Svensson 2005).

Eastern Implicit Wisdom Theories

Compared with research on Western implicit wisdom theories, studies exploring Eastern implicit wisdom theories are relatively rare. The few studies that have been conducted so far suggest that Eastern laypersons give more weight to the emotional/compassionate dimension of wisdom than Western laypersons do (Takahashi and Overton 2005). In one study, Takahashi and Bordia (2000) found that undergraduate students of Indian and Japanese descent equated wisdom more with discretion than with experience and knowledge, whereas their American and Australian counterparts equated wisdom with experience and knowledge. Yang (2001) performed an explorative factor analysis of 100 behavioral characteristics after Taiwanese Chinese adults from various age groups rated the salience of those characteristics for "a wise person." Results indicated that Taiwanese Chinese adults consider wisdom a combination of competencies and knowledge (cognitive skills), benevolence and compassion (affective abilities), and openness and profundity (reflective attributes), along with modesty and unobtrusiveness.

Culturally Inclusive Definitions of Wisdom

Takahashi and Overton (2005) recommend that wisdom be defined in a broad and culturally inclusive way that transcends cultural egocentrism. Hence, Takahashi and Overton (2002) approach wisdom as a combination of two modes:

1. The analytical mode (knowledge database and abstract reasoning abilities), which tends to be more salient in Western explicit wisdom theories
2. The synthetic mode (reflective understanding, emotional empathy, and emotional regulation), which tends to dominate in Eastern explicit wisdom theories

Therefore, a culturally inclusive definition of wisdom should contain cognitive, reflective, and emotional/compassionate components. It is noteworthy that both Western and Eastern laypersons tend to define wisdom in this culturally inclusive manner, even though Western implicit wisdom theories might emphasize the cognitive element and Eastern implicit definitions might stress the emotional/compassionate dimension of wisdom (Takahashi and Bordia 2000).

In accordance with Takahashi and Overton's (2005) advice for a culturally inclusive definition of wisdom, we conceptualize wisdom as an integration of cognitive, reflective, and affective personality characteristics, as summarized in Table 6–1 (Ardelt 2004). This relatively parsimonious definition of wisdom was originally derived from Clayton and Birren's (1980) study of Western implicit wisdom theories but has the distinct advantage that it comprises the major components of both implicit and explicit wisdom theories from the Western and the Eastern wisdom traditions (Sternberg and Jordan 2005).

TABLE 6–1. Definition and operationalization of wisdom as a three-dimensional personality characteristic

Dimension	Definition	Operationalization
Cognitive	An understanding of life and a desire to know the truth (i.e., to comprehend the significance and deeper meaning of phenomena and events, particularly with regard to intrapersonal and interpersonal matters) Includes knowledge and acceptance of the positive and negative aspects of human nature, of the inherent limits of knowledge, and of life's unpredictability and uncertainties	Items or ratings assess • Ability and willingness to understand a situation or phenomenon thoroughly • Knowledge of the positive and negative aspects of human nature • Acknowledgment of ambiguity and uncertainty in life • Ability to make important decisions despite life's unpredictability and uncertainties
Reflective	A perception of phenomena and events from multiple perspectives Requires self-examination, self-awareness, and self-insight	Items or ratings assess • Ability and willingness to look at phenomena and events from different perspectives • Absence of subjectivity and projections (i.e., the tendency to blame other people or circumstances for one's own situation or feelings)
Affective	Sympathetic and compassionate love for others	Items or ratings assess • Presence of positive, caring, and nurturing emotions and behavior toward others • Absence of indifferent or negative emotions and behavior toward others

Source. Adapted from Ardelt 2004.

The *cognitive dimension of wisdom* is characterized by a strong desire to know the truth, which leads to a more comprehensive understanding of life in general and of the deeper meaning and significance of phenomena and events, particularly the intrapersonal and interpersonal aspects of life (Osbeck and Robinson 2005). This requires knowledge and acceptance of the positive and negative aspects of human nature, of the inherent limits of knowledge, and of life's unpredictability and uncertainty. To attain such a state of deeper knowledge, it is necessary to learn how to "see through illusion" (McKee and Barber 1999) and to transcend subjectivity and projections, which is the tendency to blame other people and circumstances for one's own faults and failures (Sherwood 1981). The *reflective dimension of wisdom,* therefore, refers to the ability to perceive phenomena and events from multiple perspectives and to engage in self-examination, self-awareness, and self-insight. Self-reflection and a transcendence of one's subjectivity and projections, in turn, tend to decrease self-centeredness, and this allows for a more comprehensive understanding of life and the human condition (Levitt 1999). At the same time, reduced self-centeredness and a greater understanding of human behavior are likely to result in greater empathy and sympathetic and compassionate love for others, which describes the *affective dimension of wisdom* (Levitt 1999).

If the definitions of wisdom vary between experts and laypersons and between different researchers in the field, how is wisdom assessed by contemporary wisdom researchers? In the next section we show that the measurement of wisdom varies even more widely than the definition of this elusive concept.

Assessment of Wisdom

Although the assessment of wisdom depends to a large degree on the definition used, assessment can be further subdivided into two general approaches: ratings-based measures and self-reported questionnaire measures.

- *Ratings-based measures* are wisdom ratings based on transcribed oral or written responses to hypothetical, ill-structured problems, written responses to an open-ended question, or transcribed, semistructured qualitative interviews.
- *Self-reported questionnaire measures,* by contrast, ask respondents to rate how much they agree or disagree with certain statements or personality qualities that presumably measure the presence or absence of their own wisdom characteristics, but do not let the participants know they are responding to questions on a wisdom scale.

Ratings-Based Measures of General Wisdom–Related Performance and Personal Wisdom

The Berlin Wisdom Paradigm (Baltes and Staudinger 2000; Staudinger et al. 2005) was developed to measure general wisdom–related knowledge or wisdom-related performance rather than self-related personal wisdom. Participants are asked to "think aloud" about ill-defined hypothetical life problems in the areas of life review, life planning, or life management. The transcribed responses are scored by at least two independent raters with regard to two basic wisdom criteria (rich factual knowledge and rich procedural knowledge about the fundamental pragmatics of life) and three metacriteria of life-span contextualism (knowledge about the contexts of life and how these change over time), value relativism (knowledge that considers the relativism of values and life goals), and recognition and management of uncertainty (Baltes and Smith 2008). General wisdom–related knowledge is assessed as the average of these five wisdom criteria.

Kitchener and Brenner (1990) measure wisdom-related performance through the Reflective Judgment Interview. Participants' responses to four ill-structured problems regarding the dilemmas of knowing in history, science, religion, and everyday life are rated according to their level of reflective judgment. The highest (and wisest) stage of the reflective judgment model denotes "a recognition of the limits of personal knowledge, an acknowledgment of the general uncertainty that characterizes human knowing, and a humility about one's own judgments in the face of such limitations" (Kitchener and Brenner 1990, p. 226).

Helson and Srivastava (2002) assess wisdom-related performance by asking participants to provide written responses to an ill-structured hypothetical life problem ("What would you do if you received a phone call from a friend who had decided to commit suicide?"), which has also been used in research by the Berlin wisdom group (Baltes et al. 1995). Two psychologists rate the responses with regard to cognitive differentiation, procedural knowledge, emotional understanding, and acknowledgment of moral complexity.

In contrast to measures of general wisdom–related performance, Staudinger et al. (2005) developed a measure of personal or self-related wisdom based on a think-aloud task and rating procedure similar to the Berlin Wisdom Paradigm. High personal or self-related wisdom is characterized by rich self-knowledge, the availability of heuristics for growth and self-regulation (the expression and regulation of emotions and the development and maintenance of close social relationships), interrelating the self (insight into the nature of interdependence and the causes of one's emotions and behavior), self-relativism (reflection, self-reflection, and the acceptance of oneself and others), and tolerance of ambiguity and uncertainty.

To measure personal transcendent wisdom, Wink and Helson (1997) asked study participants to give written examples of their own wisdom and its development, which were subsequently rated by four judges. Statements that received high ratings on personal transcendent wisdom were insightful, transcended the personal, and contained major elements of wisdom, such as a recognition of the complexity and limitations of knowledge, an integration of thought and emotion, and a concern with philosophical and spiritual issues.

Ardelt (2000) assessed personal wisdom by combining cognitive, reflective, and affective items from the California Q-Sort (Block 1971) and Haan's (1969) Ego Rating Scale. All items were rated by at least two trained and clinically experienced coders based on transcribed, semistructured interviews with the study participants.

- The five items for the cognitive wisdom dimension (objectivity, intellectuality, logical analysis, concentration, and ability "to see to the heart of important problems") assess the ability and willingness to understand a situation or phenomenon thoroughly.
- The nine items of the reflective wisdom dimension (e.g., [no] projection, "is introspective," "has insight into own motives and behavior," "is [not] extrapunitive; does [not] end to transfer or project blame") measure the ability and willingness to look at phenomena and events from different perspectives.
- The 11 items of the affective wisdom dimension (e.g., empathy, "behaves in a sympathetic or considerate manner," "has warmth," "is compassionate," "has [no] hostility toward others") gauge the presence of positive, caring, and nurturant emotions and behavior toward others and the absence of negative emotions and behavior toward others.

The cognitive, reflective, and affective wisdom dimensions serve as effect indicators for latent, variable wisdom (Bollen 1989).

Similarly, Wink and Dillon (2003) used 13 cognitive and reflective items from the California Q-Sort to measure personal wisdom. The 13 items characterize a wise person as straightforward, clear thinking, introspective, insightful, philosophically concerned, and unconventional in his or her thinking.

Self-Reported Questionnaire Measures of Personal Wisdom

Self-rated wisdom measures are given to study participants in the form of self-administered mail or Internet questionnaires or face-to-face interview surveys. Participants are asked how strongly they agree or disagree with certain statements or adjectives that describe their personality, attitudes, or behavior, usually without being informed that the statements or adjectives are intended to assess their degree of wisdom.

Brugman (2000) developed the Epistemic Cognition Questionnaire (ECQ15) to measure wisdom as expertise in uncertainty. The 15 items of the ECQ15 assess acknowledgment of uncertainty (e.g., "As I come to know more and more, I realize that I know very little indeed"), emotional stability despite uncertainty (e.g., "I only feel quiet when I'm certain that my decision is the only right one. Uncertainty makes me nervous and leads to hesitations as far as what to do goes"—with scores reversed so that a high score on that item is counted as a low score for the ECQ15 and vice versa), and the ability to act in the face of uncertainty (e.g., "Although I'm never quite sure about my decisions, once made, I firmly back them up").

For Takahashi and Overton (2002), wisdom consists of an analytic mode and a synthetic mode. The analytic wisdom mode is a combination of one's knowledge database and abstract reasoning skills. Study participants' knowledge database is assessed by the vocabulary (word definition) subtest of the Wechsler Adult Intelligence Scale—Revised, whereas abstract reasoning skills are measured by the similarity subtest, which requires participants to describe the common features of paired word items. The synthetic wisdom mode contains reflective understanding, emotional empathy, and emotional regulation. Reflective understanding is assessed by the 15-item Short Index of Self-Actualization (Jones and Crandall 1986), emotional empathy by the empathetic concern subscale of the Interpersonal Reactivity Index (Davis 1980, 1983), and emotional regulation by the Negative Mood Regulation Scale (Catanzaro and Mearns 1990).

Wink and Helson (1997) measure practical wisdom through 18 cognitive, reflective, and mature self-descriptive adjectives from the Adjective Check List (a list of 300 adjectives). Fourteen of the adjectives are indicative of wisdom (e.g., *clear thinking, insightful, reasonable, reflective, fair minded, mature*) and four adjectives are contraindicative of wisdom (*immature, intolerant, reckless,* and *shallow*). Study participants are asked to check all adjectives that describe them best. Practical wisdom is assessed by the number of checked adjectives that are indicative of wisdom minus the number of checked contraindicative adjectives.

Ardelt (2003) developed a Three-Dimensional Wisdom Scale (3D-WS) based on the definition of wisdom (shown in Table 6–1) as an integration of cognitive, reflective, and affective dimensions. The scale contains 14 items for the cognitive dimension, 12 items for the reflective wisdom dimension, and 13 items of the affective wisdom dimension:

- Cognitive dimension items assess the ability and willingness to understand a situation or phenomenon thoroughly (e.g., "Ignorance is bliss"), knowledge of the positive and negative aspects of human nature (e.g., "People are either good or bad"), acknowledgment of ambiguity and uncertainty in life (e.g., "There is only one right way to do anything"), and the ability to make important decisions despite life's unpredictability and uncertainties ("I am hesitant about making important decisions after thinking about them"). It is noteworthy that all the items that make up the cognitive dimension measure the *absence* rather than the *presence* of cognitive wisdom qualities and, hence, all items are reverse scored so that low scores represent high scores on the cognitive wisdom dimension and vice versa. Items in the original pool of items that assessed the presence of cognitive characteristics (e.g., "I always try to get to the core of a problem") had to be removed from the final scale due to a social desirability bias and/or weak or even negative correlations with other items on the scale.

- Reflective wisdom dimension items measure the ability and willingness to look at phenomena and events from different perspectives (e.g., "I always try to look at all sides of a problem") and the absence of subjectivity and projections (e.g., "Things often go wrong for me by no fault of my own"—reversed scored).

- Affective wisdom dimension items assess positive, caring, and nurturing emotions and behavior toward others (e.g., "Sometimes I feel a real compassion for everyone") and the absence of indifferent or negative emotions and behavior toward people (e.g., "It's not really my problem if others are in trouble and need help"—reversed scored).

After the average of the items for each individual wisdom dimension is calculated, the cognitive, reflective, and affective dimensions of wisdom can be used as effect indicators for wisdom as a latent variable, or personal wisdom can be computed as the average of the three wisdom dimensions.

If wisdom is defined as a combination of cognitive, reflective, and affective personality qualities, items from existing personality scales and surveys might be used to assess the three dimensions of wisdom. In this vein, Ardelt and Vaillant (2007) selected cognitive, reflective, and affective items from the Lazare Personality Inventory (Lazare et al. 1970) and the Wellsprings of a Positive Life Survey conducted by the Gallup organization in 2001 to measure personal wisdom:

- The cognitive dimension of the Lazare Personality Inventory consists of seven items, which assess the recognition and acceptance of ambiguity and uncertainty in life (e.g., "I am somewhat resistant to changes"—reversed) and the ability to make important decisions despite life's unpredictability and uncertainties (e.g., "When I face a problem, I am apt to do nothing"—reversed). The 14 items of the reflective dimension measure the ability and willingness to look at phenomena and events from different perspectives (e.g., "I make decisions as rapidly as others, but only after considering a large number of other possibilities") and the absence of subjectivity and projections (e.g., "People usually let you down"—reversed). The 13 items of the affective dimension assess the absence of indifferent or negative emotions and behavior toward others (e.g., "I hold grudges for long periods of time"—reverse scored).

- The cognitive wisdom dimension of the Gallup Wellsprings of a Positive Life Survey contains five items, which measure the ability and willingness to understand a situation or phenomenon thoroughly (e.g., "My mind is always asking questions") and the ability to make important decisions despite life's unpredictability and uncertainties ("I have confidence in the choices I make"). The four items of the reflective dimension assess the ability and willingness to look at phenomena and events from different perspectives (e.g., "Others seek me out to discuss topics in depth"), and the 14 items of the affective dimension measure the presence of positive emotions and behavior toward others (e.g., "I frequently go out of my way to help people in need").

Similar to the way the 3D-WS is assessed, the individual wisdom dimensions consist of the average of their respective items. Personal wisdom is assessed either as a latent variable with the cognitive, reflective, and affective wisdom dimensions as effect indicators or as the average of the three individual wisdom dimensions.

Brown and Greene (2006) created the Wisdom Development Scale to assess the development of wisdom among college students (Brown 2004). This scale is composed of seven factors:

1. Life knowledge (nine items; e.g., "I see the interconnectedness between people and the natural world," "I reflect on my life regularly")
2. Judgment (11 items, e.g., "I understand that there are contradictions and imperfections in human nature," "I am inquisitive")
3. Self-knowledge (six items, e.g., "I know what makes me happy," "I am well aware of all my weaknesses")
4. Emotional management (nine items, e.g., "I manage uncertainty well," "I can quiet my mind")
5. Altruism (14 items, e.g., "I use my influence for the good of others," "I learn from others")
6. Inspirational engagement (11 items, e.g., "I inspire others," "I have general confidence in what I know")
7. Life skills (11 items, e.g., "I manage time effectively," "I multitask well")

Webster (2007) developed a 40-item Self-Assessed Wisdom Scale (SAWS), based on the original 30-item SAWS (Webster 2003), to measure the noncognitive components of personal wisdom. The SAWS consists of five 8-item factors that assess the following:

1. Critical life experiences (e.g., "I have lived through many difficult life transitions," "I have had to make many important life decisions")
2. Emotional regulation (e.g., "I can regulate my emotions when the situation calls for it," "It is easy for me to adjust my emotions to the situation at hand")
3. Reflectiveness/reminiscence (e.g., "I often think about my personal past," "Recalling my earlier days helps me gain insight into important life matters")
4. Openness to experience (e.g., "I'm very curious about other religious and/or philosophical belief systems," "Controversial works of art play an important and valuable role in society")
5. Humor (e.g., "I can make fun of myself to comfort others," "I am easily aroused by laughter")

Finally, Levenson and colleagues (2005) developed an 18-item Adult Self-Transcendence Inventory (ASTI) to assess self-transcendent wisdom. Study participants are asked whether their view of life is different today than it was 10 years ago. The ASTI contains two subscales, self-transcendence (e.g., "My sense of self is less dependent on other people and things," "Material things mean less to me") and alienation (e.g., "I feel that my life has less meaning," "I feel more isolated and lonely"). The alienation subscale was included to distinguish self-transcendent wisdom from withdrawal based on alienation.

Association of Personal Wisdom With Indicators of Successful Cognitive and Emotional Aging

Theoretically, wisdom should have a positive impact on successful aging given that wise elders know "the art of living," that is, how to live a life that is good for oneself, good for others, and good for society in general (Kupperman 2005). Therefore, one would expect that wisdom is positively related to mastery, purpose in life, life satisfaction, supportive social relationships, and concern for future generations (Ardelt 2003; Solomon et al. 2005). Furthermore, growing wiser might be intrinsically rewarding and joyful (Csikszentmihalyi and Nakamura 2005) due to less preoccupation with self-centered problems and concerns and the gradual transcendence of the self (Ardelt 2008). Yet because wise people have seen through illusion (McKee and Barber 1999) and are more aware of the negative aspects of life, such as life's uncertainties and the inevitability of physical deterioration and death, it might also be that wisdom has a detrimental effect on successful aging (Staudinger et al. 2005).

To determine empirically whether wisdom is related to successful cognitive and emotional aging, we need to know exactly how wisdom was defined and operationalized in a specific study, given the wide variety of wisdom definitions and measurements. For example, it is likely that general wisdom matters less to successful aging than personal wisdom does. Indeed, in a sample of 125 German adults ranging in age from 19 to 87 years (mean=45 years), general wisdom–related knowledge, measured by the Berlin Wisdom Paradigm, was not associated with autonomy, mastery of the environment, positive relations, purpose in life, or self-acceptance (Staudinger et al. 1997).

Table 6–2 summarizes research on personal wisdom and a variety of indicators of successful aging. Most of the studies found a positive association between personal wisdom and indicators of successful aging, despite variations in the definition and measurement of wisdom. Wisdom, defined and operationalized as a combination of cognitive, reflective, and affective personality dimensions, is positively related to indicators of subjective well-being and negatively related to indicators of ill-being as measured by both ratings-based and self-reported measures of wisdom. Specifically:

- Wisdom, assessed by cognitive, reflective, and affective items from the California Q-Sort and Haan's Ego Rating Scale, was positively associated with life satisfaction in a sample of 81 white women and 39 men between ages 58 and 82 years (mean, 68 years for women and 70 years for men; Ardelt 1997) and, in a study with only the 81 women, was positively related to better family relations (Ardelt 2000).
- Similarly, in a sample of 180 white and African American elders between ages 52 and 87 years (mean, 71 years), the self-administered 3D-WS was positively correlated with general well-being, purpose in life, and mastery, and negatively associated with depressive symptoms, death avoidance, and fear of death (Ardelt 2003).
- Furthermore, in a sample of 98 white, college-educated men, ranging in age from 77 to 86 years (mean, 80 years), the average of cognitive, reflective, and affective personality qualities, assessed by items from the self-administered Gallup Wellsprings of a Positive Life Survey, was positively correlated with life satisfaction, general adjustment to aging, and marital happiness (Ardelt and Vaillant 2007).

TABLE 6–2.   Bivariate correlations of personal wisdom with indicators of successful cognitive and emotional aging

Research study	N	Age of participants (years)	Wisdom measure	Indicators of successful aging	Correlation with wisdom
Operationalization of wisdom as a combination of cognitive, reflective, and affective personality qualities					
Ardelt (1997)	81 39	58–82 Women: mean, 68 Men: mean, 70	Cognitive, reflective, and affective items from the California Q-Sort and Haan's Ego Rating Scale	Life satisfaction	Women: 0.77*** Men: 0.64****
Ardelt (2000a)	81	Women only: 59–81 (mean, 68)	Cognitive, reflective, and affective items from the California Q-Sort and Haan's Ego Rating Scale	Positive family relations	0.24*
Ardelt (2003)	180	52–87 (mean, 71)	3D-WS (cognitive, reflective, and affective personality qualities)	General well-being Purpose in life Mastery Depressive symptoms Death avoidance Fear of death	0.45*** 0.61*** 0.63*** −0.60*** −0.33*** −0.56***
Ardelt and Vaillant (2007)	98	Men only: 77–86 (mean, 80)	Cognitive, reflective, and affective items from the Gallup Wellsprings of a Positive Life Survey	Life satisfaction General adjustment to aging Marital happiness	0.32*** 0.18* 0.26*

TABLE 6–2. Bivariate correlations of personal wisdom with indicators of successful cognitive and emotional aging *(continued)*

Research study	N	Age of participants (years)	Wisdom measure	Indicators of successful aging	Correlation with wisdom
Other operationalizations of wisdom					
Takahashi and Overton (2002)	68	36–59 (mean, 45)	Knowledge database	Life satisfaction	0.32***
	68	>65 (mean, 70)	Abstract reasoning		0.23***
			Reflective understanding		0.31***
			Emotional empathy		0.19**
			Emotional regulation		0.45***
Webster (2003)	85	22–78 (mean, 53)	30-item SAWS (critical life experiences, emotional regulation, reflectiveness/ reminiscence, openness to experience, and humor)	Generativity	0.44***
				Ego integrity	0.23**
Webster (2007)	171	17–92 (mean, 43)	40-item SAWS	Generativity	0.45***
Wink and Dillon (2003)	157	Late sixties to late seventies	Cognitive and reflective items from the California Q-Sort	Orientation toward personal growth	0.34***
				Generativity	0.65***

TABLE 6–2.   Bivariate correlations of personal wisdom with indicators of successful cognitive and emotional aging *(continued)*

Research study	*N*	Age of participants (years)	Wisdom measure	Indicators of successful aging	Correlation with wisdom
Other operationalizations of wisdom *(continued)*					
Helson and Srivastava (2002)	110	Women only: ~60	Combination of practical wisdom, transcendent wisdom, and wisdom-related performance	Orientation toward personal growth	0.27***
				Positive social relations	0.27***
Brugman (2000)	45	44–90 (mean, 68)	ECQ15 (acknowledgment of uncertainty, emotional stability despite uncertainty, and ability to act in the face of uncertainty)	Life satisfaction	0.27**
				Depressive symptoms	0.12
	50	64–93 (mean, 74)		Life satisfaction	0.07
Wink and Helson (1997)	138	Early to mid-fifties	Practical wisdom (cognitive, reflective, and mature adjectives from the Adjective Check List)	Life satisfaction	0.16
				Marital satisfaction	0.02
			Transcendent wisdom	Life satisfaction	0.15
				Marital satisfaction	0.00
Jennings et al. (2006)	387	Men only: 56–95 (mean, 74)	Self-transcendent wisdom subscale of the ASTI	Positive coping	0.21***
				Negative coping	–0.01

Note.   3D-WS=Three-Dimensional Wisdom Scale; ASTI=Adult Self-Transcendence Inventory; ECQ15=Epistemic Cognition Questionnaire; SAWS=Self-Assessed Wisdom Scale.
*$P<0.1$; **$P<0.05$; ***$P<0.01$.

Yet, wisdom measures based on other conceptualizations of wisdom also show a positive association with indicators of successful aging:

- Measures of Takahashi and Overton's (2002) analytical mode of wisdom (knowledge database and abstract reasoning) and synthetic mode of wisdom (reflective understanding, emotional empathy, and emotional regulation) were positively related to life satisfaction in combined samples of 68 middle-aged (36–59 years; mean=45 years) and 68 older (>65 years; mean=70 years) American and Japanese adults.
- Webster's (2003) 30-item SAWS was positively correlated with generativity (a measure of concern for and mentoring of younger generations) and ego integrity in an ethnically diverse sample of 85 Canadians, ranging in age from 22 to 78 years (mean=53 years). In a different sample of 171 primarily white Canadians between ages 17 and 92 (mean=43 years), the revised 40-item SAWS was also positively associated with generativity (Webster 2007).
- Similarly, in a sample of 157 primarily white Americans in their late sixties to late seventies from diverse socioeconomic backgrounds, wisdom, measured by cognitive and reflective items from the California Q-Sort, was positively related to generativity and orientation toward personal growth (Wink and Dillon 2003), and in a sample of 110 white, college-educated women around the age of 60, wisdom, assessed as a combination of practical wisdom, transcendent wisdom, and wisdom-related performance, was associated with greater orientation toward personal growth and positive social relations (Helson and Srivastava 2002).

However, not all measures of personal wisdom are significantly related to successful aging:

- Although expertise in uncertainty, assessed by the ECQ15, was correlated with greater life satisfaction in an educationally diverse sample of 45 Dutch adults between ages 44 and 90 years (mean, 68 years), the ECQ15 was unrelated to depressive symptoms in this sample (Brugman 2000). Moreover, in a sample of 50 highly educated Dutch older adults, ranging in age from 64 to 93 (mean, 74 years), the ECQ15 failed to correlate significantly with life satisfaction (Brugman 2000).
- Similarly, in a sample of 138 college-educated white adults in their early to mid-fifties, neither practical wisdom nor transcendent wisdom was significantly related to life satisfaction or marital satisfaction (Wink and Helson 1997).
- Finally, in a sample of 387 mostly white men between age 56 and 95 years (mean=74 years), the self-transcendent wisdom subscale of the

ASTI was significantly correlated with more positive coping behavior but was unrelated to negative coping behavior (Jennings et al. 2006).

It appears that the association between wisdom and successful aging is less consistent among highly educated and privileged study participants, such as white men. Compared with adults with lower socioeconomic status and minorities, highly educated and privileged members of society are more likely to be healthy (L.G. Martin et al. 2007) and less likely to be depressed (Aneshensel et al. 2007) and, therefore, might find it easier to engage in successful and meaningful aging (Hungerford 2007). This suggests that wisdom might be particularly valuable in unfavorable social circumstances and trying times.

Conclusion

Although a uniform definition of wisdom does not exist, most contemporary wisdom researchers would probably agree that wisdom contains cognitive, reflective, and socioemotional elements. The measurement of wisdom, however, is quite diverse, with many measures focusing more on the cognitive and reflective dimensions of wisdom than on the socioemotional/affective dimension. Still, research points to the overall positive effect of wisdom on cognitive and emotional aging. Wisdom has been positively related to life satisfaction, general subjective well-being, adjustment to aging, purpose in life, mastery, positive social relations, generativity, ego integrity, orientation toward personal growth, and positive coping, and inversely related to depressive symptoms, death avoidance, and fear of death. Moreover, it appears that wisdom becomes particularly valuable in times of hardship and life crises and, hence, might foster and also result from stress-related growth (Park and Fenster 2004).

With the passage of time, people are likely to encounter hardships and obstacles in their life. Yet growth in wisdom does not depend on *what* we experience in life but *how* we deal with difficult events (Holliday and Chandler 1986). How we manage and work through failure and loss prepares us for future challenges and hardships in later life (Elder 1991). Wisdom is the tool that makes us more resilient and able to apply what we have learned from previous experiences, but crises and hardships might also make us wiser, if we are willing to learn from our experiences and be transformed in the process (Kupperman 2005). As Pascual-Leone (2000, p. 247; emphasis as in the original) points out,

> *[U]ltimate limit situations* that cannot be undone and are nonetheless faced with consciousness and resolve—situations like death, illness, aging, irreme-

diable oppression or loss, extreme poverty, rightful resistance or rebellion, guilt, absolute failure, danger, uncontrollable fear, etc., lead to the natural emergence of a transcendental self, if they do not destroy the person first.

Our lot in life might improve. Our future might be better than the past and present. However, people who are inwardly rich do not simply pursue better lives. Rather, wise persons see life crises and happiness as two sides of the same coin: living a full life. By living a full life, we encounter life crises and hardships but also learn how to cherish our lives. Wisdom helps us to see that experiencing hardship amplifies our appreciation of happiness and wellness. As one of our relatively wise study participants said (Ardelt 2005, p. 14),

I think everything goes around like from...positive to negative[, from] negative to neutral to positive, [that] kind of thing....But you don't let it worry you. Expect that, because everything has an opposite. Otherwise, it wouldn't be...If there weren't bad, there wouldn't be good. If there [weren't] unhappiness, there wouldn't be happiness.

KEY POINTS

■ A uniform definition of wisdom does not exist in contemporary wisdom studies, yet most researchers agree that wisdom contains cognitive, reflective, and socioemotional elements.

■ Wisdom has been measured in diverse ways, ranging from ratings of wisdom characteristics by study participants to ratings of the participants' general wisdom–related performance and personal wisdom by independent judges, to self-reported questionnaire measures of personal wisdom.

■ Despite the variation in wisdom measures, wisdom tends to have positive effects on cognitive and emotional aging in most empirical studies.

■ Research has found that wisdom is positively related to life satisfaction, general subjective well-being, adjustment to aging, purpose in life, mastery, positive social relations, generativity, ego integrity, orientation toward personal growth, and positive coping, and inversely related to depressive symptoms, death avoidance, and fear of death.

■ Empirical evidence also suggests that wisdom can facilitate stress-related growth in times of crises and hardships. Stress-related growth, in turn, might result in greater wisdom.

■ To age well, it is advisable to develop the cognitive, reflective, and socio-emotional qualities that constitute wisdom early in life.

References

Achenbaum AW, Orwoll L: Becoming wise: a psycho-gerontological interpretation of the Book of Job. Int J Aging Hum Dev 32:21–39, 1991

Aneshensel CS, Wight RG, Miller-Martinez D, et al.: Urban neighborhoods and depressive symptoms among older adults. J Gerontol B Psychol Sci Soc Sci 62:S52–S59, 2007

Ardelt M: Wisdom and life satisfaction in old age. J Gerontol B Psychol Sci Soc Sci 52:P15–P27, 1997

Ardelt M: Antecedents and effects of wisdom in old age: a longitudinal perspective on aging well. Res Aging 22:360–394, 2000

Ardelt M: Development and empirical assessment of a three-dimensional wisdom scale. Res Aging 25:275–324, 2003

Ardelt M: Wisdom as expert knowledge system: a critical review of a contemporary operationalization of an ancient concept. Hum Dev 47:257–285, 2004

Ardelt M: How wise people cope with crises and obstacles in life. ReVision: A Journal of Consciousness and Transformation 28:7–19, 2005

Ardelt M: Self-development through selflessness: the paradoxical process of growing wiser, in Transcending Self-Interest: Psychological Explorations of the Quiet Ego. Edited by Wayment HA, Bauer JJ. Washington, DC, American Psychological Association, 2008, pp 221–233

Ardelt M, Vaillant GE: Wisdom as a cognitive, reflective, and affective three-dimensional personality characteristic. Paper presented at the annual meeting of the Gerontological Society of America, San Francisco, CA, November 2007

Arlin PK: Wisdom: the art of problem finding, in Wisdom: Its Nature, Origins, and Development. Edited by Sternberg RJ. Cambridge, UK, Cambridge University Press, 1990, pp 230–243

Baltes PB, Staudinger UM, Maercker A, et al.: People nominated as wise: a comparative study of wisdom-related knowledge. Psychol Aging 10:155-166, 1995

Baltes PB, Smith J: Towards a psychology of wisdom and its ontogenesis, in Wisdom: Its Nature, Origins, and Development. Edited by Sternberg RJ. Cambridge, UK, Cambridge University Press, 1990, pp 87–120

Baltes PB, Smith J: The fascination of wisdom: its nature, ontogeny, and function. Perspect Psychol Sci 3:56–64, 2008

Baltes PB, Staudinger UM: Wisdom: a metaheuristic (pragmatic) to orchestrate mind and virtue toward excellence. Am Psychol 55:122–136, 2000

Birren JE, Fisher LM: The elements of wisdom: overview and integration, in Wisdom: Its Nature, Origins, and Development. Edited by Sternberg RJ. Cambridge, UK, Cambridge University Press, 1990, pp 317–332

Birren JE, Svensson CM: Wisdom in history, in A Handbook of Wisdom: Psychological Perspectives. Edited by Sternberg RJ, Jordan J. New York, Cambridge University Press, 2005, pp 3–31

Block J: Lives Through Time. Berkeley, CA, Bancroft Books, 1971

Bluck S: Is it clever to be wise? Paper presented at the annual meeting of the Gerontological Society of America, San Francisco, CA, November 2007

Bluck S, Glück J: From the inside out: people's implicit theories of wisdom, in A Handbook of Wisdom: Psychological Perspectives. Edited by Sternberg RJ, Jordan J. New York, Cambridge University Press, 2005, pp 84–109

Bollen KA: Structural Equations With Latent Variables. New York, Wiley, 1989

Brown SC: Learning across the campus: how college facilitates the development of wisdom. Journal of College Student Development 45:134–148, 2004

Brown SC, Greene JA: The Wisdom Development Scale: translating the conceptual to the concrete. Journal of College Student Development 47:1–19, 2006

Brugman GM: Wisdom: Source of Narrative Coherence & Eudaimonia: A Life-Span Perspective. Delft, The Netherlands, Eburon, 2000

Catanzaro SJ, Mearns J: Measuring generalized expectancies for negative mood regulation: initial scale development and implications. J Pers Assess 54:546–563, 1990

Clayton VP, Birren JE: The development of wisdom across the life-span: a reexamination of an ancient topic, in Life-Span Development and Behavior, Vol. 3. Edited by Baltes PB, Brim OG Jr. New York, Academic Press, 1980, pp 103–135

Csikszentmihalyi M, Nakamura J: The role of emotions in the development of wisdom, in A Handbook of Wisdom. Psychological Perspectives. Edited by Sternberg RJ, Jordan J. New York, Cambridge University Press, 2005, pp 220–242

Davis MH: A multidimensional approach to individual differences in empathy. Catalog of Selected Documents in Psychology 10:85, 1980

Davis MH: Measuring individual differences in empathy: evidence for a multidimensional approach. J Pers Soc Psychol 44:113–126, 1983

Elder GH Jr: Making the best of life: perspectives on lives, times, and aging. Generations 15:12–17, 1991

Fromm E: To Have or to Be? New York, Harper & Row, 1976

Glück J, Bluck S, Baron J, et al: The wisdom of experience: autobiographical narratives across adulthood. Int J Behav Dev 29:197–208, 2005

Haan N: A tripartite model of ego functioning: values and clinical research applications. J Nerv Ment Dis 148:14–30, 1969

Helson R, Srivastava S: Creative and wise people: similarities, differences and how they develop. Pers Soc Psychol Bull 28:1430–1440, 2002

Holland D: Contemplative education in unexpected places: teaching mindfulness in Arkansas and Austria. Teach Coll Rec 108:1842–1861, 2006

Holliday SG, Chandler MJ: Wisdom: Explorations in Adult Competence. Basel, S Karger, 1986

Hungerford TL: The persistence of hardship over the life course. Res Aging 29:491–511, 2007

Jennings PA, Aldwin CM, Levenson MR, et al: Combat exposure, perceived benefits of military service, and wisdom in later life: findings from the Normative Aging Study. Res Aging 28:115–134, 2006

Jeste DV, Vahia IV: Comparison of the conceptualization of wisdom in ancient Indian literature with modern views: focus on the Bhagavad Gita. Psychiatry 71:197–209, 2008

Jones A, Crandall R: Validation of a short index of self-actualization. Pers Soc Psychol Bull 12:63–73, 1986

Kekes J: Wisdom. Am Philos Q 20:277–286, 1983

Kitchener KS, Brenner HG: Wisdom and reflective judgment: knowing in the face of uncertainty, in Wisdom: Its Nature, Origins, and Development. Edited by Sternberg RJ. Cambridge, UK, Cambridge University Press, 1990, pp 212–229

Kupperman JJ: Morality, ethics, and wisdom, in A Handbook of Wisdom: Psychological Perspectives. Edited by Sternberg RJ, Jordan J. New York, Cambridge University Press, 2005, pp 245–271

Lazare A, Klerman GL, Armor DJ: Oral-obsessive and hysterical personality patterns: replication of factor analysis in an independent sample. J Psychiatr Res 7:275–290, 1970

Levenson MR, Jennings PA, Aldwin CM, et al: Self-transcendence: conceptualization and measurement. Int J Aging Hum Dev 60:127–143, 2005

Levitt HM: The development of wisdom: an analysis of Tibetan Buddhist experience. Journal of Humanistic Psychology 39:86–105, 1999

Martin LG, Schoeni RF, Freedman VA, et al: Feeling better? Trends in general health status. J Gerontol B Psychol Sci Soc Sci 62:S11–S21, 2007

Martin LL, Kleiber DA: Letting go of the negative: psychological growth from a close brush with death. Traumatology 11:221–232, 2005

McKee P, Barber C: On defining wisdom. Int J Aging Hum Dev 49:149–164, 1999

Meacham JA: The loss of wisdom, in Wisdom: Its Nature, Origins, and Development. Edited by Sternberg RJ. Cambridge, UK, Cambridge University Press, 1990, pp 181–211

Moody HR: Late life learning in the information society, in Education and Aging. Edited by Peterson DA, Thornton JE, Birren JE. Englewood Cliffs, NJ, Prentice-Hall, 1986, pp 122–148

Ñanamoli B: The Life of the Buddha: According to the Pali Canon. Seattle, WA, BPS Pariyatti Editions, 2001

Osbeck LM, Robinson DN: Philosophical theories of wisdom, in A Handbook of Wisdom: Psychological Perspectives. Edited by Sternberg RJ, Jordan J. New York, Cambridge University Press, 2005, pp 61–83

Park CL, Fenster JR: Stress-related growth: predictors of occurrence and correlates with psychological adjustment. J Soc Clin Psychol 23:195–215, 2004

Pascual-Leone J: Mental attention, consciousness, and the progressive emergence of wisdom. J Adult Dev 7:241–254, 2000

Riegel J: Confucius, in The Stanford Encyclopedia of Philosophy [electronic resource]. Edited by Zalta EN. Stanford, CA, Metaphysics Research Lab, Center for the Study of Language and Information, Stanford University, 2006

Sherwood GG: Self-serving biases in person perception: a reexamination of projection as a mechanism of defense. Psychol Bull 90:445–459, 1981

Solomon JL, Marshall P, Gardner H: Crossing boundaries to generative wisdom: an analysis of professional work, in A Handbook of Wisdom: Psychological Perspectives. Edited by Sternberg RJ, Jordan J. New York, Cambridge University Press, 2005, pp 272–296

Staudinger UM, Lopez DF, Baltes PB: The psychometric location of wisdom-related performance: intelligence, personality, and more? Pers Soc Psychol Bull 23:1200–1214, 1997

Staudinger UM, Dörner J, Mickler C: Wisdom and personality, in A Handbook of Wisdom: Psychological Perspectives. Edited by Sternberg RJ, Jordan J. New York, Cambridge University Press, 2005, pp 191–219

Sternberg RJ: Implicit theories of intelligence, creativity, and wisdom. J Pers Soc Psychol 49:607–627, 1985

Sternberg RJ: Wisdom and its relations to intelligence and creativity, in Wisdom: Its Nature, Origins, and Development. Edited by Sternberg RJ. Cambridge, UK, Cambridge University Press, 1990a, pp 142–159

Sternberg RJ (ed): Wisdom: Its Nature, Origins, and Development. Cambridge, UK, Cambridge University Press, 1990b

Sternberg RJ: A balance theory of wisdom. Review of General Psychology 2:347–365, 1998

Sternberg RJ, Jordan J (eds): A Handbook of Wisdom: Psychological Perspectives. New York, Cambridge University Press, 2005

Takahashi M: Toward a culturally inclusive understanding of wisdom: historical roots in the East and West. Int J Aging Hum Dev 51:217–230, 2000

Takahashi M, Bordia P: The concept of wisdom: a cross-cultural comparison. Int J Psychol 35:1–9, 2000

Takahashi M, Overton WF: Wisdom: a culturally inclusive developmental perspective. Int J Behav Dev 26:269–277, 2002

Takahashi M, Overton WF: Cultural foundations of wisdom: an integrated developmental approach, in A Handbook of Wisdom: Psychological Perspectives. Edited by Sternberg RJ, Jordan J. New York, Cambridge University Press, 2005, pp 32–60

Taranto MA: Facets of wisdom: a theoretical synthesis. Int J Aging Hum Dev 29:1–21, 1989

Webster JD: An exploratory analysis of a self-assessed wisdom scale. J Adult Dev 10:13–22, 2003

Webster JD: Measuring the character strength of wisdom. Int J Aging Hum Dev 65:163–183, 2007

Wink P, Dillon M: Religiousness, spirituality, and psychosocial functioning in late adulthood: findings from a longitudinal study. Psychol Aging 18:916–924, 2003

Wink P, Helson R: Practical and transcendent wisdom: their nature and some longitudinal findings. J Adult Dev 4:1–15, 1997

Yang S-Y: Conceptions of wisdom among Taiwanese Chinese. J Cross Cult Psychol 32:662–680, 2001

Zaehner RC: The Bhagavad-Gita, With a Commentary Based on the Original Sources. Oxford, UK, Clarendon, 1969

Recommended Readings and Web Sites

Age-ing to Sage-ing: http://www.allaboutaging.com/index.html

Bianchi EC: Elder Wisdom: Crafting Your Own Elderhood. New York, Crossroad, 1994

Birren JE, Feldman L: Where to Go From Here: Discovering Your Own Life's Wisdom in the Second Half of Your Life. New York, Simon & Schuster, 1997

Collective Wisdom Initiative: http://www.collectivewisdominitiative.org/

Macdonald C: Toward Wisdom: Finding Our Way to Inner Peace, Love & Happiness. Willowdale, ON, Canada, Hounslow, 1993

Schachter-Shalomi Z, Miller RS: From Age-ing to Sage-ing: A Profound New Vision of Growing Older. New York, Warner Books, 1997

Wisdom Factors International: http://www.wisdomfactors.com/

The Wisdom Page: http://www.wisdompage.com/index.html

7

Cognition and Emotion in Centenarians

Leonard W. Poon, Ph.D.
Peter Martin, Ph.D.
Jennifer Margrett, Ph.D.

It may be surprising to some that centenarians are the fastest-growing population in most industrialized countries. The U.S. Census Bureau (2004) reported that there were about 22 centenarians per 100,000 residents in the United States as of 2004. Most industrial countries report a range of 10–20 per 100,000, and some prefectures in Japan such as Okinawa report as many as 50 per 100,000 (Japan Ministry of Health, Labour and Welfare 2009). Logical questions for both scientists and laypersons alike focus on factors that contribute to centenarians' adaptation and longevity. Unfortunately, answers about the biological, psychological, and sociological contributors are still elusive (for review, see Poon and Perls 2008). However, it is quite clear that studies have shown two unambiguous findings:

1. Women have the advantage of living longer. Of the 10 oldest living persons in the world, all are women, and it is well known that the female-

---

This work was supported by National Institute on Aging Grant 1P01 AG17553.

superiority longevity phenomenon increases with increasing age (Gerontology Research Group 2009).

2. There is no one dominating contributor to longevity. Twenty years of systematic research associated with the Georgia Centenarian Study (Poon and Perls 2008) has shown there is much diversity among centenarians in their behaviors, functioning, and environment and the individualized contributors to their longevity.

The latter finding may be encouraging and uplifting for some in that there may be different pathways to longevity for different persons, so not only a select few may have the opportunity to live to an extreme old age. Our purpose in this chapter is to focus on two attributes among centenarians—emotion, which consists of personality, coping, and affect, and cognition—and to share our reflections on how they may be pathways to longevity and adaptation.

This chapter focuses on the findings of the Georgia Centenarian Study (1988–2009), with particular attention to the domains of cognition and personality/emotion among centenarians who are cognitively intact and reside in the community. After a discussion of the heterogeneity of centenarians, we describe the study methods and procedures, then summarize the study findings, and conclude the chapter with a discussion of how these domains could contribute to extreme old age.

A Matter of Diversity

Research examining adult development and aging demonstrates that heterogeneity between individuals increases with age, as genetic and environmental factors play increasingly differential roles. The lack of homogeneity among centenarians contributes to the paradox in identifying potential contributors to longevity. For the purpose of discussion about cognition in this chapter, for example, it may be difficult to speculate that greater cognitive ability is a prerequisite for extreme longevity, owing to the diversity of cognitive functioning. Some centenarians can perform cognitively at the level of 60-year-old adults (Poon et al. 1992b), but it is estimated that 40%–80% of centenarians experience dementia (Gondo and Poon 2007). Nevertheless, the review by Gondo and Poon (2007) shows that greater cognitive abilities can contribute to longevity in centenarians as well as in the general population. Similarly, some centenarians are physically functional to the extent that they live independently in the community (Poon et al. 1992b), although about half of American centenarians live in care facilities (Perls et al. 1999). Hence the ranges of abilities, health, and functioning are large among centenarians. On the other hand, even though there is much diversity among centenarians, we have uncovered some personality factors and coping strategies (Martin et al. 2001) that seem to differentiate centenarians from octogenarians and sexagenarians. Although there is much we need to learn about survival factors among the oldest of the old, this research area is on the verge of breakthrough discoveries that will be useful in aiding successful adaptation in very old age.

The Georgia Centenarian Study

The Georgia Centenarian Study (Poon and Perls 2008; Poon et al. 1992a) was a collaborative effort among researchers from different disciplines to examine characteristics and attributes of long-lived individuals. Phase I (1988–1992) examined the unique adaptation characteristics of community-dwelling and cognitively intact centenarians, octogenarians, and sexagenarians in Georgia. Phase II (1992–1998) was a longitudinal study of the same cohorts. Building on lessons learned in the first two phases, Phase III (2001–2008) was a population-based study designed to do the following:

- Identify and isolate longevity genes
- Describe the neuropathology of dementia
- Assess neuropsychological and physical functioning
- Characterize the resources and adaptations of centenarians

This chapter includes selected cognitive and personality and emotion findings from Phases I, II, and III of the study. The selection of appropriate control groups in centenarian studies is problematic (Poon and Perls 2008) owing primarily to the increasing diversity of functions and environments with age. From this perspective, Phase I was unique in that only cognitively intact and community-dwelling participants in their hundreds, eighties, or sixties were compared in order to reduce potential confounding factors in functioning and cognition. The weakness in this design is that findings from these convenience samples may not be representative of the overall population of centenarians. To investigate this possibility, we are currently comparing Phase III findings from convenience samples with findings from population-based samples to evaluate the generalization of results.

Phase I of the study included 321 cognitively intact and community-dwelling participants: 38 male and 53 female sexagenarians, 31 male and 62 female octogenarians, and 35 male and 102 female centenarians. Octogenarians and sexagenarians exceeded a score of 23 on the Mini-Mental State Examination (MMSE; Folstein et al. 1975) and were rated as no greater than stage 2 on the Global Deterioration Scale, which is indicative of normative age-related memory impairment (Reisberg et al. 1982). Owing to a greater prevalence of sensory problems among centenarians and a reflection of sensory limitations in MMSE scoring, the centenarian MMSE minimum score was 21. Centenarians were tested individually in their homes over four sessions. Additional sessions were scheduled in order to complete all testing. Octogenarians and sexagenarians were tested in groups in community centers nearby (except octogenarians with physical limitations, who were tested individually in their homes), and all testing was completed in 1 day.

Phase III of the study is ongoing (Poon and Perls 2007) and has included 287 centenarian (i.e., 98 years and older) and 88 octogenarian participants: 30 male and 58 female octogenarians, and 51 male and 236 female centenarians. This population-based sample has included participants from skilled nursing facilities and personal care homes in a 44-county area in northern Georgia. Voter registration lists have been used to identify additional centenarians residing in the community or in care facilities. Not all participants have been able to answer questions regarding personality and emotion. More specifically, of the original sample, 137 centenarians and 71 octogenarians have participated in the survey on individual and social resources.

Figure 7–1 displays hypothetical models of the variables under investigation as well as the direct and indirect influences of these variables toward successful adaptation and longevity. Cognitive instruments included the following:

- Assessments and ratings of global cognitive functioning
- Tests of primary and secondary recall
- Four tests covering crystallized and fluid intelligence from the Wechsler Adult Intelligence Scale (WAIS)
- Solutions to everyday problems

Personality and emotion instruments included:

- Selected traits and facets from the Revised NEO Personality Inventory
- Coping Indices from the Health and Daily Living Manual (Moos et al. 1985)
- Bradburn Affect Balance Scale

Cognitive Functions Among Cognitively Intact Participants

Turning first to indicators of global cognitive functioning, as expected, age differences on global indicators of cognitive functioning were evident. Three major clusters of specific cognitive functions were compared among the three groups of participants separated by 20 years of age in Phase I (Holtsberg

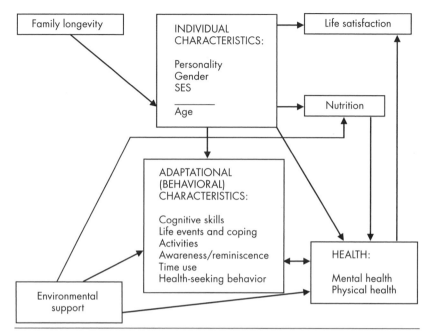

FIGURE   7–1. Georgia   Centenarian   Adaptation   Model: study constructs and influences on successful adaptation.

Source.   Reprinted from Poon LW, Clayton GM, Martin P, et al.: "The Georgia Centenarian Study." *International Journal on Aging and Human Development* 34:1–17, 1992. Used with permission.

et al. 1995; Poon et al. 1992b, 2007). The first cluster focused on memory and learning functions: retrieval from primary (newly presented information) and secondary (learned information) memory was assessed with a paired-associate learning procedure; tertiary memory of well-known and memorized information, such as the names of U.S. presidents, was also tested (Hamsher and Roberts 1985; Poon 1985). The second cluster of specific cognitive functions examined exemplars of fluid intelligence (e.g., Block Design and Picture Arrangement) and crystallized intelligence (e.g., Vocabulary and Arithmetic) in the WAIS (Wechsler 1981). The third cluster examined the everyday problem-solving abilities needed to handle problems and issues one would encounter in day-to-day life (Denney et al. 1982).

The patterns of age-related differences from the 100-, 80-, and 60-year-old groups in Phase I parallel the findings from normative samples of younger and older adults in the cognitive aging literature (e.g., Craik 1977; Hoyer and Verhaeghen 2006; Poon 1985). That is, smaller and minimal age differences in primary and tertiary memory were found, whereas a significant age difference in secondary memory was found. Although the centenarians performed worse on all psychometric intelligence tests compared with octogenarians and sexagenarians, the magnitude of age differences was significantly smaller on crystallized intelligence tests than on fluid intelligence tests. The findings reflected significant cohort influences in these standardized psychometric tests, in that none of the participants from the three age groups had likely been exposed to this type of testing since they were in formal schooling. The centenarians had perhaps never been exposed to these tests at all, and, hence, they were the most handicapped in responding to them. Indeed, education was shown to have a profound positive effect that modulated the level of performance for all participants, especially the centenarians.

It is most interesting that when these community-dwelling 60-, 80-, and 100-year-old participants were asked to list solutions to problems and issues encountered in everyday life, there were minimal or no differences in number and quality of solutions (Poon et al. 1992a, 1992b). Taken together, these findings show that although community-dwelling and dementia-free centenarians are lower in psychometric abilities, their crystallized intelligence and cumulative experience tend to compensate in situations involving everyday problem solving. Thus, when one considers the role cognition plays in later-life adaptation and survival, it is important to distinguish among various indicators of cognition (e.g., self-reported functioning, global cognitive measures such as the MMSE, specific abilities, and everyday problem-solving skills) because they possess differential trajectories and predictive utility. In the population-based samples in Phase III a greater proportion of centenarians (68%) compared with octogenarians (15%) scored below the typical impairment cutoff score on the MMSE (i.e., <23). Of the oldest participants scoring 23 and greater on the MMSE, octogenarians (mean score= 27.63) tended to outperform centenarians (mean score= 26.32) ($t=4.40$ [$df=165$]; $P<0.001$). When self-ratings and proxy ratings of mental fatigue are considered, octogenarians were viewed as less fatigued than centenarians (self-ratings: $t=-2.12$ [$df=245$]; $P<0.05$) (proxy ratings: $t=-2.27$ [$df=285$]; $P<0.05$). Consistent with these ratings, interviewers also viewed centenarians as being more cognitively impaired than octogenarians ($t=-4.29$ [$df=285$]; $P<0.001$).

Personality and Emotion Among Cognitively Intact Participants

To survive into very late life, individuals often draw on resources that allow them to adapt to functional and cognitive changes. There are three emotional resources that tend to be important, particularly in late life: 1) personality traits related to emotional stability, 2) emotion-focused coping behaviors, and 3) states of subjective well-being as assessed by measurements of positive and negative affect. In this section, we highlight these three components of individual resources among centenarians.

Personality Traits Related to Emotional Stability

A number of studies have summarized distinct personality traits among centenarians (for a detailed summary, see Martin 2007). Results from Phase I of the Georgia Centenarian Study indicated that centenarians had higher scores for dominance, suspiciousness, and shrewdness, but their lower scores for imagination and tension were comparable to those of the two younger age groups. On retesting after approximately 20 months during Phase II, centenarians displayed decreased scores in sensitivity but increased scores in openness. It can be argued that the "robust personality" among these highly selected centenarians was not only an indication of survivorship but also an important resource that may help centenarians to adapt well to later life. Recent findings from Phase III of the Georgia Centenarian Study using the Big-5 framework suggest that centenarians overall have low levels of neuroticism and high levels of extraversion, competence (a facet of conscientiousness), and trust (a facet of agreeableness) (Martin et al. 2006).

Low levels of anxiety and neuroticism appear to be the most remarkable personality traits among centenarians. Figure 7–2 displays the relative frequencies of centenarians in Phase III of the Georgia Centenarian Study endorsing discrete emotions as measured by items of the neuroticism factor. As Chipperfield et al. (2003) pointed out, the study of specific emotions has received far less attention than it deserves, particularly among oldest-of-the-old populations. In our study, the highest endorsements were obtained for feeling "worthless" (33.1%) and "ashamed" (21.3%), whereas the lowest endorsements were obtained for feeling "sad" (6.6%) and "angry" (9.6%). The results suggest that centenarians rate highly in emotional stability but that negative emotions tend to relate to aspects of self-sufficiency. The functional limitations (e.g., vision, hearing, mobility) that often accompany very old age take their toll for a sizable number of centenarians and may be the reason for these emotions. Feelings of uselessness, however, do not automatically translate to feelings of sadness or anger.

Emotion-Focused Coping Behaviors

Assessing personality traits for emotional stability is only one component of emotions. A second aspect relates to coping behaviors used by centenarians when faced with problems or changes in life. Findings from Phase I of the Georgia Centenarian Study suggest that centenarians have relatively low lev-

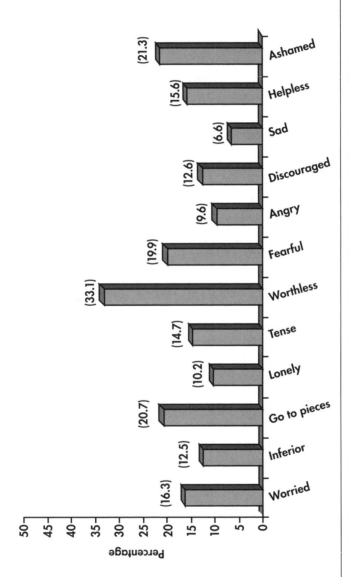

FIGURE 7–2. Profile of neuroticism among centenarians in Phase III of the Georgia Centenarian Study.

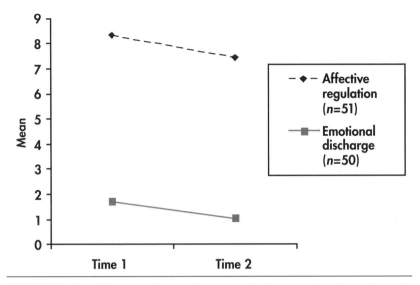

FIGURE 7–3. **Changes in emotional coping among centenarians in Phase I of the Georgia Centenarian Study.**

Note. Time 1=baseline; Time 2=20 months. Both affective regulation (n=51) and emotional discharge (n=50) were measured with six items; scores could range from 0 to 18.

els of behavioral coping but maintain high levels of cognitive coping (Martin et al. 1992, 2008). Centenarians were particularly likely "not to worry," "to rely on religious beliefs," "to take things a day at a time," and "to accept" health problems (Martin et al. 2001). Our longitudinal data on coping suggest that centenarians and octogenarians experience decreases in active behavioral coping over time, whereas sexagenarians are more likely to experience increases in this coping mode (Martin et al. 2008).

Two specific dimensions of coping measured in Phase I of the Georgia study are worth assessing in more detail: affective regulation in response to a stressful event (e.g., "I see the positive side of the situation" and "I keep busy") and emotional discharge, again in response to a stressful event (e.g., "I get angry" and "I let my feelings out somehow"). When centenarians are compared with participants in other age groups, no specific age differences on these coping dimensions were noted: $F_{2,272}=1.08$, $P=0.34$ for affective regulation and $F_{2,265}=1.49$, $P=0.23$ for emotional discharge. However, when assessing coping changes over a 20-month time frame, centenarians facing a health event had a decrease in their use of affective regulation and emotional discharge. Among these changes, only the decrease in emotional discharge was statistically significant: $t_{51}=1.50$, $P=0.14$ for affective regulation and $t_{51}=2.44$, $P<0.05$ for emotional discharge. The change patterns are shown in Figure 7–3.

Taken together, the results suggest that centenarians are more likely to use specific cognitive regulation techniques, such as religious coping or acceptance, and that emotion-focused coping may decrease in very old age. Others have pointed out that coping behaviors can help in the regulation of distress and management of problems (Folkman and Moskowitz 2000). In general, older adults are just as effective in coping with distress as are adults at younger ages (Aldwin et al. 1996). Older adults, however, tend to use fewer coping behaviors (Aldwin et al. 2006). The frequent use of religious coping indicates that this mode of coping may offer a source of personal stability and mastery when personal control is diminishing (Emery and Pargament 2004).

States of Subjective Well-Being

A final noteworthy component of emotion relates to aspects of subjective well-being among centenarians. Two dimensions are discussed here in the context of emotions: positive and negative affect as measured by the Bradburn Affect Balance Scale (Bradburn 1969). When centenarians in Phase I of the Georgia study were compared with younger age groups, results indicated that there were no differences in negative affect, whereas age-group differences in positive affect were highly significant: $F_{2,304}=0.82$, $P=0.44$, and $F_{2,304}=9.22$, $P<0.001$, respectively. The post hoc contrast suggests that all three age groups differed significantly from one another. When longitudinal changes are assessed over time, a main effect is seen in the change in positive affect—$F_{1,183}=19.79$, $P<0.001$—but not in negative affect: $F_{1,183}=1.36$, $P=0.25$. Even more noteworthy is the significant effect that the age × time interaction had on positive affect: $F_{1,183}=3.90$, $P<0.05$. The interaction results, depicted in Figure 7–4, suggest an accelerated decline in positive affect among centenarians, whereas there is only a slight change for octogenarians and no change for sexagenarians over a 60-month period. The results point to clear differences and changes in positive emotions when comparing younger-old and oldest-of-the-old populations, and are consistent with results of other studies such as the study by Kunzmann et al. (2000), which also indicated that there is a lower level of positive affect among the very oldest populations.

Cognitive Abilities, Longevity, and Adaptation

Evidence from a number of centenarian studies supports the finding that even cognitively intact centenarians without dementia tend to perform at a significantly lower level than younger control subjects on psychometric cognitive tests (Gondo and Poon 2007). The Tokyo Centenarian Study (Inagaki and Gondo 2003) reported findings comparable to those of the Georgia Cen-

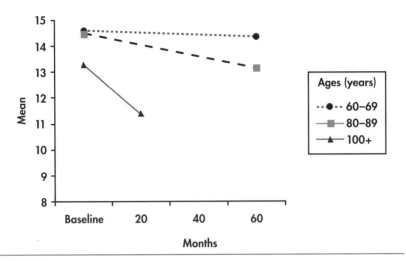

FIGURE 7–4.   Age differences and changes in positive affect in Phases I and II of the Georgia Centenarian Study.

Note.   Postive Affect was measured with few items, each ranging from 1 to 4. Centenarians (*n*=60) were assessed at baseline and at 20 months; octogenarians (*n*=56) and sexagenarians (*n*=70) were assessed at baseline and at 60 months.

tenarian Study using similar cognitive tests; centenarians scored significantly lower on the WAIS subtests of Digit Symbol, Block Design, Letter-Number Sequencing, and Vocabulary. Significantly lower scores were reported on both fluid and crystallized intelligence tests when centenarians were compared with 50- and 80-year-old control subjects. Similar results were reported in the Swedish Centenarian Study on verbal performance, reaction time, and memory tests (S.M. Samuelsson et al. 1997). On the other hand, it is interesting to note that community-dwelling centenarians in the Georgia Centenarian Study who did not have dementia maintained their everyday cognitive abilities, such as problem solving and episodic memory embedded in everyday life contexts. This finding was supported by a study by Fromholt and colleagues (2003) that compared autobiographical memory in centenarians and octogenarians; that study found no difference in the number of recalled memories and found similar patterns of frequency of memories in the two age groups. It may be logical to inquire whether psychometric tests are appropriate assessments of centenarians' cognitive abilities.

Do Cognitive Abilities Influence Adaptation?

Individuals with adequate cognitive skills and higher levels of cognitive functioning tend to demonstrate superior adaptation in later life. Cognitive skills and functioning are predictors of important outcomes such as mental health, ability to perform activities of daily living, and mortality even within nondemented samples. In the Georgia Centenarian Study, analyses examining selected demographic, cognitive, functional, and personality predictors of mental health outcomes for octogenarians and centenarians in Phase III of the study revealed that greater problem-solving ability was predictive of fewer depressive symptoms among octogenarians and greater positive affect among centenarians. Consistent with prior research linking cognitive functioning and activities-of-daily-living performance (Allaire and Marsiske 2002; Perneczky et al. 2006; Robine et al. 2003), findings from the Georgia study revealed that cognitive status and everyday problem-solving skills were significant and strong predictors of octogenarians' and centenarians' ability to perform activities of daily living in Phase III of the study.

Do Cognitive Abilities Influence Longevity?

In spite of generally lower cognitive abilities among centenarians compared with younger control subjects, there may be sufficient reserves in cognitive abilities to predict length of survival. Cognition was reported as a significant predictor of survivorship in both the Tokyo Centenarian Study (Gondo et al. 2006) and the Swedish Centenarian Study (H. Samuelsson et al. 1997). The Georgia Centenarian Study compared predictors for the number of days of survival beyond 100 years and found that cognition (as assessed by verbal intelligence) was one of four significant predictors (Poon et al. 2000). The other predictors were gender (being female), nutrition sufficiency, and father's age at death. The French Centenarian Study reported that the MMSE significantly predicted length of survival in addition to residential status (institutional dwelling), health status, and basic and instrumental activities of daily living (Robine et al. 2003).

In addition to studies among centenarians, large-scale longitudinal studies also point to the importance of cognition in terms of mortality. For example, in the Terman Cohort Study (Friedman and Markey 2003), cognitively gifted young individuals with high IQs tended to have a lower mortality rate than the general population. Similar findings were reported in the Scottish Mental Survey of 11-year-old children performed in 1932, in which the rates of mortality and morbidity at age 79 were associated with cognitive status (Deary et al. 2004). Two measures of linguistic abilities (grammatical complexity and idea density) were found to inversely correlate with the risk of mortality in the Nun Study (Snowden et al. 1999). Finally, a review of nine studies on the relationship between the rate of cognition decline and death (Bosworth and Siegler 2002) found that level of cognitive abilities predicted mortality.

Personality, Emotional Factors, Longevity, and Adaptation

The emotional profile of centenarians suggests that on the trait level, these survivors have high scores of emotional stability, and emotional stability may indeed be an important characteristic of survivorship (Martin 2007). Centenarians do not worry much, are fairly relaxed, and show very low levels of sadness and anger. Another adaptive survivorship mechanism is on the behavioral coping level: emotion-focused coping behaviors are used fairly infrequently. Third, on the subjective well-being level, centenarians show lower levels of positive emotions than younger adults. The relatively low levels of positive emotions may be a by-product of the ailments and limitations inherent to such old age.

Do Personality and Coping Influence Adaptation?

There is ample evidence that personality traits contribute to adaptation or maladaptation in later life. Personality traits have been linked to cognitive impairment (Crowe et al. 2006), health-related quality of life (Chapman et al. 2007), functional capacity (Duberstein et al. 2003), and perceived health (Chapman et al. 2006). For centenarians who experience many life changes, such as increased sensory impairment, decreased functional capacity, and the loss of family and friends, a robust personality contributes to a continued sense of self that may be preserved until the very end of life. Centenarians are unique because of their individual characteristics and because of their configuration of traits that allow them to be seen not only in cognitive, physical, and functional decline, but also in their own special way. A continuous robust personality can overshadow developmental decline.

In a similar vein, coping behaviors allow centenarians to adapt well to significant changes in their lives. Although behavioral modes of coping are increasingly diminished, centenarians maintain relatively high levels of cognitive coping. Perhaps it is because of their restricted mobility that centenarians are more likely to use their thoughts and reflections when coping with adversity. It is this contemplative mode of reflection that adds to the fascination of this population. Some centenarians write poetry and books to share their life stories (Poon et al. 1991), and most readily offer their advice to interviewers and visitors. Finally, other centenarians turn toward religious coping (e.g., praying and relying on religious beliefs) when adapting to the many losses experienced over time.

Do Personality and Coping Influence Longevity?

Several centenarian studies have pointed out that low levels of neuroticism are found among centenarians. Other traits associated with centenarians as described in the Swedish Centenarian Study were responsible, easygoing, capable, relaxed, efficient, and not prone to anxiety (H. Samuelsson et al. 1997). A recent Japanese centenarian study (the Tokyo Centenarian Study; Masui et al. 2006) reported that centenarians scored higher in openness to experience and that female (compared with male) centenarians had higher scores in conscientiousness and extraversion when compared with younger control subjects. The most consistent personality trait found in almost every centenarian study is a low level of neuroticism (see Figure 7–2). Additional longevity traits may include relatively high levels of extraversion and conscientiousness. With increasing age, extraverted individuals are perhaps more resourceful in obtaining social support, and conscientious individuals may be able to take better care of themselves in tasks that are necessary for survival (Martin 2007).

The results from centenarian studies mirror findings reported in other longitudinal studies assessing premature mortality or survivorship. For example, low levels of conscientiousness and extraversion and high levels of neuroticism have been linked to mortality in several longitudinal studies (Almada et al. 1991; Christensen et al. 2002; Friedman et al. 1993; Kubzansky et al. 1997; Wilson et al. 2004). Mroczek et al. (2006) hypothesize that individuals high in conscientiousness engage in better health behaviors, such as eating a healthy diet and exercising, and these health behaviors may result in a longer life. The association between mortality and neuroticism, Mroczek et al. (2006) speculate, may have its roots in sensitivity to stress. Neuroticism is associated with greater exposure and reactivity to stress (Mroczek and Almeida 2004), and a continuously high level of neuroticism may cause physical damage to the cardiovascular system, contributing to premature mortality. Centenarians low in neuroticism may have escaped the noxious effects of neuroticism.

In addition to a robust personality, centenarians may have contributed to their own longevity by effectively using those coping behaviors that work in reducing the negative effects of stress. Cognitive coping is an effective mode of working through one's problems, and if a situation cannot be changed easily, acceptance may well prompt these survivors to simply move on. Finally, religious coping may provide comfort, understanding, and meaning and can relieve the stress experienced by older adults (Pargament 1997).

Conclusion

Intuitively, it is logical to conclude that a higher level of cognition and more adaptive personality and emotional affect would contribute to longevity and survivorship. Empirical evidence is available to support this conclusion. However, it is important to note that significant variability is found among centenarians. Future studies need to assess interactions between the individual and the environment as well as between genetics and the environment. Among the four predictors of the length of survival beyond 100 years in the Georgia Centenarian Study (Poon et al. 2000), two were more genetically determined (being female and father's age at death) and two were more environmentally determined (cognition and nutrition sufficiency); it may be argued that interactions were at play among these four predictors. Intraindividual variability can be assessed by measuring fluctuation in function over time; this may be a more important indicator of adaptation and survival than static mean-level assessments (e.g., Ghisletta et al. 2002; MacDonald et al. 2003; Nesselroade and Salthouse 2004). Researchers and clinicians must also attend to theoretical and practical aspects of assessment. In the cognitive realm, findings can vary depending on the nature of the cognitive assessment, and traditional psychometric assessments may not best capture the abilities of the oldest of the old. In terms of personality and emotion, distinctions must be made between various coping behaviors as well as between positive and negative affect and well-being assessments.

KEY POINTS

■ Centenarians are the fastest-growing segment of the population, and there are now about 22 centenarians per 100,000 U.S. residents.

■ In cognitive and emotional phenotypes, centenarians display a wide variability both among themselves and, over time, within themselves. Greater intraindividual variability may predict worse outcomes.

■ In the Georgia Centenarian Study, two genetically based phenotypes (female gender, father's age at death) and two more environmental phenotypes (cognitive functioning, nutrition sufficiency) predicted survival beyond age 100.

■ Emotional stability and a capacity to handle negative affect appear to be traits associated with centenarians.

References

Aldwin CM, Sutton KJ, Chiara G, et al: Age differences in stress, coping, and appraisal: findings from the Normative Aging Study. J Gerontol B Psychol Sci Soc Sci 51:179–188, 1996

Aldwin CM, Spiro A, Park CL: Health, behavior, and optimal aging: a life-span developmental perspective, in Handbook of the Psychology of Aging, 6th Edition. Edited by Birren JE, Schaie KW. Amsterdam, Elsevier Academic Press, 2006, pp 85–104

Allaire JC, Marsiske M: Well- and ill-defined measures of everyday cognition: relationship to older adults' intellectual ability and functional status. Psychol Aging 17:101–115, 2002

Almada SJ, Zonderman AB, Shekelle RB, et al: Neuroticism, cynicism and risk of death in middle-aged men: the Western Electric Study. Psychosom Med 53:165–175, 1991

Bosworth HB, Siegler IC: Terminal change in cognitive function: an updated review of longitudinal studies. Exp Aging Res 28:299–315, 2002

Bradburn NM: The Structure of Psychological Well-Being. Chicago, IL, Aldine, 1969

Chapman BP, Duberstein PR, Sörensen S, et al: Personality and perceived health in older adults: the five-factor model in primary care. J Gerontol B Psychol Sci Soc Sci 61:362–365, 2006

Chapman B, Duberstein P, Lyness JM: Personality traits, education, and health-related quality of life among older adult primary care patients. J Gerontol B Psychol Sci Soc Sci 62:343–352, 2007

Chipperfield JG, Perry RP, Weiner B: Discrete emotions in later life. J Gerontol B Psychol Sci Soc Sci 58:23–34, 2003

Christensen AJ, Ehlers SL, Wiebe JS, et al: Patient personality and mortality: a 4-year prospective examination of chronic renal insufficiency. Health Psychol 21:315–320, 2002

Craik FIM: Age differences in human memory, in Handbook of the Psychology of Aging. Edited by Birren JE, Schaie KW. New York, Van Nostrand Reinhold, 1977, pp 384–420

Crowe M, Andel R, Pedersen NL, et al: Personality and risk of cognitive impairment 25 years later. Psychol Aging 21:573–580, 2006

Deary IJ, Whiteman MC, Pattie A, et al: Apolipoprotein E gene variability and cognitive functions at age 79: a follow-up of the Scottish Mental Survey of 1932. Psychol Aging 19:367–371, 2004

Denney NW, Pearce KA, Palmer AM: A developmental study of adults' performance on traditional and practical problem-solving tasks. Exp Aging Res 8:115–118, 1982

Duberstein PR, Sörensen S, Lyness JM, et al: Personality is associated with perceived health and functional status in older primary care patients. Psychol Aging 18:25–37, 2003

Emery EE, Pargament KL: The many faces of religious coping in late life: conceptualization, measurement, and links to well-being. Ageing Int 29:3–27, 2004

Folkman S, Moskowitz JT: Positive affect and the other side of coping. Am Psychol 55:647–654, 2000

Folstein MF, Folstein SE, McHugh PR: "Mini-mental state": a practical method for grading the cognitive state of patients for the clinician. J Psychiatr Res 12:189–198, 1975

Friedman H, Markey C: Paths to longevity in the highly intelligent Terman cohort, in Brain and Longevity (Research and Perspectives in Longevity). Edited by Finch CE, Robine J-M, Christen Y. Berlin, Springer, 2003, pp 165–175

Friedman HS, Tucker JS, Tomlinson-Keasey C, et al: Does childhood personality predict longevity? J Pers Soc Psychol 65:176–185, 1993

Fromholt P, Mortensen DB, Torpdahl P, et al: Life-narrative and word-cued autobiographical memories in centenarians: comparisons with 80-year-old control, depressed, and dementia groups. Memory 11:81–88, 2003

Gerontology Research Group: Validated living supercentenarians as of January 16, 2009. Available at: http://www.grg.org/Adams/E.HTM. Accessed January 18, 2009.

Ghisletta P, Nesselroade JR, Featherman DL, et al: Structure and predictive power of intraindividual variability in health and activity measures. Swiss Journal of Psychology 61:73–83, 2002

Gondo Y, Poon LW: Cognitive function of centenarians and its influence on longevity, in Annual Review of Gerontology and Geriatrics, Vol 27: Biopsychosocial Approaches to Longevity. Edited by Poon LW, Perls T. New York, Springer, 2007, pp 129–149

Gondo Y, Hirose N, Arai Y, et al: Functional status of centenarians in Tokyo, Japan: developing better phenotypes of exceptional longevity. J Gerontol A Biol Sci Med Sci 61:305–310, 2006

Hamsher KD, Roberts RJ: Memory for recent U.S. presidents in patients with cerebral disease. J Clin Exp Neuropsychol 7:1–13, 1985

Holtsberg PA, Poon LW, Noble CA, et al: Mini-Mental Status Exam status of community-dwelling cognitively intact centenarians. Int Psychogeriatr 7:417–427, 1995

Hoyer WJ, Verhaeghen P: Memory aging, in Handbook of the Psychology of Aging, 6th Edition. Edited by Birren JE, Schaie KW. Amsterdam, Elsevier Academic Press, 2006, pp 209–232

Inagaki H, Gondo Y: Biomechanism of centenarians: functional aspect and successful aging. Journal of the Society of Biomechanisms 27(1):18–22, 2003

Japan Ministry of Health, Labour and Welfare: We Are at the Door to the Super Aged Society. Health and Welfare Bureau for the Elderly. Available at: http://www.mhlw.go.jp/english/org/policy/p32-33.html. Accessed January 19, 2009.

Kubzansky LD, Kawachi I, Spiro A 3rd, et al: Is worrying bad for your heart? A prospective study of worry and coronary heart disease in the Normative Aging Study. Circulation 95:818–824, 1997

Kunzmann U, Little TD, Smith J: Is age-related stability of subjective well-being a paradox? Cross-sectional and longitudinal evidence from the Berlin Aging Study. Psychol Aging 15:511–526, 2000

MacDonald SW, Hultsch DF, Dixon RA: Performance variability is related to change in cognition: evidence from the Victoria Longitudinal Study. Psychol Aging 18:510–523, 2003

Martin P: Personality and coping among centenarians, in Annual Review of Gerontology and Geriatrics, Vol 27: Biopsychosocial Approaches to Longevity. Edited by Poon LW, Perls TT. New York, Springer, 2007, pp 89–106

Martin P, Poon LW, Clayton GM, et al: Personality, life events, and coping in the oldest-old. Int J Aging Hum Dev 34:19–30, 1992

Martin P, Rott C, Poon LW, et al: A molecular view of coping behavior in older adults. J Aging Health 13:72–91, 2001

Martin P, da Rosa G, Siegler I, et al: Personality and longevity: findings from the Georgia Centenarian Study. Age (Omaha) 28:343–352, 2006

Martin P, Kliegel M, Rott C, et al: Age differences and changes of coping behavior in three age groups: findings from the Georgia Centenarian Study. Int J Aging Hum Dev 66:97–114, 2008

Masui Y, Gondo Y, Inagaki H, et al: Do personality characteristics predict longevity? Findings from the Tokyo Centenarian Study. Age (Omaha) 28:353–361, 2006

Moos RH, Cronkite RC, Billings AG, et al: Health and Daily Living Manual. San Francisco, CA, Stanford University Medical Centers, 1985

Mroczek DK, Almeida DM: The effects of daily stress, personality, and age on daily negative affect. J Pers 72:355–378, 2004

Mroczek DK, Spiro A 3rd, Griffin PW: Personality and aging, in Handbook of the Psychology of Aging, 6th Edition. Edited by Birren JE, Schaie KW. Amsterdam, Elsevier Academic Press, 2006, pp 363–377

Nesselroade JR, Salthouse TA: Methodological and theoretical implications of intraindividual variability in perceptual-motor performance. J Gerontol B Psychol Sci Soc Sci 59:49–55, 2004

Pargament KI: The Psychology of Religion and Coping: Theory, Research, Practice. New York, Guilford, 1997

Perls TT, Bochen K, Freeman M, et al: Validity of reported age and centenarian prevalence in New England. Age Ageing 28:193–198, 1999

Perneczky R, Pohl C, Sorg C, et al: Impairment of activities of daily living requiring memory or complex reasoning as part of the MCI syndrome. Int J Geriatr Psychiatry 21:158–162, 2006

Poon LW: Differences in human memory with aging: nature, causes, and clinical implications, in Handbook of the Psychology of Aging, 2nd Edition. Edited by Birren JE, Schaie KW. New York, Van Nostrand Reinhold, 1985, pp 427–462

Poon LW, Perls TT: The trials and tribulations of studying the oldest old, in Annual Review of Gerontology and Geriatrics, Vol 27: Biopsychosocial Approaches to Longevity. New York, Springer, 2008, pp 1–10

Poon LW, Clayton GM, Martin P: In her own words: Cecilia Payne Grove, 1889–1990. Generations 15:67–68, 1991

Poon LW, Clayton GM, Martin P, et al: The Georgia Centenarian Study. Int J Aging Hum Dev 34:1–17, 1992a

Poon LW, Messner S, Martin P, et al: The influences of cognitive resources on adaptation and old age. Int J Aging Hum Dev 34:381–390, 1992b

Poon LW, Johnson MA, Davey A, et al: Psycho-social predictors of survival among centenarians, in Autonomy Versus Dependence in the Oldest-Old. Edited by Martin P, Rott C, Hagberg B, et al. Paris, Serdi, 2000, pp 77–89, 2000

Reisberg B, Ferris SH, de Leon MJ, et al: Global Deterioration Scale for assessment of primary degenerative dementia. Am J Psychiatry 139:1136–1139, 1982

Robine JM, Romieu I, Allard M: French centenarians and their functional health status [in French]. Presse Med 32:360–364, 2003

Samuelsson H, Jensen C, Ekholm S, et al: Anatomical and neurological correlates of acute and chronic visuospatial neglect following right hemisphere stroke. Cortex 33:271–285, 1997

Samuelsson SM, Alfredson BB, Hagberg B, et al: The Swedish Centenarian Study: a multidisciplinary study of five consecutive cohorts at the age of 100. Int J Aging Hum Dev 45:223–253, 1997

Snowden DA, Greiner LH, Kemper SJ, et al: Linguistic ability in early life and longevity: findings from the Nun Study, in The Paradoxes of Longevity. Edited by Robine JM, Borette B, Francheschi C, et al. Berlin, Springer-Verlag, 1999, pp 103–113

U.S. Census Bureau: National population estimates for the 2000s. Available at: http://www.census.gov/popest/national/asrh/2004_nat_res.html. Accessed March 11, 2008.

Wechsler D: Wechsler Adult Intelligence Scale—Revised Manual. New York, Harcourt Brace Jovanovich, 1981

Wilson RS, Mendes de Leon CF, Bienias JL, et al: Personality and mortality in old age. J Gerontol B Psychol Sci Soc Sci 59:110–116, 2004

Recommended Readings

Bosworth HB, Siegler IC: Terminal change in cognitive function: an updated review of longitudinal studies. Exp Aging Res 28:299–315, 2002

Gerontology Research Group: Validated living supercentenarians as of January 16, 2009. Available at: http://www.grg.org/Adams/E.HTM. Accessed January 18, 2009

Gondo Y, Hirose N, Arai Y, et al: Functional status of centenarians in Tokyo, Japan: developing better phenotypes of exceptional longevity. J Gerontol A Biol Sci Med Sci 61:305–310, 2006

Poon LW, Perls TT: The trials and tribulations of studying the oldest old, in Annual Review of Gerontology and Geriatrics, Vol 27: Biopsychosocial Approaches to Longevity. New York, Springer, 2008, pp 1–10

PART II

Biological Aspects

8

Neuroimaging of Successful Cognitive and Emotional Aging

Lisa T. Eyler, Ph.D.
Sanja Kovacevic, Ph.D.

Preservation of cognitive abilities and of emotional well-being in old age are two features that are widely cited as important for successful aging both by researchers (Depp and Jeste 2006) and by seniors themselves (Reichstadt et al. 2007). Cognitive performance in most domains declines with age, although some abilities, such as word knowledge, are stable or may improve into late life. Emotional well-being and outlook also appear to change with age; in this case, the trend is toward greater positivity in elders than in younger individuals. Against the backdrop of these general trends, however, there is a great deal of variability from individual to individual. The trajectories of cognitive change with age vary widely among older adults (Wilson et al. 2002), and there is also evidence that not all seniors experience positive emotional changes to the same degree. A better understanding of the neurobiology underlying these individual differences is likely to inform efforts to improve the quality of life for all individuals of advanced age.

In the past decade, there has been an increased interest in using powerful neuroscientific techniques to help understand both the average changes in cognition and emotion with age and the variability among individuals in these domains. A large amount of literature has focused on brain changes associated with age-related neurological conditions, such as Alzheimer disease and mild cognitive impairment. Although these studies address important public health issues, they are less informative about the processes of normal biological aging that may occur outside of disease states. Fewer studies have attempted to examine age-related brain changes in samples of older adults who are psychologically and neurologically healthy. Most of the healthy aging literature consists of cross-sectional studies that compare various measures of brain structure and function between a young adult group and an older adult group. A handful of studies have examined longitudinal changes in the brain with age. Such studies have been made possible by the development of relatively noninvasive and high-resolution brain imaging methods such as magnetic resonance imaging (MRI), electroencephalography, magnetoencephalography, positron emission tomography (PET), and functional MRI (fMRI). Although this review focuses on individual differences in emotion and cognition and how they relate to brain imaging measures, we start by briefly summarizing what is known about how the brain typically changes with age.

Brain Changes in Aging

A consistent finding from both cross-sectional and longitudinal studies of aging is that brain volume, both globally and regionally, declines throughout adulthood, although the rate of change seems to vary among structures and the shapes of the age-related curves seem to differ as well (Jernigan and Gamst 2005). In addition to, or perhaps related to, these decreases in volume, the amount of cerebrospinal fluid increases and the degree of white matter abnormalities increases (Raz and Rodrigue 2006). Decreases in volume and increases in white matter abnormalities both appear to be particularly steep in the frontal lobes.

Age-related changes in brain function have also been investigated in healthy individuals, primarily through cross-sectional comparisons of old and young participants. Localized age-related changes in resting blood flow and metabolism have been identified using PET, with studies generally finding decreased metabolism and blood flow at rest among older individuals, particularly in the frontal cortex (Dennis and Cabeza 2007; Meltzer et al. 2003). More recent studies of functional brain changes with age have focused on brain response during cognitive or emotional challenge as measured by PET or fMRI (Dennis and Cabeza 2007). These investigations revealed decreased brain response in some regions among older individuals compared with younger individuals; however, greater brain response in some regions in older participants was commonly observed. In some, but not all, studies, this *overactivation* occurred in a homologous region in the hemisphere opposite from the region that was typically responsive in the younger adults. This has led some researchers to formulate a model of decreased hemispheric asymmetry with age known as HAROLD: hemispheric asymmetry reduction in older adults (Cabeza 2002). Furthermore, response in posterior regions is often weaker in older adults, whereas anterior regions show greater response than in younger individuals (posterior-anterior shift with aging; Dennis and Cabeza 2007).

There is therefore ample evidence that the brain changes significantly with age, even among healthy individuals. What is less clear is how these changes relate to observed changes in cognition and emotion that impact quality of life in the later years. In this chapter, we review studies that are relevant to this issue. Specifically, we highlight investigations that have examined the correlation of cognitive and emotional performance with brain measures among healthy older adults (generally those older than 65 years). We begin with an examination of brain structure, including volumetrics and white matter integrity, and then move on to review functional imaging studies that have examined brain–behavior relationships. Finally, we briefly discuss evidence from neuroimaging studies about brain plasticity in old age, point out some limitations of the existing literature, and make suggestions for future research.

Brain Structure

Cognition and Brain Volume

As mentioned in the previous section, reduced volume of cortical and subcortical structures has been consistently observed in older adults compared with young adults and also in longitudinal studies of aging. We conducted a review (unpublished data) of 48 studies that directly examined the correlation between brain volume and cognitive performance among older adults and found that most studies supported the general finding that "bigger is better." That is, older individuals with a relatively larger volume of brain structures also have better cognitive performance. Positive correlations were not found in every study, however, nor in every brain region, nor for every cognitive domain. Most of the studies included in the review focused on the prefrontal cortex and medial temporal lobe and the associated cognitive domains of memory, executive function, attention, and working memory. The few longitudinal studies have shown less support for a strong prospective relationship between brain size and cognitive change over time, but the follow-up periods were relatively short. Only a few studies also examined the volume–behavior correlation among younger adults, and those that did generally found a weaker relationship among the younger adults or found different regions where volume was associated with good performance in older individuals than in younger individuals. In one study (Fjell et al. 2006), a subsample of elders with a high level of performance had greater cortical thickness in posterior cingulate regions than even high-performing young adults, raising the question of whether these older individuals had always had thicker cortices or whether, through experience and "exercising" their brains, they increased their cortical thickness, leading to preserved abilities in old age.

Cognition and White Matter Integrity

White matter abnormalities increase with age in an exponential fashion even in cognitively healthy individuals. The relationship of these changes to cognition has been reviewed by Gunning-Dixon and Raz (2000). In this meta-analysis of 23 studies, a modest negative relationship between cognitive performance and white matter abnormalities was observed, with significant relationships in the subdomains of processing speed, immediate memory, delayed memory, and executive functioning. These relationships were not attenuated when age was accounted for, suggesting that cognition has an independent relationship with white matter abnormality. Studies of individuals with older mean ages reported slightly weaker relationships between white matter abnormalities and cognition than studies of individuals with younger mean ages. A noted limitation of the reviewed studies was their use of global, and often qualitative, measures of white matter pathology, precluding an examination of how regional abnormalities might relate to specific cognitive abilities.

Newer techniques, such as diffusion tensor imaging (DTI), may be more sensitive to declines in white matter organization and integrity, and have the ability to reveal localized changes in myelination. Although studies have consistently shown that older individuals have more evidence of myelin breakdown and white matter disorganization than young adults (Sullivan and Pfefferbaum 2006), few have examined how this relates to cognitive performance. In general, it has been shown that performance on motor tasks that require transfer of information across hemispheres is significantly related to white matter structural integrity as measured by DTI (Sullivan and Pfefferbaum 2006). Although white matter microstructural changes appear to be particularly pronounced in the frontal cortex, little is known about how these changes influence complex cognitive tasks that require frontal lobe integrity. Also, it is unclear whether the relationship between DTI measures and cognition differs depending on the age of the sample.

Emotion and Brain Volume

Research indicates that regional declines in brain volume with aging occur in several structures that support emotional functioning, including the medial and lateral frontal cortex, anterior cingulate, basal ganglia, and amygdala (although the amygdala findings have been somewhat equivocal) (see, e.g., Fjell et al. 2006; Jernigan and Gamst 2005; Kalpouzos et al. 2009). Emotional well-being has been indicated as an important feature of successful aging. Thus, a question of particular relevance to successful aging is whether emotional stability or resilience to stress is related to regional brain atrophy. Although there is a limited amount of research in this area, existing evidence hints that emotional stability may be associated with less atrophy. For example, Lupien et al. (1998) found that abnormal response to stress measured by basal plasma cortisol level was related to hippocampal atrophy in otherwise healthy older individuals. In addition, evidence from studies of mood disorders, such as chronic depression, suggests that the prefrontal cortex and amygdala undergo atrophy during a prolonged period of stress (as reviewed by McEwen [2005]). In a recent study of healthy participants with a wide range of ages (12–79 years), reduced gray matter density in the medial prefrontal cortex was associated with reduced accuracy of recognizing fearful facial expressions (Williams et al. 2006). However, emotional stability measured by level of neuroticism was not associated with gray matter density in this region or the amygdala. Future research with samples of older adults is necessary to further clarify how individual differences in emotional well-being relate to the degree of regional brain atrophy.

Emotion and White Matter Integrity

Little is known about how white matter integrity relates to normal variability in emotion processing and stability in old age. A wealth of evidence suggests, however, that late-life depression is associated with increased numbers of white matter hyperintensities in the frontal deep white matter and basal ganglia (reviewed by Malloy et al. [2007]). In addition, white matter hyperintensities have been associated with depressive symptoms in older people (Teodorczuk et al. 2007). For example, a large study of older subjects reported that frontal and temporal white matter hyperintensities predicted scores on the Geriatric Depression Scale and that temporal white matter hyperintensity rating was an important predictor even in those without hypertension (O'Brien et al. 2006).

DTI studies of healthy older individuals commonly report disruptions of white matter integrity (particularly in frontal regions), which presumably would influence emotional stability as well (Sullivan and Pfefferbaum 2006). As mentioned earlier (see subsection "Cognition and White Matter Integrity"), disruption of white matter integrity has been associated with impaired cognitive function in a number of studies of normal aging; however, research is lacking on how white matter integrity relates to emotional functioning in healthy individuals.

In summary, although more research is needed in the area of emotional function in successful aging and white matter integrity, research thus far suggests that emotional stability might be associated with lower levels of white matter hyperintensities and preserved white matter tracts in the frontal regions.

Brain Function

Brain Function and Cognitive Performance

Resting blood flow or metabolism studies.   Numerous studies of glucose metabolism or resting blood flow have reported that metabolic differences related to aging are most prominent in the anterior brain regions. The most common finding is that frontal regions and the anterior cingulate show reduced metabolism with increased age (Dennis and Cabeza 2007). In addition, the caudate shows marked hypometabolism, while the amygdala shows less change (e.g., Beason-Held et al. 2008; Kalpouzos et al. 2009). The brain regions showing age-related metabolic differences seem to overlap well with the regions showing volume reduction described previously (see subsections "Cognition and Brain Volume" and "Emotion and Brain Volume"), suggesting that metabolic changes occur due to structural changes in these regions. However, studies that utilized partial volume correction methods (e.g., Kalpouzos et al. 2009) still noted metabolic changes in these regions, suggesting that volume reductions cannot fully explain observed changes in metabolism. The link between reduced resting function of these regions and cognition has been less thoroughly investigated. Most studies that examined this relationship, however, found that lower blood flow and metabolism were related to poorer performance on neuropsychological measures (Persson and Nyberg 2006).

Challenge studies.   Given the findings of widespread decreases in brain volume and resting brain metabolism, it is somewhat surprising to find that when the brains of older adults are challenged with a cognitive task, brain response (e.g., level of blood oxygenation–dependent signal or regional blood flow) is not universally reduced compared with younger individuals. In fact, as summarized above, brain response as measured by both PET and fMRI has often been found to be greater among older adults, perhaps particularly on the side of the brain not typically engaged in younger adults. It is not altogether clear, however, how this overactivation relates to cognitive performance and success in old age. Two main possibilities have been suggested and discussed in the literature:

1.   First, overactivation could reflect an attempt to compensate for other areas of deficit. This view suggests that additional brain regions not typi-

cally involved in younger adults are recruited by the aging brain in order to provide additional resources in an effort to overcome processing deficits in areas where function has declined. This *compensation* may or may not be complete (i.e., raise the level of performance to youthful levels) but, in general, if the compensatory view is correct, then cognitive performance should correlate positively with brain response in the regions of overactivation.

2. An alternative view is that extraneous activation seen in old age is reflective of *dedifferentiation* of neural resources. That is, aging confers less specificity in the neural systems involved in a task, so that activity spreads to other regions not typically involved in cognitive performance. In this view, extra activation is generally seen as reduced efficiency of processing and should therefore be negatively related to performance or not related to performance at all.

Recently, interest in trying to disentangle these possibilities has increased. Some studies have done so by examining subgroups of older individuals who have a high or low level of performance on a particular domain and comparing them to young adults. Other studies have directly examined the correlation of cognitive performance measures (during scanning or from separate testing) to brain response measures. Findings from these studies are summarized below.

Cross-sectional studies. We have reviewed 41 studies that examined how cognitive performance relates to brain function among healthy older individuals. All but two studies were cross-sectional in design. Studies were selected to include a sample of older individuals (mean age of the older samples ranged from 59 to 82 years), and many also included a sample of younger individuals (mean age ranged from 20 to 33 years). The studies were split between those using PET (19 studies) and those using fMRI (22 studies), and the sample sizes were typical of those in many functional neuroimaging investigations (median = 12 participants in each group). The great majority of studies used medical, neurological, and psychiatric screening criteria to assure that the samples were healthy; most employed some sort of cognitive screening (e.g., Mini-Mental State Exam or full neuropsychological battery), about half also excluded individuals based on medication usage, and a smaller number had an additional criterion that the structural magnetic resonance images be free of abnormalities. Education level, when reported, was generally quite high (median of study means for young and old groups = 16 years) and well matched between the groups. Sex ratio was matched across groups in most studies, although in about half of the studies there was an imbalance within groups (slightly more often in favor of women). A range of cognitive paradigms were tested: episodic learning and memory tasks were the most frequently employed, followed by working memory tasks and visual attention, go/no-go, motor, and language paradigms. Group comparison of mean brain response was generally conducted either across the entire brain in each voxel in the image or in a priori regions of interest determined by previous studies or by a conjunction analysis of the response in both groups.

The examination of brain–behavior correlations, however, was frequently only conducted in regions in which an age difference in mean level of brain response was observed. This leaves open the possibility that other regions could have been sensitive to individual differences in performance among older individuals, but were not explored because average brain response in the area was not age dependent. The behavioral measure used to correlate with the brain response varied but was most often accuracy of task performance, followed in frequency by mean reaction time. Some studies, however, used a battery of neuropsychological tests conducted outside the scanner as the index of performance. To be included in this review, the study had to have calculated the relationship of a performance measure to brain response separately for the older group. Most cross-sectional studies also reported brain–behavior relationships within the young group, but few of these studies statistically tested the reliability of any observed differences in correlation between the two groups.

All but five studies found at least one positive association between cognition and brain response among the individuals in the older groups. That is, across many different types of tasks and experiments, elders with a higher level of performance (as measured by accuracy and/or speed) had greater brain response in at least one brain region compared with elders with a lower level of performance. In most of these studies, however, significant negative correlations with performance also were observed in other brain regions. When positive correlations were observed, there was a tendency for them to be found in the frontal lobes, although this is also the region where most studies examined correlations and age-related effects. Negative correlations were slightly more likely to be found in more posterior regions. There was no striking hemispheric laterality to the location of positive and negative correlations with performance, although some studies that specifically examined this issue found bilateral or left-lateralized positive correlations in the older group. The studies that found only negative correlations (i.e., greater brain response in less successful elders) assessed reaction time to incongruent versus congruent visual distracters (Colcombe et al. 2005), go/no-go task accuracy in the basal ganglia (Langenecker et al. 2007) and when evaluated across the entire brain (Nielson et al. 2002), and the relationship of cognitive reserve to age-differential networks of response during nonverbal learning and recognition of difficult versus easy word lists (Stern et al. 2005).

Longitudinal studies. In the one truly longitudinal study of the relationship of brain function to cognitive performance (Beason-Held et al. 2008), 25 adults with a mean age of 68 years at baseline were followed yearly and, at baseline and at the follow-up assessment in the ninth year of the study, were assessed with PET imaging during a recognition memory test for words and figures. In terms of mean changes over 8 years, cognitive performance did not change significantly, but both longitudinal increases and decreases in brain activity were observed across and within each task. When the degree of change in accuracy and reaction time over 8 years was correlated to the degree of longitudinal change in brain response, several regions, including the inferior temporal and parietal region, pre- and postcentral gyri, and parahippocampal gyrus, showed a positive relationship for the verbal task, and other regions, the insula and superior and middle temporal gyri, showed a positive relationship for the figural task. However, those individuals whose performance slowed or became less accurate had increased brain response over time in other regions, including the superior temporal gyrus in the verbal task and the precentral gyrus and middle frontal gyrus in the figural task. Thus, over an 8-year period, there was an apparent reorganization of cortical networks among older individuals in the face of overall preservation of cognitive performance, with some changes appearing to benefit performance and some not. This study did not follow a comparable group of young adults to see whether there would be similar changes in brain response over the same time period.

In a quasi-longitudinal, retrospective study, Persson et al. (2006) compared the fMRI response related to incidental encoding of words during a semantic categorization task in groups of individuals who had either stable or declining memory performance across the previous decade (although all were still cognitively normal at the time of scanning). Within the frontal regions activated by both groups during the task, those individuals whose memory performance had declined showed greater response in the right ventral prefrontal region than those whose performance had remained stable. Those who had declined from a moderate to a low level of performance had the greatest response in this region, but those who had declined from a high to a moderate level of performance also showed greater response than those who had remained stable at a moderate level of performance. This study contradicts many cross-sectional studies by suggesting that overactivation is more likely among those whose cognitive performance is declining with age.

Comparison to brain-behavior relationship in younger adults. Many of the cross-sectional studies examined the correlation of cognitive performance with brain response in the younger group as well, although not all of these directly compared the magnitude of the correlations between the younger and older groups. Comparison of the correlations in the two age groups is important, because it helps to understand whether the associations are general (e.g., related to cognitive endowment regardless of age) or whether the relationships change with age (e.g., because of functional reorganization). We identified several different categories of findings in our review. Some studies found strong correlations in both the younger group and the older group. Most of these found some regions where the correlations were similar in the two age groups (Lustig and Buckner 2004), but many also identified regions in which the correlations were significant only in one group or the other (Bernard et al. 2007; Grady et al. 2002; Iidaka et al. 2002). Interestingly, several studies identified regions in which the relationship between performance and brain response was opposite in direction in the two age groups. For example, Rypma and colleagues, across several replication studies (e.g., Rypma et al. 2005), found a positive association between working memory performance and prefrontal brain response among older individuals but a negative relationship among younger adults. Thus, greater brain response was related to greater cognitive success in the elders but to worse performance among the young adults. The same pattern was also observed by other groups using other types of cognitive tasks (Stern et al. 2005), although there were also some findings (particularly in posterior regions) of positive correlations among the young adults and negative correlations among the elders (van der Veen et al. 2006). In a handful of studies, brain-behavior correlations were much more pronounced in the older group, but the opposite (no correlations in the old and widespread correlations in the young) was not seen in any study.

Dedifferentiation or compensation?. Our literature review suggests support for both the compensatory and dedifferentiation hypotheses. Extraneous activation might be particularly detrimental in tasks that require inhibitory processes, but posterior activation also may be related to poor performance in other types of tasks. Even within the frontal lobes, however, activation of some regions seems to support higher performance whereas other regional activation may be reflective of dedifferentiation (Rajah and D'Esposito 2005). Further research is needed to understand the biological processes that might explain these different patterns in the brain-behavior relationship that are regionally or hemisphere specific.

Brain Function and Emotion

Resting blood flow or metabolism studies.   How changes in metabolism during resting relate to emotional functioning or emotional well-being in elderly individuals has not yet been investigated directly. However, studies that have investigated mood disorders commonly report hypometabolism in the prefrontal cortex and hypermetabolism in the limbic regions (e.g., Mayberg et al. 1999), which may be modulated by psychotherapy or pharmacotherapy (e.g., Goldapple et al. 2004; Kennedy et al. 2007). In addition, higher resting glucose metabolism in the amygdala was associated with dispositional negative affect in depressed patients in one study (Abercrombie et al. 1998), whereas hypometabolism in frontal regions has been associated with depressive symptoms in patients with Alzheimer disease (e.g., Holthoff et al. 2005). This suggests that emotional well-being in aging might be associated with relatively preserved metabolism in the prefrontal regions. Future studies are needed to elucidate how resting metabolism is related to emotion constructs such as emotional regulation or wisdom, both of which are observed to improve with age.

Challenge studies.   Unlike cognitive abilities, such as memory and executive functioning, emotional functions tend to improve with advancing age. As reviewed by Carstensen and Lockenhoff (2003), behavioral studies have reported less negativity, reduced emotional intensity and trait neuroticism, and better emotional stability with increasing age. A shift in emotional bias occurs with aging; whereas young adults show better memory for negatively valenced information, older adults show better memory for positive information (for review, see Mather and Carstensen 2005). It has been suggested that reduction in daily stress influences, such as during retirement, may contribute to reduction in negativity (Carstensen and Lockenhoff 2003). In addition, structural and metabolic changes in the regions responsible for emotional processing may contribute to better emotional stability with advancing age. The underlying neural mechanisms of improved emotional functioning in older age are an area that has only recently started to receive attention.

Emotional processing. Numerous studies of emotional processing in young adults suggest involvement of a network of regions, including the prefrontal cortex, amygdala, insula, basal ganglia, and anterior cingulate (for review, see Phan et al. 2002). Several studies have focused on age-related changes in functional activation during emotional tasks, typically contrasting negative versus neutral facial expressions or negative emotion-inducing stimuli versus neutral stimuli. The most common finding in older participants compared with younger participants is that responses in the visual cortices and amygdala are lesser to negative stimuli than to neutral stimuli, whereas responses in the frontal regions are greater to negative stimuli than to neutral stimuli. Interestingly, Wright et al. (2006) showed that amygdalar responses were preserved in older adults when novel fearful faces were compared with familiar neutral faces, suggesting that novelty and emotion activate the amygdala to the same level in older adults despite smaller amygdala volume. However, some researchers have also suggested that reduced responses to negative emotional stimuli in the amygdala may be explained by a shift in the type of information to which it is most responsive, which may be due to reduced bias toward negative stimuli and greater capacity for emotional control of negative information. In a study by Mather et al. (2004), responses in older adults were stronger for positive than for negative stimuli—a pattern that is reversed from the pattern of amygdalar response found in younger adults. In addition, differences in patterns of activation across age might be due to changes in emotional responsiveness. Older adults typically show reduced arousal ratings and physiological responses to emotional stimuli compared with younger adults (Tsai et al. 2000). When stimuli used were such that arousal ratings were similar across young and old age groups, observed age-related differences in amygdala activation were no longer present (Mather et al. 2004). Similarly, St. Jacques et al. (2008) found that the right amygdala was commonly engaged by both young and old adults when participants' own classifications of negative and neutral stimuli were used in the analyses.

Stress, well-being, and brain function. Individual differences in medial frontal and amygdala responses have also been found to be related to emotional stability, psychological well-being, and stress. It has been suggested that prefrontal regions play an important role in the regulation of emotion. Kern et al. (2008) reported that in healthy young adults, higher cortisol levels in response to psychosocial stress were associated with reduced glucose metabolism in the medial prefrontal regions, and response in the medial prefrontal regions correlated negatively with response in the amygdala during a stress-inducing task. This negative correlation between the medial prefrontal regions and amygdala response has also been observed in older adults during trials in which negative information was perceived as neutral (St. Jacques et al. 2008) and during regulation of negative affect (Urry et al. 2006). Individuals showing less activation in the amygdala and more activation in the ventromedial prefrontal cortex while they actively reduced their negative affect in response to negative pictures (pictures likely to induce negative reactions) also had a more normative decline in salivary cortisol levels over the course of the day, suggesting better emotional regulation and less perceived stress (Urry et al. 2006).

In a recent study, Williams and collaborators (2006) found that across a wide range of ages (12–79 years), a decreased level of neuroticism—that is, improved emotional stability—was predicted by lesser medial prefrontal cortex responses to happy facial expressions and greater responses to fearful facial expressions. In addition, medial prefrontal responses also predicted reduced ratings of perceived emotional intensity. Finally, another recent study (van Reekum et al. 2007), which focused on adults in their early sixties, reported that psychological well-being was associated with greater ventral anterior cingulate responses to negative pictures than to neutral pictures. Subjects with higher responses in the ventral anterior cingulate to negative pictures also had higher psychological well-being scores and evaluated negative stimuli more slowly. It has been suggested that the ventromedial prefrontal cortex might play a role in top-down regulation of the amygdala and fast recovery from negative stimuli (Williams et al. 2006). With increasing age, more control over negative emotion is exerted, and emotional well-being is improved.

Cognition and Plasticity

Given the evidence that the functional organization of the brain seems to change with age in ways that may or may not correlate positively with cognitive performance and emotional well-being, there has been some recent interest in directly examining short-term functional plasticity. By examining the response of neural systems to training, we can observe whether successful training leads to a pattern of brain response that is more youthful (less dedifferentiated) or whether it leads to even greater overactivation (is more compensatory) than is seen in untrained older adults. Thus, the results of training studies can inform the debate about the compensatory versus dedifferentiation hypotheses of overactivation in older persons. In the realm of cognitive training, there have been relatively few neuroimaging studies, but these studies have consistently observed brain changes that parallel beneficial effects on cognition in older adults.

In one study (Erickson et al. 2007), training (five 1-hour sessions over a 2- to 3-week period) on a dual visual choice reaction time task improved reaction times and accuracy on the task to a similar degree in old and young participants and, among the older adults, resulted in greater task-related activity in the left ventrolateral prefrontal cortex, less activity in the right ventrolateral prefrontal cortex, and less activity in the bilateral dorsolateral prefrontal cortex. Training-related change in activity in these regions was correlated with magnitude of behavioral improvement among older adults, and the change in response after training made the older adults' activation levels similar to the younger adults' posttraining levels. These results were interpreted as evidence in favor of training-related plasticity in the frontal cortex in older adults, and against the compensatory hypothesis of overactivation. Specifically, training led to brain patterns that were more like those of younger adults (including becoming more lateralized), which is inconsistent with the prediction of the compensatory hypothesis that improved performance should be associated with more bilateral and widespread activation. It should be noted, however, that the time scale of training studies (days or weeks) is very different from the time scale of most cross-sectional studies that have examined the issue of compensation (decades), so this might explain the conflicting interpretations.

In sum, there appears to be plasticity of brain function with acute training, which therefore leads to optimism that interventions can be designed to help maintain cognitive performance in the face of aging. What is not known, however, is how lasting these changes are, and how well they may generalize to other cognitive domains outside of those targeted for training (see Chapter 17, "Cognitive Training").

Emotion and Plasticity

Perhaps the most interesting research area that needs further exploration is whether emotion regulation training can induce plasticity in the aging brain. Could people be trained to be better at regulating their emotions, and would this training lead to more enduring changes in the patterns of brain activation? Initial findings showing differential effects on brain activity with various training programs aimed at improving emotional well-being are encouraging. Studies in depressed patients have shown that patients who underwent cognitive-behavioral therapy showed changes in regional brain metabolic activity comparable to those produced by medication (Kennedy et al. 2007). In addition, regular practitioners of Zen meditation show less age-related gray matter volume loss in the putamen (Pagnoni and Cekic 2007) than nonpractitioners. Finally, subjects who practiced mindfulness meditation for 8 weeks had larger increases in left-sided anterior frontal activation along with higher antibody titers to influenza compared with their counterparts in the control group (Davidson et al. 2003). Little is known, however, about whether such interventions would be helpful in older adults.

Conclusion: Limitations of Current Literature and Future Directions

One of the biggest limitations of the existing literature examining brain correlates of successful cognitive and emotional aging is that the majority of studies have been designed and powered primarily to investigate mean differences between young and old individuals. Because the relationship between cognitive or emotional performance and brain measures was not the focus of the studies, several features that would help us understand this relationship were often lacking. For example, a larger sample size in each group is needed for correlational analyses than for detection of mean differences between groups. In addition, adequate variability in each measure is helpful in order to observe important relationships. The older adults in many of the studies discussed in this chapter were very highly educated and the participants were therefore usually all performing quite well. The high education level of the participants in most brain imaging studies also raises the issue of representativeness of the samples and the subsequent generalizability of the results to the average elder. Another feature that is lacking from many of the studies is a direct comparison of the brain-behavior relationships in the younger and older subjects. If we are to learn anything about brain systems related to successful *aging* as opposed to just about those related to successful cognitive performance and emotional stability in general, we need to focus on those factors that are uniquely predictive of good cognitive and emotional functioning in older age.

Finally, most of the reviewed studies are cross-sectional in design, which raises the question of whether observed differences in the magnitude or direction of brain–behavior relationships between the younger and older groups may have to do with cohort or survival effects. Indeed, in the few longitudinal studies, results were more mixed than or less supportive of the fairly consistent results from cross-sectional studies. Only through further longitudinal studies can we hope to understand how some elders manage to maintain functioning with progressing years and then to develop effective interventions to help other seniors to maximize their cognitive and emotional health. In the area of successful emotional aging, there is a dearth of studies examining the relationship between emotional functioning and brain function in healthy older adults. Further research is needed to understand brain systems related to variability in emotional responses, as well as how neural processes related to cognition and emotion may interact to help maintain functioning and well-being in old age.

KEY POINTS

- Neuroimaging provides a sensitive way to explore individual differences in cognitive performance and emotional well-being among older adults.

- As a group, healthy older individuals have smaller volumes of gray matter structures, larger amounts of cerebrospinal fluid, greater abnormality of white matter connections, lower metabolic rates at rest, and both increased and decreased brain responses to cognitive and emotional challenge tasks compared with younger individuals. Similar, but more dramatic, changes with age are observed when the same person is studied across time.

■ Older adults who perform the best on cognitive tasks tend to have larger gray matter volumes, fewer white matter abnormalities, and more intact white matter connections.

■ Emotional well-being in old age may be associated with larger brain volumes in areas important for emotional regulation (perhaps mediated by a deleterious effect of stress on brain volume) and with fewer white matter abnormalities (which appear to play a role in late-life depression), but further studies of emotionally healthy seniors are needed.

■ Cognitive success in old age is associated with greater resting metabolism and, at least for some types of cognitive challenges, with more widespread brain responses, particularly in the prefrontal cortex. Further work is needed to determine when, how, and under what circumstances such compensatory responses develop.

■ Older individuals with the best emotional functioning may have more preserved prefrontal resting metabolism, and greater prefrontal and anterior cingulate responses and lesser amygdaloid responses to emotional stimuli.

■ In initial studies, interventions designed to improve cognition and emotional well-being seem to have short-term benefits and may positively alter brain physiology, but how lasting and general the gains may be among older adults has yet to be explored.

References

Abercrombie HC, Schaefer SM, Larson CL, et al: Metabolic rate in the right amygdala predicts negative affect in depressed patients. Neuroreport 9:3301–3307, 1998

Beason-Held LL, Kraut MA, Resnick SMI: Longitudinal changes in aging brain function. Neurobiol Aging 29:483–496, 2008

Bernard FA, Desgranges B, Eustache F, et al: Neural correlates of age-related verbal episodic memory decline: a PET study with combined subtraction/correlation analysis. Neurobiol Aging 28:1568–1576, 2007

Cabeza R: Hemispheric asymmetry reduction in older adults: the HAROLD model. Psychol Aging 17:85–100, 2002

Carstensen LL, Lockenhoff CE: Aging, emotion, and evolution: the bigger picture. Ann NY Acad Sci 1000:152–179, 2003

Colcombe SJ, Kramer AF, Erickson KI, et al: The implications of cortical recruitment and brain morphology for individual differences in inhibitory function in aging humans. Psychol Aging 20:363–375, 2005

Davidson RJ, Kabat-Zinn J, Schumacher J, et al: Alterations in brain and immune function produced by mindfulness meditation. Psychosom Med 65:564–570, 2003

Dennis NA, Cabeza R: Neuroimaging of healthy cognitive aging, in The Handbook of Aging and Cognition, 3rd Edition. Edited by Craik FIM, Salthouse TA. New York, Psychology Press, 2007, pp 1–54

Depp CA, Jeste DV: Definitions and predictors of successful aging: a comprehensive review of larger quantitative studies. Am J Geriatr Psychiatry 14:6–20, 2006

Erickson KI, Colcombe SJ, Wadhwa R, et al: Training-induced plasticity in older adults: effects of training on hemispheric asymmetry. Neurobiol Aging 28:272–283, 2007

Fjell AM, Walhovd KB, Reinvang I, et al: Selective increase of cortical thickness in high-performing elderly—structural indices of optimal cognitive aging. Neuroimage 29:984–994, 2006

Goldapple K, Segal Z, Garson C, et al: Modulation of cortical-limbic pathways in major depression: treatment-specific effects of cognitive behavior therapy. Arch Gen Psychiatry 61:34–41, 2004

Grady CL, Bernstein LJ, Beig S, et al: The effects of encoding task on age-related differences in the functional neuroanatomy of face memory. Psychol Aging 17:7–23, 2002

Gunning-Dixon FM, Raz N: The cognitive correlates of white matter abnormalities in normal aging: a quantitative review. Neuropsychology 14:224–232, 2000

Holthoff VA, Beuthien-Baumann B, Kalbe E, et al: Regional cerebral metabolism in early Alzheimer's disease with clinically significant apathy or depression. Biol Psychiatry 57:412–421, 2005

Iidaka T, Okada T, Murata T, et al: Age-related differences in the medial temporal lobe responses to emotional faces as revealed by fMRI. Hippocampus 12:352–362, 2002

Jernigan TL, Gamst AC: Changes in volume with age—consistency and interpretation of observed effects. Neurobiol Aging 26:1271–1274; discussion 1275–1278, 2005

Kalpouzos G, Chételat G, Baron JC, et al: Voxel-based mapping of brain gray matter volume and glucose metabolism profiles in normal aging. Neurobiol Aging 30:112–124, 2009

Kennedy SH, Konarski JZ, Segal ZV, et al: Differences in brain glucose metabolism between responders to CBT and venlafaxine in a 16-week randomized controlled trial. Am J Psychiatry 164:778–788, 2007

Kern S, Oakes TR, Stone CK, et al: Glucose metabolic changes in the prefrontal cortex are associated with HPA axis response to a psychosocial stressor. Psychoneuroendocrinology 33:517–529, 2008

Langenecker SA, Briceno EM, Hamid NM, et al: An evaluation of distinct volumetric and functional MRI contributions toward understanding age and task performance: a study in the basal ganglia. Brain Res 1135:58–68, 2007

Lupien SJ, de Leon M, de Santi S, et al: Cortisol levels during human aging predict hippocampal atrophy and memory deficits. Nat Neurosci 1:69–73, 1998

Lustig C, Buckner RL: Preserved neural correlates of priming in old age and dementia. Neuron 42:865–875, 2004

Malloy P, Correia S, Stebbins G, et al: Neuroimaging of white matter in aging and dementia. Clin Neuropsychol 21:73–109, 2007

Mather M, Carstensen LL: Aging and motivated cognition: the positivity effect in attention and memory. Trends Cogn Sci 9:496–502, 2005

Mather M, Canli T, English T, et al: Amygdala responses to emotionally valenced stimuli in older and younger adults. Psychol Sci 15:259–263, 2004

Mayberg HS, Liotti M, Brannan SK, et al: Reciprocal limbic-cortical function and negative mood: converging PET findings in depression and normal sadness. Am J Psychiatry 156:675–682, 1999

McEwen BS: Glucocorticoids, depression, and mood disorders: structural remodeling in the brain. Metabolism 54 (suppl 1):20–23, 2005

Meltzer CC, Becker JT, Price JC, et al: Positron emission tomography imaging of the aging brain. Neuroimaging Clin N Am 13:759–767, 2003

Nielson KA, Langenecker SA, Garavan H: Differences in the functional neuroanatomy of inhibitory control across the adult life span. Psychol Aging 17:56–71, 2002

O'Brien JT, Firbank MJ, Krishnan MS, et al: White matter hyperintensities rather than lacunar infarcts are associated with depressive symptoms in older people: the LADIS study. Am J Geriatr Psychiatry 14:834–841, 2006

Pagnoni G, Cekic M: Age effects on gray matter volume and attentional performance in Zen meditation. Neurobiol Aging 28:1623–1627, 2007

Persson J, Nyberg L: Altered brain activity in healthy seniors: what does it mean? Prog Brain Res 157:45–56, 2006

Persson J, Nyberg L, Lind J, et al: Structure-function correlates of cognitive decline in aging. Cereb Cortex 16:907–915, 2006

Phan KL, Wager T, Taylor SF, et al: Functional neuroanatomy of emotion: a meta-analysis of emotion activation studies in PET and fMRI. Neuroimage 16:331–348, 2002

Rajah MN, D'Esposito M: Region-specific changes in prefrontal function with age: a review of PET and fMRI studies on working and episodic memory. Brain 128:1964–1983, 2005

Raz N, Rodrigue KM: Differential aging of the brain: patterns, cognitive correlates and modifiers. Neurosci Biobehav Rev 30:730–748, 2006

Reichstadt J, Depp CA, Palinkas LA, et al: Building blocks of successful aging: a focus group study of older adults' perceived contributors to successful aging. Am J Geriatr Psychiatry 15:194–201, 2007

Rypma B, Berger JS, Genova HM, et al: Dissociating age-related changes in cognitive strategy and neural efficiency using event-related fMRI. Cortex 41:582–594, 2005

Stern Y, Habeck C, Moeller J, et al: Brain networks associated with cognitive reserve in healthy young and old adults. Cereb Cortex 15:394–402, 2005

St Jacques P, Dolcos F, Cabeza R: Effects of aging on functional connectivity of the amygdala during negative evaluation: a network analysis of fMRI data. Neurobiol Aging May 2, 2008 (Epub ahead of print)

Sullivan EV, Pfefferbaum A: Diffusion tensor imaging and aging. Neurosci Biobehav Rev 30:749–761, 2006

Teodorczuk A, O'Brien JT, Firbank MJ, et al: White matter changes and late-life depressive symptoms: longitudinal study. Br J Psychiatry 191:212–217, 2007

Tsai JL, Levenson RW, Carstensen LL: Autonomic, subjective, and expressive responses to emotional films in older and younger Chinese Americans and European Americans. Psychol Aging 15:684–693, 2000

Urry HL, van Reekum CM, Johnstone T, et al: Amygdala and ventromedial prefrontal cortex are inversely coupled during regulation of negative affect and predict the diurnal pattern of cortisol secretion among older adults. J Neurosci 26:4415–4425, 2006

van der Veen FM, Nijhuis FA, Tisserand DJ, et al: Effects of aging on recognition of intentionally and incidentally stored words: an fMRI study. Neuropsychologia 44:2477–2486, 2006

van Reekum CM, Urry HL, Johnstone T, et al: Individual differences in amygdala and ventromedial prefrontal cortex activity are associated with evaluation speed and psychological well-being. J Cogn Neurosci 19:237–248, 2007

Williams LM, Brown KJ, Palmer D, et al: The mellow years? Neural basis of improving emotional stability over age. J Neurosci 26:6422–6430, 2006

Wilson RS, Beckett LA, Barnes LL, et al: Individual differences in rates of change in cognitive abilities of older persons. Psychol Aging 17:179–193, 2002

Wright CI, Wedig MM, Williams D, et al: Novel fearful faces activate the amygdala in healthy young and elderly adults. Neurobiol Aging 27:361–374, 2006

Recommended Readings

Cabeza R: Hemispheric asymmetry reduction in older adults: the HAROLD model. Psychol Aging 17:85–100, 2002

Raz N, Rodrigue KM: Differential aging of the brain: patterns, cognitive correlates and modifiers. Neurosci Biobehav Rev 30:730–748, 2006

Williams LM, Brown KJ, Palmer D, et al: The mellow years? Neural basis of improving emotional stability over age. J Neurosci 26:6422–6430, 2006

9

Cognitive and Brain Reserve

Adam M. Brickman, Ph.D.
Karen L. Siedlecki, Ph.D.
Yaakov Stern, Ph.D.

In the quest to determine exactly how the brain produces behavior, few consistent observations have emerged. Among the most perplexing problems is the apparent disconnection between pathological changes that occur in the brain and their clinical manifestations. Why, for example, might two people with a stroke of similar size and location have very different degrees of associated cognitive impairment? Why does mild head trauma result in a great amount of cognitive impairment in one person, but severe head trauma result in little cognitive impairment in another? This disconnection is perhaps most evident in studies of Alzheimer disease, which have shown that about one-quarter of individuals who have the hallmark neuropathology for Alzheimer disease at autopsy did not have the characteristic cognitive impairment during life (Ince 2001).

The concept of *reserve* has been proposed to help account for the discrepancy between amount of brain damage—due to measurable pathology—and the expression of that damage. In our conceptualization, reserve takes two forms: *brain reserve* and *cognitive reserve*. Although these two concepts are often conflated and the terms used interchangeably (e.g., Ropacki and Elias 2003), they refer to distinct, albeit related, mechanistic constructs. Individual differences in both brain reserve and cognitive reserve can account for the apparent disconnection between brain damage and the symptoms it produces. In this chapter, focusing on aging and dementia as an example, we explore the concept of reserve and discuss evidence of its existence, its neural implementation, and potential treatment targets.

Brain Reserve

An intuitive explanation for why the same degree of brain damage can cause varying severities of cognitive symptoms across individuals is that some people can afford to sustain greater insults to the brain than others. This idea was codified by Satz in 1993 with his idea of brain reserve or *brain reserve capacity*. Brain reserve is a *threshold model* of individual differences in clinical expression of brain pathology. That is, only once a critical threshold of brain damage is sustained do the clinical symptoms associated with that damage emerge. Although brain reserve itself is not a measurable variable, it can be operationalized as brain size, neural density, or amount of synaptic connectivity. Increases in any one of these factors can increase the amount of brain reserve.

Brain reserve provides a testable framework, and there are many positive examples of its existence in the literature. One of the most widely cited studies on the topic comes from Katzman and colleagues (1989), who described 10 cases of cognitively normal elderly women discovered to have advanced Alzheimer disease pathology in their brains at autopsy. These individuals were also noted to have greater brain volume than average, which the authors speculated was the reason for their lack of symptoms during life. In terms of the brain reserve theory, these women may have had greater amounts of brain tissue or neurons than others with similar amounts of Alzheimer disease pathology and required greater amounts of Alzheimer disease–related damage before reaching the critical threshold required for cognitive impairment.

Quantifying Brain Reserve

Brain reserve can be estimated through the calculation of brain volume or head size. In the context of aging, head size provides an estimate of premorbid brain volume. That is, the brain at its healthiest, most mature point is restricted to the size of the cranial vault, which does not shrink with aging. Reliable measurements of the head or cranial vault thus represent the largest size the brain has ever been, and degree of brain atrophy can be estimated cross-sectionally by taking the ratio of brain volume to cranial size. Research emerging from our center's community-based longitudinal studies of aging and dementia has shown that those with the smallest head circumference are most likely to have Alzheimer disease, even after several relevant variables were controlled for (Schofield et al. 1997). Another population-based study (Graves et al. 1996) showed a similar effect: individuals with Alzheimer disease had smaller cranial volumes than their counterparts without dementia.

Stern (2002) conceptualized brain reserve as a *passive model* of reserve. That is, the theoretical threshold for impairment is fixed and clinical symptoms emerge only after enough brain damage (or pathology) has accumu-

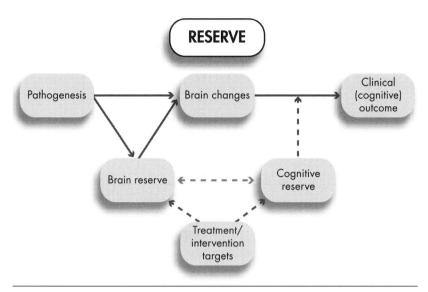

FIGURE 9–1. Schematic representation of the reserve hypothesis.

lated. Unlike cognitive reserve, discussed below, no active compensation occurs. Conceptualized in a slightly different manner, brain reserve can be thought of as a mediator between some pathogenic process and the amount of brain changes that result from that process (Figure 9–1). The degree (or percentage) of brain changes associated with pathology depends on how much brain reserve is available.

Correlates of Brain Reserve

What accounts for individual differences in brain reserve? Because brain reserve is considered to be "hardwired," factors that contribute to the development of the brain's structural integrity may be most important. These factors may include genetic contributions, nutritional quality, and access to health care during early childhood. Furthermore, there is evidence that attainment of formal education may increase brain reserve through the growth of synapses (Katzman 1993) or through increased dendritic branching (Jacobs et al. 1993). Using diffusion tensor magnetic resonance imaging, recent work by McCandliss and colleagues, which demonstrated region-specific positive relationships between reading ability and white matter tract integrity in children, is consistent with this idea (Niogi and McCandliss 2006; for a review, see Schlaggar and McCandliss 2007).

Despite its passive nature and the clear importance of developmental factors in its establishment, brain reserve can be modified through environmental manipulation throughout the life span. For example, there is emerging evidence that aerobic fitness or engagement in aerobic activity is associated with better cognitive functioning (Hillman et al. 2008). perhaps due to the direct effect of aerobic activity on the integrity of the brain (see below). Among children, increased levels of aerobic fitness and amount of physical activity are associated with better academic achievement (Castelli et al. 2007), including better mathematics, reading, and better academic grades (California Department of Education 2001). Beneficial effects of exercise on memory, processing speed, and reasoning have also been noted among young adults following sustained regimens (Young 1979), and on executive control processes after acute exercise (Hillman et al. 2008), although little work in the latter area has been done among young adults specifically. In recent years, there has been much more research addressing the effects of aerobic exercise on cognition during older adulthood. Correlational data from epidemiological studies show that engagement in physical activities maintains cognitive function in later life and may have protective effects against dementia (Wilson et al. 2002). Intervention trials, in which sedentary older adults are randomized to engage in varying levels of aerobic exercise, have shown increased executive abilities, motor function, and auditory attention and delayed memory function associated with aerobic exercise (Colcombe and Kramer 2003).

Effects of Interventions on Brain Reserve

Intervention and epidemiological studies suggest that aerobic exercise may have beneficial effects on cognition, but are these effects due to increases in or development of brain reserve? Evidence from both human and nonhuman studies suggests that exercise directly enhances the physical and functional integrity of the brain through increased perfusion or vascularization, through increases in levels of brain-derived neurotrophic factors (Cotman and Berchtold 2002), and/or through modification of catecholaminergic or monoaminergic neurotransmitters (Blomstrand et al. 1989). Further, a recent structural neuroimaging study showed that older adults who were randomly assigned to engage in aerobic exercise had significantly larger gray and white matter volumes following the trial (Colcombe et al. 2006). Aerobic exercise may increase angiogenesis and synaptogenesis, particularly in regions critical for the maintenance of memory function throughout the life span (Pereira et al. 2007).

It is unclear whether mental stimulation, through engagement in paper-and-pencil tasks or computerized gaming software, boosts brain reserve and has a beneficial effect on cognition. There has been a commercial explosion of *cognitive calisthenics* technology that has been marketed directly to con-

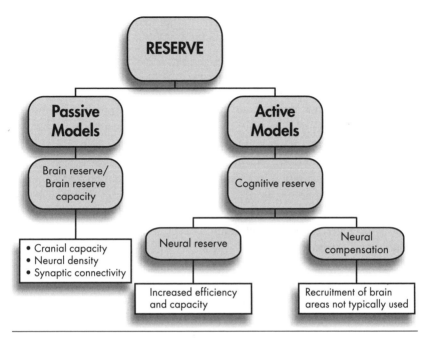

FIGURE 9–2. Schematic representation of passive and active models of reserve.

sumers, but sufficient empirical testing is lacking (Mahncke et al. 2006). Given the profound public interest and theoretical potential for efficacy, well-designed nonpharmacological interventions for boosting cognition or modifying age-associated cognitive decline are clearly warranted. Furthermore, identification of the mechanisms through which these interventions may operate is critical for development of the most effective strategies. Similar to aerobic exercise interventions, cognitive stimulation paradigms may work directly on brain reserve, increasing structural plasticity or synaptogenesis. Or, alternatively, they may benefit cognitive aging through a more active process of enhancing compensatory strategies and mental flexibility, as in the case of cognitive reserve.

Cognitive Reserve

Unlike brain reserve, *cognitive reserve* is considered an *active model* (Stern 2002) (Figure 9–2). The cognitive reserve concept is grounded in the repeated observation that individuals with higher intelligence and greater educational or occupational attainment are able to sustain more brain damage before demonstrating a cognitive or functional deficit. This idea is theoretically different than that of brain reserve. Rather than postulating that those with greater reserve have a fundamentally distinct anatomy that can sustain more brain damage, the cognitive reserve hypothesis posits that they are able to cope better with existing brain damage. In other words, cognitive reserve does not protect the brain against a pathological process (e.g., Alzheimer disease), but rather it moderates the association between pathology and the expression of that pathology (see Figure 9–1)—the clinical/cognitive result of brain pathology varies as a function of the level of cognitive reserve.

In a further explication of the hypothesis, Stern et al. (2005) suggested that the neural implementation of cognitive reserve can take two forms: neural reserve and neural compensation. *Neural reserve* refers to the *efficiency* or *capacity* of existing brain systems that is in place prior to the onset of any brain pathology and is relatively impermeable to disruption. On the other hand, *neural compensation* refers to the ability to utilize alternative brain systems (and thus cognitive strategies) in the face of pathology to offset the demands normally placed on the faulty areas. One way to conceptualize the difference between neural reserve and neural compensation is to consider that *neural reserve* may refer to use of the same or additional networks in response to task demand, whereas *neural compensation* refers to the use of additional networks that are not typically used in response to pathological changes. As opposed to the brain reserve model, which assumes that there is a critical threshold for clinical expression, the cognitive reserve model depends on the efficiency and compensation strategies employed at the neural level.

Defining Cognitive Reserve

Operational definitions for cognitive reserve usually include variables that reflect some cumulative lifetime experiences, such as occupational attainment, or the amount of time engaged in cognitively stimulating activities. The number of years of formal education is often used as a proxy measure for cognitive reserve, most likely because it is a relatively uniform metric and it is easy information to obtain through historical interview. Years of education, as a variable, however, may not be ideal. Educational experiences might vary from person to person, by region, or by socioeconomic status. Manly and colleagues (2005) proposed that literacy measures or reading ability may be a "purer" reflection of the quality of education, thereby providing a more valid measure of reserve. Reading ability or literacy level may more accurately reflect the quality of education and better reflect the actual educational experience. Estimates of current or premorbid IQ have also been proposed as proxy measures for cognitive reserve (Alexander et al. 1997). Such estimates may reflect innate or genetically determined abilities but do not necessarily capture other cumulative life experiences that may impart cognitive reserve.

Cognitive reserve may best be defined or estimated by some sort of summary measure of several differing experiences and abilities. For example, higher education, occupational attainment, and engagement in cognitively stimulating leisure activities may independently or synergistically contribute to cognitive reserve (Richards and Sacker 2003; Stern et al. 1994, 1995). Recent work in our laboratory that examined the relations among variables hypothesized to reflect cognitive reserve indicates that the variables (i.e., education level, vocabulary, National Adult Reading Test results) may represent a distinct dimension of individual differences. That is, the variables hypothesized to represent a latent cognitive reserve construct are significantly, and highly, correlated with one another (Siedlecki et al., in press). Furthermore, the cognitive reserve construct is generally distinct from constructs of other cognitive abilities, with the notable exception of executive functioning. Executive functioning tasks characteristically capture the ability to engage in flexible strategies to solve novel problems (Siedlecki et al., in press). Likewise, cognitive reserve is hypothesized to reflect the cumulative effect of life experiences that may provide individuals with the ability to use compensatory (or flexible) strategies to better manage the effects of brain pathology. It is therefore unsurprising that the construct of cognitive reserve would be highly related to that of executive functioning.

It is important to note that the variables used to estimate cognitive reserve are both proxies for reserve and reflections of experiences that, themselves, may furnish additional reserve. For example, the amount or quality of formal education an individual has pursued is both a reflection of and a contributor to reserve. Ultimately, the theory of cognitive reserve is concerned with a certain flexibility the brain may have in the face of dysfunction or pathology. Furthermore, variables that are proxies for cognitive reserve may also relate directly to brain reserve. This possibility most likely reflects how the two constructs interact. For example, having high levels of education may reflect high cognitive reserve. But those with high education are also more likely to have had better nutritional exposure, better access to health care, and better overall development—all factors that may contribute to brain reserve—than those with lower levels of education.

Correlates of Cognitive Reserve

In the context of aging and dementia, several predictions can be made that would support the cognitive reserve hypothesis. Individuals with Alzheimer disease pathology who have high levels of cognitive reserve may not evidence the syndrome of dementia until later than individuals with Alzheimer disease pathology and low levels of cognitive reserve. Indeed, several international and community-based epidemiological studies suggest a lower incidence of dementia among those with higher reserve. The observation that more highly educated participants have a lower incidence of dementia has been made in at least seven cohorts in France (Letenneur et al. 1994), Sweden (Qiu et al. 2001), Finland (Anttila et al. 2002), China (Zhang et al. 1990), and the United States (Evans et al. 1997; Stern et al. 1994; White et al. 1994) and in a pooled analysis of four European prospective studies of older adults (Launer et al. 1999).

Similar relationships have been observed with other proxies of cognitive reserve. For example, a reduced risk for developing dementia was found among older adults who engaged in more social and leisure activities, such as doing odd jobs, knitting, traveling, and gardening (Fabrigoule et al. 1995). In work in our laboratory (Scarmeas et al. 2001), monthly engagement in leisure activities was quantified on a 13-point scale among 1,772 community-dwelling individuals. Those who engaged in more leisure activities were up to 38% less likely to have developed Alzheimer disease on follow-up than those who engaged in fewer leisure activities. The finding of an association between greater amounts of engagement in leisure activities, particularly those that are cognitive in nature, and a lower incidence of dementia has now been replicated in other longitudinal studies (Wilson et al. 2002).

In studies that have examined the impact of cognitive reserve among patients with prevalent dementia, the findings have been, on first consideration, counterintuitive, with many showing that higher cognitive reserve is associated with a *faster* rate of cognitive decline (Scarmeas et al. 2006; Stern et al. 1999). Further, Alzheimer disease patients with higher cognitive reserve, estimated by education level or occupational attainment, died sooner than those with lower estimates of cognitive reserve (Stern et al. 1995). Findings such as these are actually consistent with the cognitive reserve hypothesis, which, again, stipulates that reserve moderates the association between brain pathology and expression of that pathology. Thus, for any given level of cognitive or clinical function (i.e., the expression of brain pathology), those with higher cognitive reserve should have greater amounts of brain pathology than those with lower levels of reserve.

In Alzheimer disease, the clinical disease may emerge when the pathology is more severe among those with higher cognitive reserve; at some point Alzheimer disease pathology becomes too severe to support the brain processes that allow the flexibility to compensate for that pathology. The cognitive reserve hypothesis argues that this point should arrive at an earlier stage of clinical severity in patients with higher cognitive reserve because their underlying Alzheimer disease pathology is more severe than in those with lower reserve.

In contrast, in the absence of significant brain pathology, which ultimately ravages the brain of most cognitive abilities, individuals with higher cognitive reserve have been found to have a slower rate of normal age-related cognitive decline than those with lower reserve. However, this finding has been generally observed only across fairly short time intervals of 1 year (Farmer et al. 1995) or 2½ years (Albert et al. 1995), using nonspecific measures of cognition such as the Mini-Mental State Examination or a composite score on a set of neuropsychological variables. Studies that have examined differences across specific cognitive variables suggest that reserve may only be protective against normal age-related differences in more knowledge-based measures like language (Christensen et al. 1997) or vocabulary (e.g., Salthouse 2006).

Neuroimaging and Cognitive Reserve

There has been particular interest in the examination of cognitive reserve using functional neuroimaging approaches. Neuroimaging approaches make it possible to address two critical issues around the cognitive reserve hypothesis:

1. *Neuroimaging may provide a more direct measurement of brain pathology than other clinical signs or symptoms.* When testing whether the cognitive reserve hypothesis is operative, it is essential to have a reliable estimate of three components for each individual: 1) the amount of cognitive reserve, 2) an estimate of the severity of brain pathology, and 3) a measurement reflecting clinical expression of that pathology. When one of these factors is held constant (e.g., statistically or through subject matching), the relationship between the other two can be tested. For example, the cognitive reserve hypothesis would predict that higher cognitive reserve would be associated with greater amounts of brain pathology when the clinical outcome is held constant. Using the amount of regional cerebral blood flow as an estimate of Alzheimer disease pathology, early neuroimaging work from our laboratory was consistent with this hypothesis. That is, among Alzheimer disease patients matched for overall severity of dementia, parietal-temporal blood flow deficits were greater in those with more years of education (Stern et al. 1992). This finding was replicated in a positron emission tomography study (Alexander et al. 1997), in which higher education was related to a reduction in cerebral metabolism in the prefrontal cortex, premotor areas, and superior parietal association areas after clinical dementia severity was controlled for, and again with occupational attainment (Stern et al. 1995) and leisure activities (Scarmeas et al. 2003) as estimates of cognitive reserve. Definitive confirmation of this association came from Bennett and colleagues (2003),

who showed that higher levels of education were associated with better cognitive function at the same degree of Alzheimer disease brain pathology, measured in postmortem tissue.

2. *Functional activation studies can be used to understand the neural instantiation of cognitive reserve by testing neural reserve and neural compensation hypotheses.* A relatively consistent observation from the functional neuroimaging literature is that functional activation increases in response to increasing cognitive task demand (Rypma et al. 1999). Individuals with greater skill tend to recruit additional brain resources less, suggesting greater efficiency. Work from our laboratory showed differential relationships between an estimated measure of IQ and regional brain activity as a cognitive stimulation task varied from a low demand to a high demand condition (Stern et al. 2003).

Compared with normally aging control subjects, patients with Alzheimer disease evidence greater degrees of more widely distributed brain activation during increasingly difficult cognitive tasks (Becker et al. 1996), suggesting that the brain is attempting to compensate for pathological changes. This pattern is also seen in studies of normal aging, in which more brain areas are activated during a cognitive task among older adults compared with younger adults (Cabeza et al. 2002). Regardless of whether recruitment of additional brain areas to perform the same cognitive task results in better performance, the phenomenon may still be considered compensatory because it varies as a function of the presence of pathology (e.g., Alzheimer disease) or aging. A *dedifferentiation* hypothesis has also been proposed to help account for increased brain activation in aging and dementia (Zarahn et al. 2007). Briefly, this explanation specifies that additional brain region activation may reflect an age-associated difficulty in selecting the appropriate, specific neural mechanism to successfully complete a task.

Many studies that have shown differential brain activation across groups of different clinical status or age did not address the problem of task difficulty. That is, the same cognitive task may be more difficult for individuals with Alzheimer disease than for control subjects, and it may be the increased demands of the task that account for greater activation. To address this issue, Stern and colleagues (2000) used a verbal recognition task and controlled for task difficulty by titrating the study list size so that the accuracy level was 75% for both patients and control subjects. Thus, the absolute study list size varied across individuals, but the overall accuracy (or estimated difficulty level) remained constant. In the healthy control subjects, brain areas, including the anterior cingulate, insula, and basal ganglia, were activated during the task. Greater study list size was associated with greater activation of these regions. Only 3 of the 14 Alzheimer disease patients expressed this pattern in a similar manner. Stern and colleagues interpreted this observation as an indication of neural reserve, because the recruitment of the network seemed to be in response to increasing task difficulty. On the other hand, the majority of the Alzheimer disease patients utilized a different brain pattern, including patterns involving the posterior temporal cortex, calcarine cortex, posterior cingulate, and vermis, during performance of the task. This differential network activation could indicate neural compensation (i.e., in response to Alzheimer disease pathology) whereby patients used brain networks that were not used by individuals without dementia to perform the task.

Effects of Interventions on Cognitive Reserve

As with physical exercise and brain reserve, the idea that mental exercise, or cognitive stimulation, may improve cognition and stave off dementia by boosting cognitive reserve has generated a lot of commercial excitement. Although the fundamental idea is compelling and a number of products are currently available, evidence for the "use it or lose it" idea is far from definitive. Correlational and epidemiological studies certainly support the idea that a greater amount of cumulative lifetime experiences, particularly those that are cognitively stimulating (e.g., leisure activities, education), is associated with a lower incidence of dementia and perhaps a slower rate of age-associated cognitive decline, but how these observations translate into a prescribed intervention has yet to be determined. In fact, the results of cognitive intervention trials are mixed. The Advanced Cognitive Training for Independent and Vital Elderly (ACTIVE) study, in which a national sample of 2,802 older adults were randomly assigned to receive memory training, processing speed training, reasoning training, or no training (i.e., the no-contact control group) over ten 60- to 75-minute training sessions, reported domain-specific improvements in cognitive function. Specifically, 26% of the participants who received memory training improved their memory scores; 74% of those who received processing speed training improved their processing speed scores; and 87% of those who received reasoning training improved their reasoning scores (Ball et al. 2002). These domain-specific training effects were durable and continued through 5 years of follow-up (Willis et al. 2006). However, the improvements did not transfer to other domains (e.g., receiving training in processing speed did not also confer improvements in reasoning scores), nor were they associated with improvements in the participants' ability to perform everyday tasks such as preparing food, driving, or handling their medications (Ball et al. 2002).

Although the results of the ACTIVE study are encouraging in many ways (in the form of domain-specific improvements that are durable over the course of 5 years), the evidence for the applicability to, and impact on, real-world functioning is less persuasive. There is evidence that the reasoning training group was afforded some protection against self-reported functional declines in instrumental activities of daily living at 5-year follow-up, compared with the no-contact control group (Willis et al. 2006). However, the lack of a significant general improvement in all domains of cognition suggests that the key to promoting cognitive flexibility may lie elsewhere. For example, it may be that training that promotes the use of flexible strategies for solving novel problems may confer the most benefits for cognition and function.

Conclusion

Research on the impact of aging on the brain and on cognition has led us to question why some individuals show preservation of function despite having evidence of structural changes. We have described two models, one passive (brain reserve) and the other active (cognitive reserve), portraying how cognitive aging can be preserved in later life. In this conceptualization, brain reserve mediates the association between a pathogenic process and its impact on the brain directly, such that the amount of brain damage that is sustained varies as a function of reserve. On the other hand, cognitive reserve moderates the association between brain pathology and the clinical expression of that pathology. Increased cognitive reserve does not prevent brain damage; rather, it modifies the degree to which brain damage is expressed clinically. Brain reserve and cognitive reserve may interact (e.g., the influence of nutritional factors on brain reserve during early life), and this may also predict the amount of education one receives. Both brain reserve and cognitive reserve are reasonable therapeutic targets for disease-related and age-related changes in cognition.

KEY POINTS

- The concept of *reserve* has been proposed to help account for the discrepancy between amount of brain damage—due to measurable pathology—and expression of that damage.

- Brain reserve is a passive model of reserve. That is, the theoretical threshold for impairment is fixed and clinical symptoms emerge only after enough brain damage (or pathology) has accumulated.

- Cognitive reserve is an active model of reserve. Cognitive reserve does not protect the brain against a pathological process (e.g., Alzheimer disease); rather, it moderates the association between pathology and the expression of that pathology.

▌ It may be possible to increase brain reserve; evidence from both human and nonhuman studies suggests that exercise directly enhances the physical and functional integrity of the brain.

▌ Cognitive reserve seems to be related to greater educational attainment and lifetime exposure to cognitively demanding activities. "Brain training" interventions to enhance flexibility offer promise in enhancing cognitive reserve, but more research needs to be done to enable them to have a lasting impact on individuals in their everyday performance.

References

Albert MS, Jones K, Savage CR, et al: Predictors of cognitive change in older persons: MacArthur studies of successful aging. Psychol Aging 10:578–589, 1995

Alexander GE, Furey ML, Grady CL, et al: Association of premorbid intellectual function with cerebral metabolism in Alzheimer's disease: implications for the cognitive reserve hypothesis. Am J Psychiatry 154:165–172, 1997

Anttila T, Helkala EL, Kivipelto M, et al: Midlife income, occupation, APOE status, and dementia: a population-based study. Neurology 59:887–893, 2002

Ball K, Berch DB, Helmers KF, et al: Effects of cognitive training interventions with older adults: a randomized controlled trial. JAMA 288:2271–2281, 2002

Becker JT, Mintun MA, Aleva K, et al: Compensatory reallocation of brain resources supporting verbal episodic memory in Alzheimer's disease. Neurology 46:692–700, 1996

Bennett DA, Wilson RS, Schneider JA, et al: Education modifies the relation of AD pathology to level of cognitive function in older persons. Neurology 60:1909–1915, 2003

Blomstrand E, Perrett D, Parry-Billings M, et al: Effect of sustained exercise on plasma amino acid concentrations and on 5-hydroxytryptamine metabolism in six different brain regions in the rat. Acta Physiol Scand 136:473–481, 1989

Cabeza R, Anderson ND, Locantore JK, et al: Aging gracefully: compensatory brain activity in high-performing older adults. Neuroimage 17:1394–1402, 2002

California Department of Education: California physical fitness test: report to the governor and legislature. Sacramento, CA, California Department of Education Standards and Assessment Division, 2001

Castelli DM, Hillman CH, Buck SM, et al: Physical fitness and academic achievement in third- and fifth-grade students. J Sport Exerc Psychol 29:239–252, 2007

Christensen H, Korten AE, Jorm AF, et al: Education and decline in cognitive performance: compensatory but not protective. Int J Geriatr Psychiatry 12:323–330, 1997

Colcombe S, Kramer AF: Fitness effects on the cognitive function of older adults: a meta-analytic study. Psychol Sci 14:125–130, 2003

Colcombe SJ, Erickson KI, Scalf PE, et al: Aerobic exercise training increases brain volume in aging humans. J Gerontol A Biol Sci Med Sci 61:1166–1170, 2006

Cotman CW, Berchtold NC: Exercise: a behavioral intervention to enhance brain health and plasticity. Trends Neurosci 25:295–301, 2002

Evans DA, Hebert LE, Beckett LA, et al: Education and other measures of socioeconomic status and risk of incident Alzheimer disease in a defined population of older persons. Arch Neurol 54:1399–1405, 1997

Fabrigoule C, Letenneur L, Dartigues JF, et al: Social and leisure activities and risk of dementia: a prospective longitudinal study. J Am Geriatr Soc 43:485–490, 1995

Farmer ME, Kittner SJ, Rae DS, et al: Education and change in cognitive function: the Epidemiologic Catchment Area Study. Ann Epidemiol 5:1–7, 1995

Graves AB, Mortimer JA, Larson EB, et al: Head circumference as a measure of cognitive reserve: association with severity of impairment in Alzheimer's disease. Br J Psychiatry 169:86–92, 1996

Hillman CH, Erickson KI, Kramer AF: Be smart, exercise your heart: exercise effects on brain and cognition. Nat Rev Neurosci 9:58–65, 2008

Ince P: Pathological correlates of late-onset dementia in a multicenter community-based population in England and Wales. Lancet 357:169–175, 2001

Jacobs B, Schall M, Scheibel AB: A quantitative dendritic analysis of Wernicke's area in humans, II: gender, hemispheric, and environmental factors. J Comp Neurol 327:97–111, 1993

Katzman R: Education and the prevalence of dementia and Alzheimer's disease. Neurology 43:13–20, 1993

Katzman R, Aronson M, Fuld P, et al: Development of dementing illnesses in an 80-year-old volunteer cohort. Ann Neurol 25:317–324, 1989

Launer LJ, Andersen K, Dewey ME, et al: Rates and risk factors for dementia and Alzheimer's disease: results from EURODEM pooled analyses. EURODEM Incidence Research Group and Work Groups: European Studies of Dementia. Neurology 52:78–84, 1999

Letenneur L, Commenges D, Dartigues JF, et al: Incidence of dementia and Alzheimer's disease in elderly community residents of south-western France. Int J Epidemiol 23:1256–1261, 1994

Mahncke HW, Connor BB, Appelman J, et al: Memory enhancement in healthy older adults using a brain plasticity–based training program: a randomized, controlled study. Proc Natl Acad Sci USA 103:12523–12528, 2006

Manly JJ, Schupf N, Tang MX, et al: Cognitive decline and literacy among ethnically diverse elders. J Geriatr Psychiatry Neurol 18:213–217, 2005

Niogi SN, McCandliss BD: Left lateralized white matter microstructure accounts for individual differences in reading ability and disability. Neuropsychologia 44:2178–2188, 2006

Pereira AC, Huddleston DE, Brickman AM, et al: An in vivo correlate of exercise-induced neurogenesis in the adult dentate gyrus. Proc Natl Acad Sci USA 104:5638–5643, 2007

Qiu C, Bäckman L, Winblad B, et al: The influence of education on clinically diagnosed dementia incidence and mortality data from the Kungsholmen Project. Arch Neurol 58:2034–2039, 2001

Richards M, Sacker A: Lifetime antecedents of cognitive reserve. J Clin Exp Neuropsychol 25:614–624, 2003

Ropacki MT, Elias JW: Preliminary examination of cognitive reserve theory in closed head injury. Arch Clin Neuropsychol 18:643–654, 2003

Rypma B, Prabhakaran V, Desmond J, et al: Load-dependent roles of frontal brain regions in the maintenance of working memory. Neuroimage 9:216–226, 1999

Salthouse TA: Mental exercise and mental aging. Perspect Psychol Sci 1:68–87, 2006

Satz P: Brain reserve capacity on symptom onset after brain injury: a formulation and review of evidence for threshold theory. Neuropsychology 7:273–295, 1993

Scarmeas N, Levy G, Tang MX, et al: Influence of leisure activity on the incidence of Alzheimer's disease. Neurology 57:2236–2242, 2001

Scarmeas N, Zarahn E, Anderson KE, et al: Association of life activities with cerebral blood flow in Alzheimer disease: implications for the cognitive reserve hypothesis. Arch Neurol 60:359–365, 2003

Scarmeas N, Albert SM, Manly JJ, et al: Education and rates of cognitive decline in incident Alzheimer's disease. J Neurol Neurosurg Psychiatry 77:308–316, 2006

Schlaggar BL, McCandliss BD: Development of neural systems for reading. Annu Rev Neurosci 30:475–503, 2007

Schofield PW, Logroscino G, Andrews HF, et al: An association between head circumference and Alzheimer's disease in a population-based study of aging and dementia. Neurology 49:30–37, 1997

Siedlecki KL, Stern Y, Reuben A, et al: Construct validity of cognitive reserve in a multiethnic cohort: the Northern Manhattan Study. J Int Neuropsychol Soc (in press)

Stern Y: What is cognitive reserve? Theory and research application of the reserve concept. J Int Neuropsychol Soc 8:448–460, 2002

Stern Y, Alexander GE, Prohovnik I, et al: Inverse relationship between education and parietotemporal perfusion deficit in Alzheimer's disease. Ann Neurol 32:371–375, 1992

Stern Y, Gurland B, Tatemichi TK, et al: Influence of education and occupation on the incidence of Alzheimer's disease. JAMA 271:1004–1010, 1994

Stern Y, Tang MX, Denaro J, et al: Increased risk of mortality in Alzheimer's disease patients with more advanced educational and occupational attainment. Ann Neurol 37:590–595, 1995

Stern Y, Albert S, Tang MX, et al: Rate of memory decline in AD is related to education and occupation: cognitive reserve? Neurology 53:1942–1947, 1999

Stern Y, Moeller JR, Anderson KE, et al: Different brain networks mediate task performance in normal aging and AD: defining compensation. Neurology 55:1291–1297, 2000

Stern Y, Zarahn E, Hilton HJ, et al: Exploring the neural basis of cognitive reserve. J Clin Exp Neuropsychol 25:691–701, 2003

Stern Y, Habeck C, Moeller J, et al: Brain networks associated with cognitive reserve in healthy young and old adults. Cereb Cortex 15:394–402, 2005

White L, Katzman R, Losonczy K, et al: Association of education with incidence of cognitive impairment in three established populations for epidemiologic studies of the elderly. J Clin Epidemiol 47:363–374, 1994

Willis SL, Tennstedt SL, Marsiske M, et al: Long-term effects of cognitive training on everyday functional outcomes in older adults. JAMA 296:2805–2814, 2006

Wilson RS, Mendes De Leon CF, Barnes LL, et al: Participation in cognitively stimulating activities and risk of incident Alzheimer disease. JAMA 287:742–748, 2002

Young RJ: The effect of regular exercise on cognitive functioning and personality. Br J Sports Med 13:110–117, 1979

Zarahn E, Rakitin B, Abela D, et al: Age-related changes in brain activation during a delayed item recognition task. Neurobiol Aging 28:784–798, 2007

Zhang MY, Katzman R, Salmon D, et al: The prevalence of dementia and Alzheimer's disease in Shanghai, China: impact of age, gender, and education. Ann Neurol 27:428–437, 1990

Recommended Readings

Cotman CW, Berchtold NC: Exercise: a behavioral intervention to enhance brain health and plasticity. Trends Neurosci 25:295–301, 2002

Stern Y: What is cognitive reserve? Theory and research application of the reserve concept. J Int Neuropsychol Soc 8:448–460, 2002

Stern Y: Cognitive reserve. Neuropsychologia 47:2015–2028, 2009

10

Stress, Resilience, and the Aging Brain

Ruth O'Hara, Ph.D.
Sherry A. Beaudreau, Ph.D.
Avinoam Luzon, B.S.
Mina Hah, M.D.
Jeffrey T. Hubbard, B.A.
Barbara Sommer, M.D.

Aging is a multi-faceted process, often complicated not only by an individual's genetic endowment but also by the culture and politics of the environment. It is thought that environmental factors may account for as much as 65% of the variance in lifespan (Finch and Tanzi 2003). In the United States, aging is generally considered to begin at around 65, when Medicare services become available (Kane et al. 2003). Although associations among stressful life events, psychiatric disorders, and medical illnesses have been well described over the years, the neurobiological mechanisms underlying these complex relationships are not clearly understood. Geriatric mental health researchers have become increasingly interested in the complicated interactions between stress and the neurobiology of late-life disorders. Although psychosocial stressors, such as major life events and perturbing daily situations and hassles, are generally just as common among older adults as they are in other age groups (Hunt et al. 2003), the elderly may be particularly vulnerable to the neurobiological consequences of stress due to age-related declines in brain function (McEwen 2003).

Older adults appear to experience significant difficulty coping with age-associated stressors such as decline in health (Krause 1998), reduced autonomy, and fewer financial resources (Britton et al. 2008). Stress among the elderly can precipitate or exacerbate physical and psychiatric symptoms or disorders, cognitive impairment and decline, and excessive physical disability, and, in extreme cases, can hasten mortality (Karp et al. 2008). Yet, despite past speculations that the elderly are more vulnerable to loss, not all older adults seem to be equally vulnerable to the negative effects of stress. Some older adults appear to be quite resilient to any negative effect of stress, and exhibit excellent coping abilities, which protect them both physiologically and psychologically (Hildon et al. 2008).

The overarching purpose of this chapter is to discuss the continuum of stress vulnerability to stress resiliency in aging from a biological perspective, emphasizing the role of the human brain. In particular, our objective is to describe 1) those biological factors that may place an elderly individual at increased risk for the negative consequences of stress and 2) those factors that appear to confer increased resiliency to stressful life experiences.

We accomplish this by first reviewing the diathesis stress paradigm, and concepts of allostasis and allostatic load, which have been proposed to explain age-related stress response and resiliency. Potential mechanisms by which the brain and stress may interact to create a diathesis for a range of neuropsychiatric and neurocognitive outcomes in older adults are reviewed. Biological mechanisms, such as reduced homeostatic regulation of neuroendocrine function, inflammation, and immune function, are discussed. We also describe potential risk factors or moderators (i.e., genetic markers) and stressful life experiences (e.g., early childhood trauma and abuse) that may increase an individual's vulnerability to stress. Finally, we close with a discussion of future directions for stress and resiliency research on the aging brain and clinical implications of this research, including potential prophylactic measures for vulnerable older adults.

Diathesis Stress Model of Psychiatric Illness

Regardless of age, a dominant view in both the psychiatric and psychological literature has been the *diathesis stress model*—that stress is likely to trigger mental illness, particularly in the presence of a neurobiological or genetic vulnerability. Well supported is the view that stressful life events are robust predictors of the onset or recurrence of a broad range of physical, neurocognitive, and psychiatric disorders (see Table 10–1; McEwen 1998; Reiche et

TABLE 10–1. Physiological and psychological sequelae to stress

Physiological

    Hypothalamic-pituitary-adrenal dysregulation

    Cardiovascular disease

    Insulin resistance

    Diabetes mellitus

    Hypertension

    Cancer

    Increased muscle atrophy

    Suppression of anabolic processes

Psychiatric

    Cognitive impairment

    Dementia

    Posttraumatic stress disorder

    Panic disorder

    Depressive disorder

    Generalized anxiety disorder

    Schizophrenia

    Substance abuse disorders

al. 2004). Different types of stress, such as acute stress, chronic stress, or early childhood trauma, may differentially influence the type and severity of a neurocognitive or neuropsychiatric disorder that an individual may develop with age, or may increase the risk of developing comorbid medical psychiatric conditions (Kendler et al. 2005).

Allostasis and Allostatic Load

Allostasis refers to the integrated response of the neuroendocrine, autonomic, and immune systems to stress in order to achieve physiological stability in the wake of change. McEwen (2003) describes the construct of *allostatic load,* in which physiological impairment results from an overactivated or dysregulated allostatic response. In a sense, *allostatic load* refers to the physiological price of effective adaptation and has evolved to be a key construct in explaining the age-related stress response. McEwen (2003) suggests that an overactivated or dysregulated physiological response to stress may occur in response to stressful life events and may be exacerbated by genetic risk factors for the development of medical disorders common in late life, such as cardiovascular disease and diabetes. He argues that individual differences in the aging process may represent an accumulation of the "wear and tear" of daily hassles, major stressful life events, early childhood trauma, and genetic risk factors. Shared genetic and dispositional vulnerabilities to the negative effects of stress are postulated to be involved in the risk of developing mental disorders, such as generalized anxiety disorder (Mackintosh et al. 2006), as well as in medical disorders such as those affecting cardiovascular function (McEwen 2003). Yet, the complexity of the stress response is such that effective allostasis may, in fact, enhance the capacity for resilience to stress. Across the life span, individuals lacking specific biological and dispositional vulnerabilities to stress may represent the subset that we refer to as *resilient.*

Personality, Behavior, and Physiology of Resiliency

Resiliency has been defined as the capacity to continue with one's normal functioning following stress or loss (Bonanno 2004). This construct has steadily garnered interest over the past few years, particularly in the arena of stress and trauma research. The increased focus on resiliency stems from the recognition that some individuals exhibit a normal trajectory of functioning even after the most extreme stressful events. Most compelling are studies demonstrating that some older adult survivors of the Nazi Holocaust (Kahana et al. 1998) report positive well-being because of their traumatic experiences. There are anecdotal reports of less stress and greater psychological resiliency in older compared with younger survivors of Hurricane Katrina (Harden 2005). In addition, the prevalence of posttraumatic stress disorder among those who have experienced a proximal crime or accident is lowest among older age groups (Norris 1992). A central focus of current resiliency research is identifying whether there are genetic or personality traits or special environmental experiences that are specific to those who have survived trauma and have lived to an older age, given recent evidence that older prisoner of war survivors without posttraumatic stress disorder have psychological and neuroimaging profiles similar to those of age- and education-matched control subjects (Freeman et al. 2006). How might resilience even in extremely stressful circumstances such as these best be characterized?

Lamond et al. (2008) propose that resilience is the ability to adapt positively to adversity, and found that in 1,395 community-dwelling women over age 60, higher emotional well-being, optimism, and social engagement and fewer cognitive complaints were most strongly associated with resiliency. Of course, older adults face continual attrition of their social networks with age, often experiencing the loss of their spouse, other family members, or friends due to a wide range of reasons, from death to geographical distance.

Wagnild (2003) defines resilience as a personality characteristic that moderates the negative effects of stress and promotes adaptation and that is associated with better health in terms of the vigor of the mind, body, and spirit into middle age and beyond. Certainly, an individual's perceptions, social support, self-esteem, and response to stress have all been found to impact the disease process (Benight and Harper 2002). Individual differences in response to stress have, in part, been attributed to differences in ongoing life stressors and social resources. Adaptive coping strategies, social support, and financial security are just some of the examples of social resources that are thought to buffer or moderate the impact of chronic stress on the physiological and psychological stress response.

However, rather than presuming that some older adults are buffered by external factors, Resnick (2008) suggests that resilience in older adults may be the ability to use available resources and skills to accept inevitable psychosocial and physical changes. She proposes that individuals resilient to the negative effects of stress may use such skills to sustain involvement in those aspects and activities of life that are most important. As such, she states, resilience may be the avoidance of such affective states as self-pity, anger, and depression.

Stress-Related Pathophysiological Mechanisms and the Aging Brain

But is the stress response purely a state of mind? In an excellent review of the relationship of stress to physiological functioning, McEwen (2008) emphasizes the central role played by the brain in modulating the stress response. The brain not only identifies that which is stressful but also controls our physiological and behavioral responses to the stressful experience. Recent basic science investigations suggest that brain development and subsequent response to stress may reflect both early childhood trauma and genetic risk factors (Radant et al. 2001) (Figure 10–1). Indeed, as McEwen (2008) points out, one's affect and perception of stress are likely influenced by a combination of one's experiences, genetics, and behavior. Some of the key pathophysiological mechanisms implicated in resiliency and vulnerability to stress include the neuroendocrine, autonomic, and immune systems—specifically, the action of glucocorticoids, catecholamines, and cytokines.

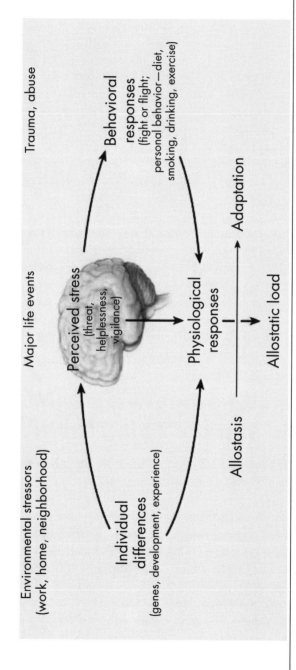

FIGURE 10–1. Central role of the brain in physiological and behavioral response to stress.

Hypothalamic-Pituitary-Adrenal Axis and Aging

Acute stress is known to negatively affect neuroendocrine function via the hypothalamic-pituitary-adrenal (HPA) axis. When stimulated, this feedback loop results in the secretion, sustained during chronic stress, of glucocorticoids such as cortisol, enabling the organism to perform with a heightened sense of alertness. The HPA response to stress is a basic adaptive mechanism in mammals, and the resultant elevations in glucocorticoids secreted by the adrenal cortex account for a significant amount of the physiological response to stimuli that may threaten homeostasis. Although an adaptive, well-functioning stress response is essential to survival, sustained elevated levels of glucocorticoids can present a serious health risk, leading to a suppression of anabolic processes, increased muscle atrophy, and hypertension.

Studies of older animals and humans have long demonstrated an age-associated impairment in HPA response to acute stress. In general, the evidence does not suggest that basal cortisol levels increase with age, but rather indicates that a significant age-related overresponsivity of the HPA axis to stressors and reduced HPA axis sensitivity to glucocorticoid feedback occur (McEwen 2008).

Within the brain, hippocampal regions appear particularly vulnerable to negative effects of HPA dysregulation—specifically, chronically elevated levels of glucocorticoids. In groundbreaking work, Sapolsky and colleagues (1985) found in an animal model that chronically administered glucocorticoids resulted in hippocampal damage. This damage in turn altered hippocampal regulation of HPA activity, resulting in a forward cascade effect whereby the hippocampal damage resulting from elevated cortisol levels led to further HPA impairment (Sapolsky 1985). A cyclical deleterious effect has been hypothesized in this regard in which damaged hippocampal neurons, normally facilitators in the downregulation of cortisol, interfere with a glucocorticoid negative feedback loop of the HPA axis, resulting in further increases in cortisol levels and damage to hippocampal neurons (for review, see Sapolsky 2000). Animal studies find elevations in cortisol are associated with hippocampal neuronal injury and loss, inhibited synaptic transmission, and decreased dendritic branching (Sapolsky 1996; Sapolsky et al. 1985). Most recently, animal studies have suggested that differential regions of the hippocampal formation, namely the CA1 and CA3 of the hippocampus, are most prominently affected by heightened cortisol levels (Zhao et al. 2007).

Constant hippocampal volume loss is well documented in normal and pathological aging (Jack et al. 2000). Thus, individuals suffering from hippocampal degeneration as a result of normal aging changes, or as a consequence of neurodegenerative disorders such as dementia, may be rendered particularly susceptible to the deleterious effect of stress-related glucocorticoids within hippocampal regions. As such, the brain aging process itself may significantly increase vulnerability to the negative effects of stress with age, and the interaction of stress and age-related brain processes, such as impairments in the brain's response to stress, may further exacerbate and contribute to impaired brain function with age.

HPA dysregulation has been implicated in several late-life disorders, including anxiety (Mantella et al. 2008), major depression (Aihara et al. 2007), and cognitive impairment and decline (O'Hara et al. 2007). Elevated levels of cortisol and other measures of dysregulated HPA activity are consistently associated with impaired cognitive function, particularly poorer memory function. Although there are fewer neuroimaging studies of the relationships between the brain and HPA function in older adults, several implicate elevated glucocorticoids in reduced hippocampal volume and deficits in memory performance (O'Hara et al. 2007). Impaired hippocampal and medial temporal lobe function are implicated in stress-related disorders such as posttraumatic stress disorder, late-life depression, and anxiety.

HPA dysregulation is also well documented in depression (Coryell et al. 2006; Schatzberg and Rothschild 1988). Although the results of studies about generalized anxiety disorder and HPA dysfunction are less conclusive (Marshall et al. 2002), HPA dysregulation is gaining support as a negative consequence of anxiety disorders such as posttraumatic stress disorder and panic disorder. It is theorized that cumulative exposure to the stress associated with being depressed or anxious results in hypersecretion of cortisol, which in turn results in neuronal death within the hippocampus, increasing vulnerability to cognitive impairment and psychiatric disorders such as anxiety and depression (Starkman 2003).

The medial temporal lobe is not the only brain region implicated in the stress response. A significant amount of literature links fear and the stress response to the amygdala (for review, see Davis et al. 1994), with several functional magnetic resonance imaging studies indicating an increased physiological response of the human amygdala to fearful and threatening faces (Gentili et al. 2008). Marked reductions in both hippocampal and amygdaloid volumes have been observed in Alzheimer disease patients and older adults with mild cognitive impairment, suggesting that amygdaloid volume contributes to the predictive value of hippocampal volume as a precursor to mild cognitive impairment and dementia (Apostolova et al. 2006). Amygdalar and hippocampal volumes have been identified as important factors in the development and progression of late-life depression (Lesch and Gutknecht 2005). Traditionally, studies on late-life disorders often neglected the amygdala and brain regions other than the medial temporal lobes, and although stress is suggested to impact additional brain regions such as the prefrontal cortex, as yet there has been limited consideration of the HPA involvement with the structure and function of other brain regions in older adults.

Although sustained increases in glucocorticoid levels are implicated in a range of neurocognitive and psychiatric disorders and physical illnesses such as cardiovascular disease, hypertension, and muscle and bone mineral loss, recent evidence suggests that some stress-related disorders, including cancer, may in fact be marked by a flattened diurnal rhythm of cortisol secretion or a hypocortisolemic response to stress (Mason et al. 1998; Spiegel et al. 2006). Indeed, flattened diurnal rhythm of cortisol secretion has been associated with mortality in both breast cancer and stroke patients (Surtees et al. 2008), and the evidence supports a role for chronic insufficiency of glucocorticoids in inflammation and an increased autoimmune response (Chrousos 1995).

Autonomic Nervous System

The autonomic nervous system is integrally associated with the stress response, with epinephrine and norepinephrine controlling significant physiological functions, from emotional state to metabolism, body temperature, and fluid and electrolyte balance—all functions that are increasingly vulnerable with age. Epinephrine and norepinephrine are both catecholamines that increase alertness. Epinephrine also exerts profound effects on myocardial excitability and increases heart rate, arterial blood pressure, and cardiac output. Norepinephrine, by contrast, decreases heart rate and cardiac output. Subjectively, epinephrine seems to induce more fear and anxiety, perhaps associated with the "fight or flight" response (Ganong 2005). McEwen (2003) suggested that circulating catecholamines constitute another key component of allostasis and can have synergistic and oppositional effects on the actions of glucocorticoids, which in turn influence epinephrine synthesis; increased levels of catecholamines have been associated with increased vigilance and arousal and also with the formation of memories attached to strong emotions.

Inflammatory Cytokines

Stress-related inflammation and alterations in peripheral immune function have long been implicated in late-life depression, anxiety, cognitive decline, and Alzheimer disease (Reale et al. 2008). The effects of proinflammatory genes may increase with age (Brüünsgaard et al. 2003; Wyss-Coray et al. 2006). Proinflammatory cytokines, such as interleukin-1 (IL-1), interleukin-2 (IL-2), and interleukin-6 (IL-6), tumor necrosis factors, and interferons, are heavily involved in the acute-phase response to stress, contributing to proinflammatory immunopathology and increased oxidative stress (Black 2006). Anti-inflammatory cytokines interleukin-4 (IL-4) and interleukin-10

(IL-10) may actually confer resilience to stress, and a protective role for the immune system, involving anti-β-amyloid antibodies, microglia, and macrophage phagocytosis of dying neurons or β-amyloid precipitates, has been proposed in several late-life disorders, including cognitive decline (Di Iorio et al. 2003). These inflammatory cytokines may be particularly important in conferring increased resilience to the inflammatory stress response.

Psychosocial Stress and the Aging Brain

Although the deleterious role of stress on neuronal integrity and function is well documented, it is as yet unclear whether physiological response to stress, such as elevations in glucocorticoid levels or an overzealous inflammatory response, directly reflects the number, magnitude, or severity of stressful experiences. Certainly, older adults appear to exhibit a heightened physiological response to an acute psychological stressor, such as public speaking or performance on the Trier Social Stress Test (Lupien and McEwen 1997). Researchers suggest that the aging process results in the gradual erosion of an appropriate physiological stress response, which in turn leads to increased neuronal impairment if the individual encounters a significant number of stressful events (McEwen 2008; Wilkinson et al. 1997).

Nevertheless, it is not at all clear from the literature whether chronic levels of psychosocial stressors are also associated with, for example, abnormal or increasing cortisol response in older adults, or how sustained levels of chronic psychosocial stress may affect the physiological stress response over time. Under conditions of chronic psychosocial stress, the physiological stress response may become dysregulated. Yet, it may also be that the individual habituates to the stress and that homeostasis is achieved more quickly, with levels of stress hormones normalizing over time. Such habituation may represent a form of resiliency, and it has been suggested that a certain amount of ongoing exposure to stress can produce *stress inoculation,* increasing the ability of an individual to more effectively respond physiologically and indeed psychologically to the stressful experience (Luecken et al. 2009). Others argue that impairments in HPA activity that occur in response to acute levels of stress, such as the death of a spouse, may negatively affect the individual's subsequent HPA response to milder levels of psychosocial stress (McEwen 2008).

To date, only a limited number of studies have investigated the relationship between psychosocial stressors and cortisol response. Few have observed a relationship between basal cortisol level and measures of lifetime stress and perceived stress (Bremner et al. 2003; Yehuda et al. 1995), and

O'Hara et al. (2007) found no relationship between lifetime stress and cortisol levels on awakening in older adults.

Genetics, Stress, and Aging

So the key question remains, why do some older adults appear to cope so effectively with stress, and others appear to mount an overzealous stress response, leading to increased risk for negative health consequences? As McEwen (2008) points out, genetic factors also may play a role in accounting for some of the individual variation in susceptibility to stress. In the past decade we have seen an enormous increase in the number of genetic studies being conducted, from consideration of candidate genes for all sorts of disorders and phenotypes, to the more recent genomewide association studies. Such investigations are in their infancy, and no systematic genomewide study of stress has been conducted. Nevertheless, certain established genetic markers have already been explored in consideration of the stress response.

The apolipoprotein E genotype (*APOE*E/*E*) is one genetic marker proposed to impact the response of the brain to stress (Roses et al. 1996). Apolipoprotein E (ApoE) is a plasma protein that is involved in the transport of cholesterol and other lipids. It is implicated in the growth and regeneration of nerves during development and/or following injury. The ApoE protein is present in senile plaques, neurofibrillary tangles, and cerebrovascular amyloid, the major neuropathological signs of Alzheimer dementia. It is expressed by a gene on chromosome 19. There are three allelic variants of *APOE* (**E2, *E3,* and **E4*), resulting in six possible genotypes. Many studies have demonstrated that the APOE*E4 allele is a genetic risk factor for the development of Alzheimer dementia and have demonstrated *APOE* status to be predictive of performance on a variety of cognitive tests in populations of individuals with and without dementia (e.g., Adamson et al. 2008; Reiman et al. 1996).

With regard to human studies, Roses et al. (1996) point out that environmental stress may differentiate "genetic differences in repair mechanisms." Individuals with the **E4* allele exhibit poorer outcome following intracerebral hemorrhage (Alberts et al. 1995), display greater cognitive decline following cardiac surgery (Newman et al. 1995), are at greater risk for brain injury associated with boxing (Jordan et al. 1997), and are at greater risk for adverse sequelae following head injury (Nicoll et al. 1995). Roses et al. (1996) concluded that regardless of the source of the stress, the **E4* allele may not protect against resultant metabolic stress as well as the **E2* and **E3* alleles do. Presence of the **E2* allele, on the other hand, may indeed confer greater resiliency to stressful events, and recent evidence suggests that the presence of this allele is protective against cognitive impairment (Blacker et al. 2007).

Some studies have suggested there may be interplay between ApoE and HPA activity. Gordon et al. (1996) found that the elevation of plasma corticosterone levels in *APOE* knockout mice undergoing restraint stress was significantly lower than the levels observed in control mice. They suggested that the reduction in the density of hippocampal synapses typically observed in *APOE*-deficient mice resulted in increased hippocampal inhibition of the HPA stress response. Because *APOE* knockout mice are considered analogous to *E4 allele carriers, these animal studies may suggest a mechanism whereby *E4 allele carriers show lower cortisol levels and a dissociation between cortisol levels and rate of cognitive decline. However, investigations of the relationships among *APOE* status, stress, and HPA function in humans have yielded inconsistent findings (Freeman et al. 2005; Peavy et al. 2007).

Kheirandish et al. (2005) examined effects of chronic hypoxia, a significant source of stress, on spatial memory performance in 24 *APOE*-deficient mice (*APOE*–/*–) compared with 24 wild-type littermates (*APOE*+/*+). Not only did the chronic intermittent hypoxia induce more cognitive impairment in the *APOE*-deficient mice; the researchers also observed increased hippocampal lipid peroxidation and cyclooxygenase-2 activity following the hypoxic exposure, which was exacerbated in the *APOE*-deficient mice. This provides evidence for the involvement of hypoxia-associated oxidation and inflammatory responses in neurocognitive dysfunction as well as increased *E4-associated vulnerability to physiological stress.

5-HTT Promoter Region Polymorphism

A significant amount of stress-related research has recently focused on the role of genetic variations in the 5-hydroxytryptamine (5-HT; serotonin) transporter promoter region polymorphism (5HTTLPR) in depressive symptomatology, anxiety, and personality traits (Lesch and Gutknecht 2005). This polymorphism is a 44–base pair allelic insertion (long, or *L, allele) or deletion (short, or *S, allele) variant that regulates the transcription of the 5-HT transporter. The *S allele is associated with lower levels of 5-HT uptake and transcriptional efficiency of the 5-HT transporter (5-HTT) (Lesch and Gutknecht 2005). As described below, several studies support the hypothesis of an interaction between stressful life events, the 5HTT*/5HTT* genotype, and psychiatric outcomes such as depression and anxiety. Recent evidence suggests that the 5HTT*S allele may increase vulnerability to stress.

Caspi et al. (2003) were the first to find that stressful life events occurring early in life predict subsequent onset of depressive symptoms in individuals with one or two copies of the *S allele of the 5-HTT promoter polymorphism. In an investigation of 549 male and female middle-aged twins, Kendler et al. (2005) found that individuals homozygous for the *S allele were more sensitive to the depressogenic effects of stressful life events compared with carriers of an *L allele.

Although the moderating impact of psychological stressors on the risk for depression in individuals with the 5HTT*S allele has been widely investigated, the vulnerability of 5HTT*S allele carriers to physiological markers of stress, such as cortisol, has only recently been considered (Gotlib et al. 2008; O'Hara et al. 2007). Our group found that the 5HTT*S allele was associated with higher waking cortisol levels, and that a negative interaction of the 5HTT*S allele and cortisol resulted in poorer memory and lower hippocampal volume in older adults than was observed in *L allele carriers (O'Hara et al. 2007). Pezawas et al. (2005) also found 5HTT*S allele carriers to be more prone to anxiety and to exhibit increased amygdaloid reactivity to stress.

The 5HTT*S allele may impact the normal aging process by increasing vulnerability to neuropsychiatric outcomes secondary to factors such as stress and medical illness. Additionally, the neurotoxic effects of chronic illness–associated stress may be due to neurodegeneration mediated by glucocorticoid modulation via the serotonergic system (O'Hara et al. 2007). As such, the 5HTT*S allele may interact with HPA activity and stress to underlie the cognitive deficits associated with a range of disorders in older adults, including depression and anxiety, particularly in individuals with documented impairments in HPA function (O'Hara and Hallmayer 2007).

The mechanism by which this occurs may involve the impact of 5-HT on brain development. The serotonergic system is implicated in hippocampal regulation of HPA axis activity, increasing hippocampal glucocorticoid receptors, specifically during certain developmental periods. It has been suggested that developmental modification of the ascending serotonergic system results in long-term dysregulation of HPA function and impaired brain plasticity that may become exacerbated with increasing age (Tralongo et al. 2005). Some have suggested that there are potential developmental effects of the 5HTTLPR on neural circuitry mediating stress reactivity, and there is growing evidence that early life trauma plays a key role in modulating stress response on behavioral outcomes and hippocampal volume (Lesch and Gutknecht 2005).

Other Potential Genetic Moderators of the Stress Response

Recently investigators have begun to move beyond the construct of stress neurotoxicity to consider the construct of brain plasticity as a significant modulator of the stress response. Brain plasticity both reflects and protects against stress. Brain neuronal plasticity may be a particularly important component of stress resiliency with age and is likely the result of environmental and genetic factors.

Just as multiple systems within the brain influence the stress response, there are genetic markers other than the APOE*E genotype and the 5-HTT polymorphism that may moderate the negative effects of stress:

- Given the relationship of HPA function to stress response, researchers have looked to glucocorticoid receptor genes as potential targets; some examples are the glucocorticoid receptor polymorphism Bcl1 (Canli et al. 2005) and the N363S (ASN363ser) polymorphism (Andrews et al. 2004).
- Others have suggested the involvement of tumor necrosis factor–α (TNF-α), a proinflammatory cytokine with functions in nerve cell growth, differentiation, and apoptosis. The gene for TNF-α has several polymorphisms in the promoter region, and these polymorphisms may impact its transcription (Hayashi et al. 2008).
- With respect to resiliency, investigators have increasingly speculated a role for brain-derived neurotrophic factor (BDNF). The gene for BDNF, a neurotrophin involved in neuronal survival, proliferation, and activity-dependent plasticity of cholinergic, dopaminergic, and serotonergic neurons in the central nervous system, is speculated to be involved in protecting the brain from stress (Bergström et al. 2008).

Despite the burgeoning of genomewide association studies to identify markers for a range of physical and mental disorders, the yield has been far less than expected. This has underscored what many have suspected: that it is not the presence of specific genes alone but rather significant gene × environment interactions that are most likely to increase an individual's vulnerability to stress.

Psychosocial Stress and Stressful Life Events

There is compelling evidence for the influence of environmental factors on how an individual responds to stress, but to date our understanding of the interface between physiological and psychological responses to stress is limited. The complexity of age-related stress responses reflects, in part, the fact that stress itself remains a nebulous construct. It is not always clear whether investigators are speaking of the same thing when they discuss "stress." There is significant variability among stressors, and the stress response of an individual may depend on the type (e.g., everyday hassle vs. traumatic event), frequency (single event vs. chronic), duration (e.g., minutes vs. days), and proximity (recent vs. remote) of stressful life events. Even when there is consensus regarding the stress construct under investigation, how stress is measured can vary tremendously. It is as yet unknown whether psychological stresses such as verbal abuse or intimidation elicit the same stress response that physiological stresses such as illness, concussion, or surgery do. Indeed, a significant complication in understanding the impact of stress is that stress-related activation of physiological systems can result in dramatic changes in cardiovascular function, immune function, and sleep patterns, raising the possibility that any deleterious effect of stress on mental and physical disorders is in fact mediated by associated impairments in medical status, which are all too common in older adults.

Measures of psychosocial stress have been associated with cognitive decline, but the contribution of life stressors to age-related psychiatric and psychological disorders remains unclear. One of the early studies of this issue found significantly lower cognitive functioning in older women who had experienced the death of a spouse, those who had an inactive lifestyle, and those who lived in relatively inaccessible areas compared with control subjects who did not have these stressors (Gribbin et al. 1980). However, others have found that a similar degree of cognitive decline occurs with age regardless of stressful life events, with the exception of the death of a spouse or child, which was found to be associated with greater cognitive decline (Grimby and Berg 1995). Several studies have examined populations of combat veterans and prisoners of war to investigate the relationship between stress in young adulthood and cognitive decline with age (Gollier et al. 2002; Yehuda et al. 2007). In one of the earliest extensive longitudinal studies, Thygesen et al. (1970) followed concentration camp survivors for years after their release to determine their physical and psychological health status, and noted that greater extent of physical disability during internment was associated with more intellectual than physical deterioration later in life.

A recent longitudinal study (Britton et al. 2008), established in 1985 to follow socioeconomic status in health and disease, followed 5,823 men and women in the aging cohort of the study, beginning at age 43.8±5.5 years for men (n=4,140) and 44.3±5.9 years for women (n=1,683). The average age at follow-up for those who had successfully aged versus those who had not was 57.5 versus 60.8 for men and 57.3 versus 61.3 for women. Other factors that contributed to a favorable older-life adjustment were height, education, not smoking, diet, exercise, moderate alcohol consumption, and work support. Lower socioeconomic status may be a significant proxy marker for increased stress.

No matter the source, severity, or duration of a stressful experience, one's ability to cope may have a significant impact on ameliorating any negative impact of the stress. Yet there is even variability among coping strategies, and not all coping styles appear to work equally well. Mausbach et al. (2006) found that among spousal caregivers of Alzheimer disease patients, escape/avoidance coping styles (wishing the problem would go away) with respect to problem behaviors in the patient resulted in higher levels of depressive symptoms in the caregiver, compared with levels in those who did not engage in this kind of coping strategy. The authors suggested that individual differences in avoidant coping approaches to stressful situations may mediate the relationship of stress to psychiatric outcomes in older adults. Increased knowledge regarding differences in how individuals cope with stress can help identify individuals who are most in need of psychosocial interventions. Similarly, knowing whether trait variables such as gender and ethnicity increase vulnerability to stress with age can also provide important information regarding individuals to whom interventions should be targeted.

The taxonomy of stressful events still needs significant work, and distinctions between acute versus chronic stressors and physical versus psychological stressors need much more consideration in the literature.

Developmental Risk of Early Childhood Adversity

There is growing evidence that traumatic and stressful events occurring in early childhood elevate a person's risk for the development of subsequent psychiatric and medical disorders. The Adverse Childhood Experiences Study (Dube et al. 2001) demonstrated, in large surveys involving thousands of subjects, a dose-dependent-like effect of abuse, witnessing violence, and serious family problems on the development of a variety of substance abuse disorders, behavioral disorders, and depression. Yet to date there has been limited consideration of the impact that negative effects of childhood trauma have on the brain and behavior in older adults. In a study of more than 250 older adults (mean age=79.8±2.1 years; 73.9% women), the Rush Memory and Aging Project found that traumatic experiences in childhood adversely impacted critical components of psychosocial functioning in old age (Wilson et al. 2006). Specifically, childhood adversity resulted in greater levels of negative emotion, smaller social networks, and more emotional isolation. In another investigation, of more than 1,000 Australian twins ages 19–78 years, stressful life events predicted depression in all age groups (Gillespie et al. 2005).

However, not all studies report a negative impact of early childhood trauma in older adults. In our own work with older adults (O'Hara et al. 2007), we observed no interactive effects of early traumatic events (assessed retrospectively via self-reports) across the life span, but we did observe a negative impact of cortisol on both hippocampal volume and memory performance. This may reflect the fact that HPA activity is a more sensitive measure of the stress response than any self-report measure. Alternatively, distal traumatic events may be less relevant for the elderly than ongoing chronic stressors. Memory for traumatic childhood events may simply be less reliable with increased age. Others have argued that due to exposure to a broad range of stressful events across the life span, the ability of middle-aged and older adults to cope with more traumatic events may be greater than that of children and young adults, suggesting an age-related resiliency to stressful events.

Conclusion and Future Directions

Complex relationships among traumatic experiences, ongoing chronic stress, physiological responsivity, genetic susceptibilities, and coping strategies conspire to increase stress responsivity and affect many neuropsychiatric, neurocognitive, and physical outcomes in older adults. The combination of variables that put patients at risk for negative stress-related outcomes, such as the 5HTT*S allele or the APOE*E4 allele, along with many of the other factors discussed in this chapter may predispose older adults to cognitive impairment or intractable anxiety or depression. One such factor alone may not pose such risk. Learning which individuals are most susceptible to hippocampal damage from the stress of elevated glucocorticoids as seen on imaging may be very valuable. For example, if subjects with the APOE*E4 allele are the most susceptible to hippocampal damage from stress, and they have dysregulated HPA activity, they may be the individuals most susceptible to posttraumatic stress disorder.

There is an increasing focus on those factors that may serve to modify or protect against the onslaught of stress. Physiological factors such as brain plasticity and genetic markers, and also psychosocial buffers, may be extremely important. Because many elderly adults will likely have experienced some traumatic stress during the course of their life, further emphasis needs to be placed on preventive strategies to minimize the negative consequences of such stressors on physical and mental health in old age. Increased understanding of which pathophysiological mechanisms underlie these negative effects and how different characteristics of an individual, state, or trait determine the stress response would go a long way toward illuminating the pathway to valuable interventions to ameliorate the negative influences of stress. It is important to study those older adults who are considered to have achieved optimal cognition and emotional well-being, surpassing norms for their age, in order to determine what it is they might do differently, or what predisposing characteristics or genetics may set them apart.

Although interventions exist for both psychological and physiological stress, their implementation is hampered by limited knowledge about which types and aspects of stress most strongly impact the older adult. Interventions for minimizing the negative impact of stress may be pharmacological or nonpharmacological, such as enumerated in Table 10–2. Future pharmacological approaches might call for investigations on the effects of anticortisolemic drugs, among others. If personality traits confer resilience, perhaps we can identify the components of these traits and teach better coping skills to those with a tendency to become more easily stressed. Investigators are already researching the benefits of relaxation techniques for reducing both physiological and psychological responses to stress (Antoni et al. 2008; Austin et al. 2005).

In-depth investigations that can truly assess the complex relationships among genetic, psychosocial, biological, behavioral, and environmental factors are required to further our understanding of the interface of stress, resilience, and aging.

TABLE 10–2.   Stress management interventions

Nonpharmacological approaches

    Meditation

    Improving social support

    Regular moderate physical activity

    Maintaining an anti-inflammatory diet

    Improving sleep quality

Pharmacological approaches

    Anticortisolemic medications

    Antianxiety medications

    Antidepressants

    Anti-inflammatories

    Beta-blockers

    Sleep medications

KEY POINTS

▋ *Allostatic load* refers to the physiological price of adaptation to chronic stress, and has evolved to be a key construct in explaining the age-related stress response.

▋ Although an adaptive, well-functioning stress response is essential for survival, sustained elevated levels of glucocorticoids can present a serious health risk, leading to suppression of anabolic processes, increased muscle atrophy, and hypertension.

▋ Physiological factors such as brain plasticity and genetic markers, and also psychosocial buffers, may be extremely important to protecting individuals against the negative effects of stress.

▋ Interventions for minimizing the negative impact of stress might be pharmacological or psychosocial. Learning from the biological and coping mechanisms exhibited in resilient older people may help to guide development of future interventions.

References

Adamson MM, Landy KM, Duong S, et al: Apolipoprotein E varepsilon4 influences on episodic recall and brain structures in aging pilots. Neurobiol Aging August 27, 2008 (Epub ahead of print)

Aihara M, Ida I, Yuuki N, et al: HPA axis dysfunction in unmedicated major depressive disorder and its normalization by pharmacotherapy correlates with alteration of neural activity in prefrontal cortex and limbic/paralimbic regions. Psychiatry Res 155:245–256, 2007

Alberts MJ, Graffagnino C, McClenny C, et al: ApoE genotype and survival from intracerebral haemorrhage. Lancet 346:575, 1995

Andrews MH, Kostaki A, Setiawan E, et al: Developmental regulation of the 5-HT7 serotonin receptor and transcription factor NGFI-A in the fetal guinea-pig limbic system: influence of GCs. J Physiol 555 (pt 3):659–670, 2004

Antoni MH, Lechner SC, Blomberg BB, et al: Stress management intervention reduces serum cortisol and increases relaxation during treatment for nonmetastatic breast cancer. Psychosom Med 70:1044–1049, 2008

Apostolova LG, Dutton RA, Dinov ID, et al: Conversion of mild cognitive impairment to Alzheimer disease predicted by hippocampal atrophy maps. Arch Neurol 63:693–699, 2006

Austin V, Shah S, Muncer S: Teacher stress and coping strategies used to reduce stress. Occupational Therapy International 12(2):63-80, 2005

Benight CC, Harper ML: Coping self-efficacy perceptions as a mediator between acute stress response and long-term distress following natural disasters. J Trauma Stress 15:177–186, 2002

Bergström A, Jayatissa MN, Mørk A, et al: Stress sensitivity and resilience in the chronic mild stress rat model of depression; an in situ hybridization study. Brain Res 1196:41–52, 2008

Black PH: The inflammatory consequences of psychologic stress: relationship to insulin resistance, obesity, atherosclerosis and diabetes mellitus, type II. Med Hypotheses 67:879–891, 2006

Blacker D, Lee H, Muzikansky A, et al: Neuropsychological measures in normal individuals that predict subsequent cognitive decline. Arch Neurol 64:862–871, 2007

Bonanno GA: Loss, trauma, and human resilience: have we underestimated the human capacity to thrive after extremely aversive events? Am Psychol 59:20–28, 2004

Bremner JD, Vythillingam M, Vermetten M, et al: Cortisol response to a cognitive stress challenge in posttraumatic stress disorder (PTSD) related to childhood abuse. Psychoneuroendocrinology 28:733–750, 2003

Britton A, Shipley M, Singh-Manoux A, et al: Successful aging: the contribution of early life and midlife risk factors. J Am Geriatr Soc 56:1098–1105, 2008

Brüünsgaard H, Pedersen BK: Age-related inflammatory cytokines and disease. Immunol Allergy Clin N Am 23:15–39, 2003.

Canli T, Omura K, Haas BW, et al: Beyond affect: a role for genetic variation of the serotonin transporter in neural activation during a cognitive attention task. Proc Natl Acad Sci USA 102:12224–12229, 2005

Caspi A, Sugden K, Moffitt TE, et al: Influence of life stress on depression: moderation by a polymorphism in the 5-HTT gene. Science 301:386–389, 2003

Chrousos GP: The hypothalamic-pituitary-adrenal axis and immune-mediated inflammation. N Engl J Med 333:1351–1363, 1995

Coryell W, Young E, Carroll B: Hyperactivity of the hypothalamic-pituitary-adrenal axis and mortality in major depression. Psychiatry Res 142:99–104, 2006

Davis M, Rainnie M, Cassell M: Neurotransmission in the rat amygdala related to fear and anxiety. Trends Neurosci 17(5):208–214, 1994

Di Iorio A, Ferrucci L, Sparvieri E, et al: Serum IL-1beta levels in health and disease: a population-based study. The InCHIANTI study. Cytokine 22:198–205, 2003

Dube SR, Anda RF, Felitti VJ, et al: Childhood abuse, household dysfunction, and the risk of attempted suicide throughout the life span: findings from the Adverse Childhood Experiences Study. JAMA 286:3120–3125, 2001

Finch CE, Tanzi RE: Genetics of aging. Science 278:407–411, 2003

Freeman T, Roca V, Guggenheim F, et al: Neuropsychiatric associations of apolipoprotein E alleles in subjects with combat-related posttraumatic stress disorder. J Neuropsychiatry Clin Neurosci 17:541–543, 2005

Freeman T, Kimbrell T, Booe L, et al: Evidence of resilience: neuroimaging in former prisoners of war. Psychiatry Res 146:59–64, 2006

Ganong WF: The adrenal medulla and adrenal cortex, in Review of Medical Physiology, 22nd Edition. New York, McGraw-Hill, 2005

Gentili C, Gobbini MI, Ricciardi E, et al: Differential modulation of neural activity throughout the distributed neural system for face perception in patients with social phobia and healthy subjects. Brain Res Bull September 1, 2008 (Epub ahead of print)

Gillespie NA, Whitfield JB, Williams B, et al: The relationship between stressful life events, the serotonin transporter (5-HTTLPR) genotype and major depression. Psychol Med 35:101–111, 2005

Gollier JA, Yehuda R, Lupien SJ, et al: Memory performance in Holocaust survivors with posttraumatic stress disorder. Am J Psychiatry 159:1682–1688, 2002

Gordon I, Ben- Eliyahu S, Rosenne E, et al: Derangement in stress response of apolipoprotein E–deficient mice. Neurosci Lett 206:212–214, 1996

Gotlib IH, Joormann J, Minor KL, et al: HPA axis reactivity: a mechanism underlying the associations among 5-HTTLPR, stress, and depression. Biol Psychiatry 63:847–851, 2008

Gribbin K, Schaie KW, Parham IA: Complexity of life-style and maintenance of intellectual abilities. J Soc Issues 36:47–61, 1980

Grimby A, Berg S: Stressful life events and cognitive functioning in late life. Aging (Milano) 7(1):35–39, 1995

Harden B: With age comes resilience, storm's aftermath proves. The Washington Post, September 14, 2005, A24

Hayashi S, Taira A, Inoue G, et al: TNF-alpha in nucleus pulposus induces sensory nerve growth: a study of the mechanism of discogenic low back pain using TNF-alpha-deficient mice. Spine 33:1542–1546, 2008

Hildon Z, Smith G, Netuveli G, et al: Understanding adversity and resilience at older ages. Sociol Health Illn 30:726–740, 2008

Hunt S, Wisocki P, Yanko J: Worry and use of coping strategies among older and younger adults. J Anxiety Disord 17:547–560, 2003

Jack CR Jr, Petersen RC, Xu Y, et al: Rates of hippocampal atrophy correlate with change in clinical status in aging and AD. Neurology 55:484–489, 2000

Jordan BD, Relkin NR, Ravdin LD, et al: Apolipoprotein E epsilon4 associated with chronic traumatic brain injury in boxing. JAMA 278:136–140, 1997

Kahana E, Kahana B, Harel Z, et al: Survivors of the Nazi Holocaust face old age. Paper presented at the annual meeting of the Gerontological Society of America, Philadelphia, PA, November 1998

Kane RL, Ouslander JG, Abrass IB (eds): Essentials of Clinical Geriatrics, 5th Edition. New York, McGraw-Hill, 2003, pp 5–14

Karp JF, Shega JW, Morone NE, et al: Advances in understanding the mechanisms and management of persistent pain in older adults. Br J Anaesth 101:111–120, 2008

Kendler KS, Kuhn JW, Vittum J, et al: The interaction of stressful life events and a serotonin transporter polymorphism in the prediction of episodes of major depression: a replication. Arch Gen Psychiatry 62:529–535, 2005

Kheirandish L, Row BW, Li RC, et al: Apolipoprotein E–deficient mice exhibit increased vulnerability to intermittent hypoxia-induced spatial learning deficits. Sleep 28:1412–1417, 2005

Krause N: Early parental loss, recent life events, and changes in health among older adults. J Aging Health 10:395–421, 1998

Lamond AJ, Depp CA, Allison M, et al: Measurement and predictors of resilience among community-dwelling older women. J Psychiatr Res 43:148–154, 2008

Lesch KP, Gutknecht L: Pharmacogenetics of the serotonin transporter. Prog Neuropsychopharmacol Biol Psychiatry 29:1062–1073, 2005

Luecken LJ, Kraft A, Appelhans BM, et al: Emotional and cardiovascular sensitization to daily stress following childhood parental loss. Dev Psychol 45:296–302, 2009

Lupien SJ, McEwen BS: The acute effects of corticosteroids on cognition: integration of animal and human model studies. Brain Res Rev 24:1–27, 1997

Mackintosh MA, Gatz M, Wetherell JL, et al: A twin study of lifetime generalized anxiety disorder (GAD) in older adults: genetic and environmental influences shared by neuroticism and GAD. Twin Res Hum Genet 9:30–37, 2006

Mantella RC, Butters MA, Amico JA, et al: Salivary cortisol is associated with diagnosis and severity of late-life generalized anxiety disorder. Psychoneuroendocrinology 33:773–781, 2008

Marshall RD, Blanco C, Printz D, et al: A pilot sudy of noradrenergic and HPA axis functioning in PTSD vs panic disorder. Psychiatr Res 110:219–230, 2002

Mausbach BT, Aschbacher K, Patterson TL, et al: Avoidant coping partially mediates the relationship between patient problem behaviors and depressive symptoms in spousal Alzheimer caregivers. Am J Geriatr Psychiatry 14:299–306, 2006

McEwen BS: Protective and damaging effects of stress mediators. N Engl J Med 338(3):171–179, 1998

McEwen BS: Interacting mediators of allostasis and allostatic load: towards an understanding of resilience in aging. Metabolism 52 (suppl 2):10–16, 2003

McEwen BS: Central effects of stress hormones in health and disease: understanding the protective and damaging effects of stress and stress mediators. Eur J Pharmacol 583:174–185, 2008

Newman M, Croughwell N, Blumenthal J, et al: Predictors of cognitive decline after cardiac operation. Ann Thorac Surg 59:1326–1330, 1995

Nicoll JA, Roberts GW, Graham DI: Apolipoprotein E epsilon 4 allele is associated with deposition of amyloid beta–protein following head injury. Nat Med 1:135–137, 1995

Norris FH: Epidemiology of trauma: frequency and impact of different potentially traumatic events on different demographic groups. J Consult Clin Psychol 60:409–418, 1992

O'Hara R, Hallmayer JF: Serotonin transporter polymorphism and stress: a view across the lifespan. Curr Psychiatry Rep 9:173–175, 2007

O'Hara R, Schröder CM, Mahadevan R, et al: Serotonin transporter polymorphism, memory and hippocampal volume in the elderly: association and interaction with cortisol. Mol Psychiatry 12:544–555, 2007

Peavy G, Lange K, Salmon D, et al: The effects of prolonged stress and APOE geno-type on memory and cortisol in older adults. Biol Psychiatry 62:472–478, 2007

Pezawas L, Meyer-Lindenberg A, Drabant EM, et al: 5-HTTLPR polymorphism im-pacts human cingulate-amygdala interactions: a genetic susceptibility mecha-nism for depression. Nat Neurosci 8:828–834, 2005

Radant A, Tsuang D, Peskind ER, et al: Biological markers and diagnostic accuracy in the genetics of posttraumatic stress disorder. Psychiatry Res 102:203–214, 2001

Reale M, Iarlori C, Feliciani C, et al: Peripheral chemokine receptors, their ligands, cytokines and Alzheimer's disease. J Alzheimers Dis 14:147–159, 2008

Reiche E, Nunes S, Morimoto H: Stress, depression, the immune system, and cancer. The Lancet Oncology 5(10):617–625, 2004

Reiman EM, Caselli RJ, Yun LS, et al: Preclinical evidence of Alzheimer's disease in-persons homozygous for the 4 allele for apolipoprotein E. N Engl J Med 334:752–758, 1996

Resnick B: Resilience in aging: the real experts. Geriatr Nurs 29:85–86, 2008

Roses AD, Einstein G, Gilbert J, et al: Morphological, biochemical, and genetic sup-port for an apolipoprotein E effect on microtubular metabolism. Ann NY Acad Sci 777:146–157, 1996

Sapolsky RM: A mechanism fro glucocorticoid toxicity in the hippocampus: increased neuronal vulnerability to metabolic insults. J Neurosci 5:1228–1232, 1985

Sapolsky R: Why stress is bad for your brain. Science 273:749–750, 1996

Sapolsky R: The possibility of neurotoxicity in the hippocampus in major depression: a primer on neuron death. Biol Psychiatry 48:755–765, 2000

Sapolsky RM, Krey LC, McEwen BS: Prolonged glucocorticoid exposure reduces hip-pocampal neuron number: implications for aging. J Neurosci 5:1222–1227, 1985

Schatzberg AF, Rothschild AJ: The roles of glucocorticoid and dopaminergic systems in delusional (psychotic) depression. Ann NY Acad Sci 537:462–471, 1988

Spiegel D, Giese-Davis J, Taylor CB, et al: Stress sensitivity in metastatic breast can-cer: analysis of hypothalamic-pituitary-adrenal axis function. Psychoneuroen-docrinology 31:1231–1344, 2006

Starkman MN: Psychiatric manifestations of hyperadrenocorticism and hypoadreno-corticism, in Psychoneuroendocrinology: The Scientific Basis of Clinical Prac-tice. Edited by Wolkowitz OM, Rothschild AJ. Washington, DC, American Psychiatric Publishing, 2003, pp 165–188

Surtees PG, Wainwright NW, Luben RN, et al: Psychological distress, major depres-sive disorder, and risk of stroke. Neurology 70:788–794, 2008

Thygesen P, Hermann K, Willanger R: Concentration camp survivors in Denmark persecution, disease, disability, compensation: a 23-year follow-up: a survey of the long-term effects of severe environmental stress. Dan Med Bull 17:65–108, 1970

Tralongo P, Di Mari A, Ferrau F: Cognitive impairment, aromatase inhibitors, and age. J Clin Oncol 23:619–629, 2005

Wagnild G: Resilience and successful aging: comparison among low and high income older adults. J Gerontol Nurs 29:42–49, 2003

Wilkinson CW, Peskind ER, Raskind MA: Decreased hypothalamic-pituitary adrenal axis sensitivity to cortisol feedback inhibition in human aging. Neuroendocrinology 65:79–90, 1997

Wilson RS, Krueger KR, Arnold SE, et al: Childhood adversity and psychosocial adjustment in old age. Am J Geriatr Psychiatry 14:307–315, 2006

Wyss-Coray T: Inflammation in Alzheimer disease: driving force, bystander or beneficial response? Nat Med 12:1005–1015, 2006

Yehuda R, Kahana B, Binder-Brynes K, et al: Low urinary cortisol excretion in Holocaust survivors with posttraumatic stress disorder. Am J Psychiatry 152:982–986, 1995

Yehuda R, Golier JA, Tischler L, et al: Hippocampal volume in aging combat veterans with and without post-traumatic stress disorder: relation to risk and resilience factors. J Psychiatr Res 41:435–445, 2007

Zhao H, Xu H, Xu X, et al: Predatory stress induces hippocampal cell death by apoptosis in rats. Neurosci Lett 421:115–120, 2007

Recommended Readings

Hildon Z, Smith G, Netuveli G, et al: Understanding adversity and resilience at older ages. Sociol Health Illn 30:726–740, 2008

McEwen BS: Central effects of stress hormones in health and disease: understanding the protective and damaging effects of stress and stress mediators. Eur J Pharmacol 583:174–185, 2008

O'Hara R, Hallmayer JF: Serotonin transporter polymorphism and stress: a view across the lifespan. Curr Psychiatry Rep 9:173–175, 2007

11

Influence of Dietary Factors on Brain Aging and the Pathogenesis of Alzheimer Disease

Mark P. Mattson, Ph.D.

Aging is the major risk factor for the most common sporadic forms of Alzheimer disease. It is therefore likely that cellular and molecular mechanisms that determine the rate of aging and the life span also influence Alzheimer disease–related pathogenic processes, including the production and accumulation of amyloid-β peptide (Aβ), the development of neurofibrillary tau pathology, synaptic dysfunction, and neuronal death (Cole et al. 2005; Mattson 2004). Two widely documented changes that occur during aging in many tissues, including the brain, are increased amounts of oxidative damage to cellular constituents (Floyd and Hensley 2002) and an impaired ability of cells to cope with various types of stress (Le Bourg 2003). The latter age-related changes are not immutable and, indeed, can be retarded by *dietary energy restriction* (also referred to as *caloric restriction*), a manipulation that increases

This work was supported by the National Institute on Aging Intramural Research Program of the National Institutes of Health.

the life span of many different animals, including mammals (Hunt et al. 2006). Conversely, excessive energy intake leads to obesity and is a major risk factor for many age-related diseases, including type 2 diabetes, cardiovascular disease, and cancers (Bray and Bellanger 2006). In laboratory animals, dietary energy restriction reduces the incidence of a range of age-related diseases (including diabetes, cancer, and kidney disease) and increases both average and maximum life spans (Sinclair 2005). Dietary energy restriction results in a decrease in levels of oxidative damage to proteins (carbonylation, nitration, and modification by lipid peroxidation products), lipids (peroxidation), and DNA (base modification and strand breaks) (Gredilla and Barja 2005). In this chapter, I briefly review emerging evidence that dietary energy intake influences key processes involved in the pathogenesis of Alzheimer disease.

Risk Factors for Alzheimer Disease

Dietary Energy Intake

Although the evidence is not yet as compelling as it is for cardiovascular disease and diabetes, emerging findings do suggest that excessive dietary energy intake is a risk factor for Alzheimer disease. In a prospective epidemiological study of 980 elderly subjects (mean age=75.3±5.8 years) in New York City who were free of dementia at baseline, in whom 242 incident cases of Alzheimer disease developed during more than 4,000 person-years of follow-up, individuals with the highest caloric intake had the greatest risk of developing Alzheimer disease (Luchsinger et al. 2002). In a study of 392 Swedish adults without dementia who were followed from age 70 to age 88, those who were overweight were more likely to develop Alzheimer disease than those who were not overweight, an association that was greater in women than in men (Gustafson et al. 2003).

Diabetes

Data from epidemiological studies suggest that diabetes is a risk factor for cognitive impairment and dementia (Launer 2005), which may be due to the effects of hyperglycemia and hyperinsulinemia and/or comorbidities such as hypertension and perturbed lipid metabolism. In a prospective, population-based cohort study of 6,370 elderly subjects, diabetes almost doubled the risk of dementia (Ott et al. 1999). In a community-based controlled study, the prevalence of type 2 diabetes and hyperglycemia was significantly greater in Alzheimer disease patients than in age-matched control subjects (Janson et al. 2004). A positive correlation was also seen between the duration of diabetes and the amount of diffuse and neuritic Aβ plaques in the Alzheimer disease subjects. In a longitudinal study of 1,301 subjects age 75 years and older without dementia who were examined twice over 6 years, those with diabetes were at greater risk of Alzheimer disease (Xu et al. 2004). In a study in which 683 subjects without prevalent dementia were followed for 3,691 person-years, the rate of Alzheimer disease was double in subjects with hyperinsulinemia, and those subjects also exhibited a significant decline in memory-related cognitive scores compared with subjects without hyperinsulinemia (Luchsinger et al. 2004a).

Although the vast majority of studies point to a negative impact of diabetes on the aging brain that may increase the risk of Alzheimer disease, subjects with diabetes are not destined to develop Alzheimer disease. Indeed, a study by Beeri et al. (2005), involving 268 autopsy cases, showed that individuals with diabetes who lived into their eighties exhibited fewer Alzheimer disease–related pathological alterations (neuritic plaques and neurofibrillary tangles) in the hippocampus than did age-matched nondiabetic subjects. Perhaps individuals who are resistant to the adverse effects of diabetes on the cardiovascular system (the major cause of death in patients with diabetes) are also resistant to its adverse effects on the brain.

Mouse Models of Diet's Role in Conferring Risk

Studies of mouse models of Alzheimer disease have provided evidence that high-energy, diabetes-promoting diets accelerate the Alzheimer disease process. When β-amyloid precursor protein (APP) mutant mice were maintained on a diabetes-promoting diet, γ-secretase activity, production of $A\beta_{1-40}$ and $A\beta_{1-42}$, and amyloid plaque burden increased significantly (Ho et al. 2004). This study demonstrated that the hyperinsulinemic diet also caused a decrease in levels of insulin-degrading enzyme and decreased phosphorylation of glycogen synthase kinase–3α (GSK-3α), which were associated with decreased activation of the insulin signaling pathway. Craft (2005) reported findings suggesting that excessive insulin induces increases in levels of Aβ and inflammatory cytokines that have deleterious effects on memory. Julien et al. (2008) found that a diabetogenic diet high in fat and glucose worsens performance in a triple-transgenic animal model of Alzheimer disease (mice with APP, presenilin-1, and tau mutations, as described in Oddo et al. 2003) in water maze tasks, suggesting an adverse effect of such diets on synaptic plasticity and cognitive function.

Benefits of Dietary Energy Restriction

Neuron Protection

Several laboratories have found that dietary energy restriction can protect neurons in the brains of rats and mice against insults relevant to the pathogenesis of Alzheimer disease. When rats were maintained for 3 months on an intermittent fasting/dietary restriction regimen (an alternate-day feeding regimen), pyramidal neurons in the hippocampus were more resistant to being damaged by the excitotoxin kainic acid, which correlated with preservation of learning and memory ability compared with control rats on an ad libitum diet (Bruce-Keller et al. 1999). Similar results were obtained by Sharma and Kaur (2005), who reported that the same dietary restriction regimen increased the expression of heat shock protein 70 and antioxidant enzymes in brain cells. Dietary restriction protected γ-aminobutyric acid–ergic neurons in the hippocampus and the olfactory-entorhinal cortex, and to a lesser extent protected forebrain cholinergic neurons, against excitotoxic degeneration in a study by Contestabile et al. (2004). Conversely, the hippocampal neurons of obese mice were more vulnerable to being damaged by kainic acid compared with control mice in a study by Sriram et al. (2002). Dietary energy restriction has been shown to suppress oxidative stress and inflammation caused by excitotoxic neuronal injury (Lee et al. 2003) or diabetes (Ugochukwu et al. 2006). Dietary restriction can also protect neurons in several different regions of the brain (including the cerebral cortex, striatum, hippocampus, and substantia nigra) against death caused by oxidative and metabolic stress (Z.F. Yu and Mattson 1999).

It has been reported that dietary restriction suppresses the development of amyloid pathology in mouse models of Alzheimer disease. Patel et al. (2005) found that the accumulation of Aβ plaques was significantly decreased in APP mutant and APP/presenilin-1 double-mutant mice maintained on an energy restriction diet for 6 and 14 weeks, respectively. The diet also resulted in a reduction in glial cell activation, suggesting a suppression of inflammatory processes. Wang et al. (2005) also found that dietary energy restriction reduces amyloid pathology in APP mutant mice, and suggested this was the result of enhanced activity of α-secretase, the enzyme that cleaves APP in the middle of the Aβ sequence, thereby preventing Aβ production. Halagappa and I have extended the evidence that dietary restriction can suppress pathogenic processes in Alzheimer disease by showing that both intermittent fasting and 40% dietary restriction ameliorate learning and memory deficits, and suppress amyloid pathology, in a triple-transgenic mouse model of Alzheimer disease (Halagappa et al. 2007). Dietary restriction may also protect neurons against genetic mutations that cause early-onset Alzheimer disease. For example, intermittent fasting protected hippocampal neurons against pathogenic effects of a presenilin-1 mutation in presenilin-1 mutant knock-in mice (Zhu et al. 1999).

Enhancement of Neuroplasticity

Dietary energy restriction enhances synaptic plasticity and may also influence neurogenesis. In humans, insulin resistance, high-calorie diets, and diabetes are associated with declining cognitive function (Greenwood and Winocur 2005). Age-related impairments of learning and memory are attenuated in rats and mice maintained on dietary restriction regimens during their adult life, as demonstrated by Idrobo et al. (1987). In another study, lifelong dietary energy restriction completely prevented the age-related deficits in long-term potentiation and N-methyl-D-aspartate receptor expression in rats (Eckles-Smith et al. 2000).

Dietary energy restriction may enhance neurogenesis and recovery from injury. When rats or mice were maintained on an intermittent fasting regimen, hippocampal neurogenesis increased (Lee et al. 2002). Rather than increasing the proliferation of neural progenitor cells, dietary restriction increased the survival of newly generated neurons. In another study, mice were maintained on ad libitum or energy restriction diets beginning at age 2 months; at ages 12, 18, and 24 months the mice were injected with bromodeoxyuridine to label proliferating cells. Progenitor cell proliferation decreased with advancing age, and this was not affected by caloric restriction; however, caloric restriction promoted the survival of hilar glial cells (Bondolfi et al. 2004). Other studies have provided evidence that overeating can impair neurogenesis. For example, rats rendered diabetic by treatment with streptozotocin exhibited reduced proliferation of neural progenitor cells in the dentate gyrus of the hippocampus (Jackson-Guilford et al. 2000). A subsequent study provided evidence that diabetes inhibits neurogenesis, an effect that was reversed by treatment with the antidepressant fluoxetine (Beauquis et al. 2006). My colleagues and I recently reported that hippocampal neurogenesis, synaptic plasticity, and cognitive function are impaired in animal models of type 1 and type 2 diabetes, and provided evidence that the adrenal stress hormone corticosterone mediates these adverse effects of diabetes on the hippocampus (Stranahan et al. 2008). The available data therefore suggest that dietary energy restriction can enhance neurogenesis and gliogenesis by promoting the survival of newly generated neurons and glia, whereas overeating and diabetes may adversely affect these processes.

Cellular and Molecular Mechanisms

Considerable evidence supports a pivotal role for oxidative stress in the pathogenesis of Alzheimer disease, including the following:

- Accumulation of advanced glycation end products in the cerebrospinal fluid and within neurons in Alzheimer disease patients (Luth et al. 2005)
- Increased oxidative damage to proteins, lipids, and DNA in neurons involved in the amyloid and tau pathologies in Alzheimer disease (Markesbery 1997)

- Involvement of oxidative stress in the neurotoxic effects of Aβ (Kruman et al. 1997)

A major source of free radicals in most cells, including neurons, is mitochondrial oxidative phosphorylation. Because dietary energy intake (i.e., calories) provides the fuel for oxidative phosphorylation, it is not surprising that considerable attention has been paid to the role of oxidative stress in the adverse effects of excessive energy intake on the brain and, conversely, the beneficial effects of dietary energy restriction. Dietary energy restriction suppresses age-related increases in oxidative damage to proteins, lipids, and DNA in the brain (Forster et al. 2000). Oxidative stress and inflammation were increased in the brains of diabetic rats and ameliorated by dietary energy restriction (Ugochukwu et al. 2006). Oxidative stress was increased in mitochondria from the brains of diabetic rats (Mastrocola et al. 2005), and the production of hydrogen peroxide by brain mitochondria from diabetic rats was exacerbated by Aβ (Moreira et al. 2005). Together with a decrease in oxidative stress, dietary restriction may stabilize neuronal calcium homeostasis during aging. Evidence of this was found in a study in which dietary restriction prevented the aging-related enhancement of dendritic spike–mediated calcium accumulation in CA1 pyramidal neurons of rats (Hemond and Jaffe 2005). Dietary energy restriction also prevented the aging-associated increase in the slow, postburst hyperpolarization, suggesting that it may preserve synaptic plasticity and learning ability during aging by stabilizing neuronal calcium homeostasis (Hemond and Jaffe 2005). Dietary energy restriction may also protect neurons by upregulating the expression of antiapoptotic proteins (Yu and Mattson 1999; Maswood et al. 2004). For example, dietary energy restriction increased the expression of ARC (apoptosis repressor with a caspase recruitment domain) in the brains of aged rats, an effect correlated with a reduction in age-related neuronal apoptosis (Shelke and Leeuwenburgh 2003).

A second mechanism by which dietary energy intake may affect the pathogenesis of Alzheimer disease is by modifying the ability of neurons to cope with various types of stress, including oxidative, metabolic, and excitotoxic stress (Figure 11–1). It has been established that the ability of organisms to respond adaptively to stress diminishes with advancing age, and that dietary restriction can increase stress resistance (Wan et al. 2003). This age-related susceptibility to stress is evident at the cellular level. When exposed to stress (heat, oxidative, metabolic, etc.), cells in young animals exhibit robust upregulation of the expression of protein chaperones and antioxidant pathways, whereas cells in old animals do not (B.P. Yu and Chung 2001). My colleagues and I have found that dietary restriction enhances the ability of neurons in the rat brain to resist various types of stress, including ischemia,

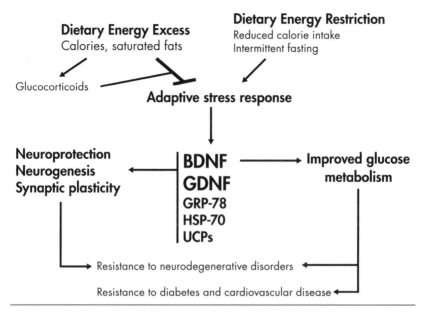

Dietary Energy Excess
Calories, saturated fats

Dietary Energy Restriction
Reduced calorie intake
Intermittent fasting

Glucocorticoids

Adaptive stress response

Neuroprotection
Neurogenesis
Synaptic plasticity

BDNF
GDNF
GRP-78
HSP-70
UCPs

Improved glucose
metabolism

Resistance to neurodegenerative disorders

Resistance to diabetes and cardiovascular disease

FIGURE 11–1. Pathways involved in the beneficial effects of dietary energy restriction, and the adverse effects of dietary energy excess, on the brain.

Dietary energy restriction stimulates neurons in ways that activate pathways leading to increased expression of genes that encode proteins that promote the survival and plasticity (synaptic function and neurogenesis) of neurons. Such proteins include brain-derived neurotrophic factor (BDNF), glial cell line–derived neurotrophic factor (GDNF), glucose-regulated protein 78 (GRP-78), heat shock protein 70 (HSP-70), and mitochondrial uncoupling proteins (UCPs). Recent findings suggest that BDNF signaling in the brain can improve peripheral glucose metabolism and cardiovascular function, and may thereby contribute to the protective effects of dietary energy restriction against diabetes and cardiovascular disease. Excessive dietary energy intake adversely affects the brain by impairing the ability of cells to respond to stress; adrenal glucocorticoids (cortisol in humans and corticosterone in rodents) may mediate, in part, the adverse effects of overeating on neuronal plasticity and vulnerability to disease.

excitotoxicity, and exposure to mitochondrial toxins (Bruce-Keller et al. 1999; Z.F. Yu and Mattson 1999). This stress resistance is associated with increased levels of certain protein chaperones (heat shock protein 70 and glucose-regulated protein 78), neurotrophic factors (brain-derived neurotrophic factor [BDNF] and glial cell line–derived neurotrophic factor), and mitochondrial uncoupling proteins (Z.F. Yu and Mattson 1999).

There is evidence to suggest that adaptive cellular stress response mechanisms may be compromised in Alzheimer disease. Levels of several neurotrophic factors and/or their receptors were reported to be diminished in

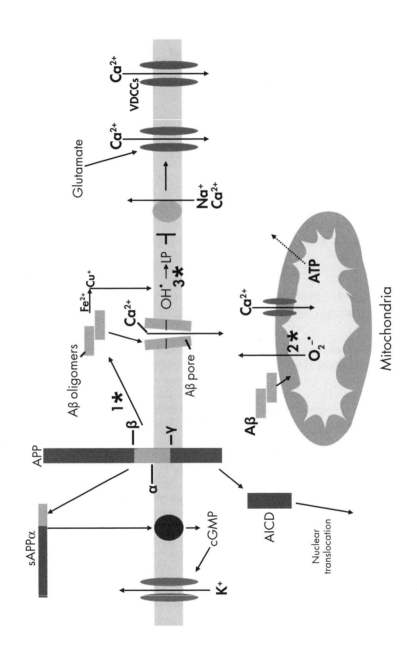

FIGURE 11–2. **Possible mechanisms by which dietary energy intake modifies the processes responsible for amyloid pathology and cognitive impairment in Alzheimer disease (*opposite*).**

Three sites at which dietary energy intake may influence the Alzheimer disease process (marked by *) are 1) proteolytic processing of the β-amyloid precursor protein (APP), 2) mitochondrial production of free radicals, and 3) membrane-associated oxidative stress. Dietary energy restriction may suppress all three processes, whereas overeating may exacerbate all three processes. Sequential cleavages of APP by β- and γ-secretases generates the amyloid-β peptide (Aβ), which can form peptide oligomers that insert into the plasma membrane and form Ca^{2+}-conducting pores. Amyloid-β peptide oligomers (Aβ oligomers) may also interact with Fe^{2+} and Cu^+ to generate hydrogen peroxide and hydroxyl radicals ($OH^{\bullet}$), resulting in membrane lipid peroxidation (LP), which impairs the function of membrane ion–motive adenosine triphosphatases (ATPases) (Na^+ and Ca^{2+} pumps). LP thereby promotes membrane depolarization and Ca^{2+} influx through glutamate receptors and voltage-dependent channels (VDCCs). Excessive caloric intake promotes mitochondrial free radical (superoxide anion radical; $O_2^{-\bullet}$) production, Ca^{2+} overload, and decreased ATP production. Nonamyloidogenic APP processing generates a secreted form of APP (sAPPα) that can activate a signaling pathway involving cyclic guanosine monophosphate (cGMP); this pathway activates K^+ channels, hyperpolarizes the membrane, and reduces Ca^{2+} influx. α=α-secretase; AICD=APP intracellular domain; β=β-secretase; γ=γ-secretase. Perpendicular lines indicate "inhibitory" and arrows indicate "stimulatory."

Source. Adapted from Bezprozvanny and Mattson 2008, p. 455.

brain tissue samples from Alzheimer disease patients compared with age-matched control subjects (Siegel and Chauhan 2000). Impaired proteasome function has been documented in analyses of brain tissue samples from Alzheimer disease patients and in cultured neurons exposed to Aβ (Ding and Keller 2003), suggesting that the protein chaperone capabilities of neurons are diminished (or overwhelmed) in Alzheimer disease. In addition, the ability of neurons to withstand excitotoxic, oxidative, and metabolic stress is compromised when they are exposed to Aβ (Goodman and Mattson 1994), suggesting that the accumulation of Aβ may render neurons vulnerable to stress during aging and in Alzheimer disease. High-energy diets also render neurons vulnerable to excitotoxic and oxidative insults, whereas dietary energy restriction protects neurons against such stressors (Bruce-Keller et al. 1999; Patel et al. 2005; Zhu et al. 1999). It is therefore likely that dietary energy excess promotes Alzheimer disease by impairing neuronal stress resistance, whereas dietary energy restriction protects against Alzheimer disease by enhancing neuronal stress resistance (Figure 11–2).

Tau is a microtubule-associated protein that dissociates from microtubules and self-aggregates to form the filamentous neurofibrillary tangles within neurons affected in Alzheimer disease (Mattson 2004). Cellular stress response pathways and oxidative stress may also be pivotal modulators of tau. In this view, high-energy diets would promote tau hyperphosphorylation and aggregation by inhibiting adaptive stress response pathways and increasing oxidative stress. There is considerable evidence that glycogen synthase kinase–3 (GSK-3) contributes to the hyperphosphorylation and aggregation of tau in neurons in Alzheimer disease (Balaraman et al. 2006). GSK-3 exhibits full kinase activity under basal (nonphosphorylated) conditions, and is inactivated when phosphorylated by Akt kinase. Interestingly, two signaling pathways that inhibit GSK-3 are those activated by insulin and BDNF. Excessive energy intake impairs insulin and BDNF signaling, whereas dietary restriction enhances these signaling pathways (Mattson et al. 2004). GSK-3 may therefore be a key mediator of the neurofibrillary tangle–promoting effects of excessive energy intake and diabetes (Freude et al. 2005). A role for the cyclin-dependent kinase CDK5 in the mechanism by which high-energy diets and diabetes promote tau pathology has been suggested (Ubeda et al. 2004). Overactivation of CDK5 has been associated with tau pathology in Alzheimer disease, and experimental findings suggest that high levels of extracellular glucose result in increased CDK5 activity (Ubeda et al. 2004).

The elevated cellular oxidative stress associated with excessive dietary energy intake and diabetes may also contribute to tau pathology in Alzheimer disease. The tau in neurofibrillary tangles is glycated, consistent with increased oxidative stress playing a role in tau pathology (Yan et al. 1994). Oxidative stress can promote tau hyperphosphorylation and aggregation. For example, covalent modification of tau by the lipid peroxidation product 4-hydroxynonenal inhibits tau dephosphorylation (Mattson et al. 1997), and peroxynitrite promotes tau aggregation and microtubule depolymerization (Reynolds et al. 2006). The available evidence suggests that Aβ promotes tau pathology by inducing oxidative stress (Markesbery 1997) and by impairing insulin and BDNF signaling (Steen et al. 2005).

Other Dietary Factors

Diets with high amounts of cholesterol and saturated fats adversely affect the brain during aging, whereas diets rich in omega-3 fatty acids such as docosahexaenoic acid (DHA) may counteract the aging process and protect against cognitive impairment (for review, see Cole et al. 2005). Epidemiological data suggest that individuals who consume foods with high amounts of cholesterol and saturated fats are at increased risk of age-related cognitive decline and Alzheimer disease (Morris et al. 2005). On the other hand, individuals who consume foods such as fish with high levels of omega-3 fatty acids may be protected against age-related memory impairment (Morris et al. 2005). In a mouse model of Alzheimer disease, compared with a regular soy-based diet, a typical Western diet with 40% saturated fatty acids and 1% cholesterol increased the accumulation of Aβ in the brain, whereas a diet supplemented with DHA decreased Aβ levels (Oksman et al. 2006). Experimental findings suggest that elevated levels of membrane-associated cholesterol can result in increased production of Aβ (Abad-Rodriguez et al. 2004), and treatment of mice with a cholesterol-lowering statin (simvastatin) improved cognitive function without affecting Aβ levels (L. Li et al. 2006).

In addition, the only genetic risk factor for Alzheimer disease that has thus far been identified involves the cholesterol transport protein apolipoprotein E (Y. Li and Grupe 2007). A diet enriched with DHA reduced the accumulation of Aβ and dystrophic changes in the dendrites of neurons in the brain in a mouse model of Alzheimer disease (Lim et al. 2005). However, the results of another study suggest that omega-6 fatty acids are associated with impaired cognitive performance, whereas elevated omega-3 fatty acid levels may not affect cognitive performance (Arendash et al. 2007). The mechanisms by which dietary lipids affect neuronal vulnerability during aging are not understood but likely involve effects on membrane-associated oxidative stress, protein processing and degradation, signal transduction, and cellular energy and ion homeostasis (Cutler et al. 2004).

The adverse consequences of dietary folic acid (folate) deficiency for the nervous system were first recognized more than 50 years ago, when it was found that babies born to folate-deficient mothers had an increased incidence of birth defects, which most often affected development of the nervous system (Sarwark 1996). However, only during the past decade has it become evident that dietary folate is also critical for the maintenance of brain function during aging. Individuals with low folate levels are at greater risk for depression, dementia, and Alzheimer disease (Mischoulon and Raab 2007). Alzheimer disease patients also exhibit elevated plasma homocysteine levels (McCaddon et al. 1998). Epidemiological findings suggest that individuals with elevated plasma homocysteine levels are at increased risk of developing Alzheimer disease (Seshadri et al. 2002), although other studies have not shown an association between homocysteine levels and Alzheimer disease risk (Luchsinger et al. 2004b).

The mechanism by which low dietary folate levels adversely affect the brain involves, at least in part, an increase in the levels of homocysteine (Mattson and Shea 2003). Folate plays a critical role in one-carbon metabolism by promoting the remethylation of homocysteine to methionine, and folate deficiency therefore causes an increase in homocysteine levels and may lead to increased amounts of damaged DNA. Studies of cell culture and animal models of Alzheimer disease have shown that folate deficiency and elevated homocysteine levels can render neurons vulnerable to Aβ toxicity by a mechanism involving DNA damage and apoptosis (Kruman et al. 2002).

Finally, emerging findings suggest the possibility that phytochemicals that have beneficial effects on the brain (and may protect against Alzheimer disease) exert their effects by activating hormetic pathways. *Hormesis* is the process in which exposure of neurons to a mild stress, such as increased synaptic activity and energetic stress, induces the expression of genes that encode neuroprotective proteins, including protein chaperones and neurotrophic factors. I have written an article on this topic that includes specific examples and references (Mattson 2008). Although much emphasis has been placed on the antioxidant activity of phytochemicals as being central to their health-promoting actions, recent findings suggest that a different, hormesis-based mechanism accounts for their ability to protect cells against disease (Mattson and Cheng 2006). Beneficial chemicals in red grapes (resveratrol), broccoli (sulforaphane), green tea and cocoa (epicatechins), and turmeric (curcumin) have each been shown to activate adaptive cellular stress response pathways. Such phytochemicals have demonstrated the ability to reduce Aβ pathology and/or protect neurons against Aβ toxicity and oxidative stress in experimental models of Alzheimer disease (van Praag et al. 2007). The pathways involve transcription factors such as Nrf-2, CREB, and NF-κB, which induce the expression of neuroprotective proteins, including antioxidant enzymes, protein chaperones, and neurotrophic factors (Mattson and Cheng 2006). It therefore appears that neurons are most healthy when they are periodically stimulated by factors that induce mild cellular stress, including dietary energy restriction and phytochemicals.

Conclusion

Environmental factors may influence the risk of Alzheimer disease, but the ways in which these factors modify the disease process at the cellular molecular level are unknown. Excessive energy intake and diabetes are associated with an increased risk of Alzheimer disease. There are two possible mechanisms by which dietary energy restriction may counteract the age-related changes that result in Aβ production and aggregation and neurofibrillary tau pathology. One mechanism involves suppression of membrane-associated oxidative stress, which stabilizes cellular energy and ion homeostasis and inhibits amyloidogenesis. A second mechanism involves hormesis (a process in which exposure of neurons to a mild stress induces the expression of genes that encode neuroprotective proteins; see "Other Dietary Factors"). There may be a central role for the latter mechanism in the Alzheimer disease risk–lowering effects of exercise, cognitive stimulation, and beneficial phytochemicals in fruits and vegetables (Adlard et al. 2005; Larson et al. 2006; Lazarov et al. 2005; Wilson et al. 2002).

KEY POINTS

▮ Data from epidemiological studies suggest that being overweight or having diabetes is a risk factor for cognitive impairment and dementia.

▮ Studies of mouse models of Alzheimer disease have provided evidence that high-energy, diabetes-promoting diets accelerate the Alzheimer disease process.

▮ Dietary energy restriction appears to protect neurons in the brains of rats and mice against insults relevant to the pathogenesis of Alzheimer disease.

▮ Dietary restriction also appears to enhance synaptic plasticity, as well as to increase neurogenesis after injury.

▮ Two possible mechanisms for the beneficial effect of dietary energy restriction on the brain are reduction of oxidative damage and enhancement of cellular resistance to stress.

▮ The latter mechanism may involve hormesis, in which exposure of neurons to a mild stress induces the expression of genes that encode neuroprotective proteins, including protein chaperones and neurotrophic factors. Hormesis may be a central mechanism in other aging-related interventions, such as cognitive stimulation and physical exercise.

References

Abad-Rodriguez J, Ledesma MD, Craessaerts K, et al: Neuronal membrane cholesterol loss enhances amyloid peptide generation. J Cell Biol 167:953–960, 2004

Adlard PA, Perreau VM, Pop V, et al: Voluntary exercise decreases amyloid load in a transgenic model of Alzheimer's disease. J Neurosci 25:4217–4221, 2005

Arendash GW, Jensen MT, Salem N Jr, et al: A diet high in omega-3 fatty acids does not improve or protect cognitive performance in Alzheimer's transgenic mice. Neuroscience 149:286–302, 2007

Balaraman Y, Limaye AR, Levey AI, et al: Glycogen synthase kinase 3beta and Alzheimer's disease: pathophysiological and therapeutic significance. Cell Mol Life Sci 63:1226–1235, 2006

Beauquis J, Roig P, Homo-Delarche F, et al: Reduced hippocampal neurogenesis and number of hilar neurones in streptozotocin-induced diabetic mice: reversion by antidepressant treatment. Eur J Neurosci 23:1539–1546, 2006

Beeri MS, Silverman JM, Davis KL, et al: Type 2 diabetes is negatively associated with Alzheimer's disease neuropathology. J Gerontol A Biol Sci Med Sci 60:471–475, 2005

Bezprozvanny I, Mattson MP: Neuronal calcium mishandling and the pathogenesis of Alzheimer's disease. Trends Neurosci 31:454–463, 2008

Bondolfi L, Ermini F, Long JM, et al: Impact of age and caloric restriction on neurogenesis in the dentate gyrus of C57BL/6 mice. Neurobiol Aging 25:333–340, 2004

Bray GA, Bellanger T: Epidemiology, trends, and morbidities of obesity and the metabolic syndrome. Endocrine 29:109–117, 2006

Bruce-Keller AJ, Umberger G, McFall R, et al: Food restriction reduces brain damage and improves behavioral outcome following excitotoxic and metabolic insults. Ann Neurol 45:8–15, 1999

Cole GM, Lim GP, Yang F, et al: Prevention of Alzheimer's disease: omega-3 fatty acid and phenolic anti-oxidant interventions. Neurobiol Aging 26 (suppl 1):133–136, 2005

Contestabile A, Ciani E, Contestabile A: Dietary restriction differentially protects from neurodegeneration in animal models of excitotoxicity. Brain Res 1002:162–166, 2004

Craft S: Insulin resistance syndrome and Alzheimer's disease: age- and obesity-related effects on memory, amyloid, and inflammation. Neurobiol Aging 26 (suppl):S65–S69, 2005

Cutler RG, Kelly J, Storie K, et al: Involvement of oxidative stress–induced abnormalities in ceramide and cholesterol metabolism in brain aging and Alzheimer's disease. Proc Natl Acad Sci USA 101:2070–2075, 2004

Ding Q, Keller JN: Does proteasome inhibition play a role in mediating neuropathology and neuron death in Alzheimer's disease? J Alzheimers Dis 5:241–245, 2003

Eckles-Smith K, Clayton D, Bickford P, et al: Caloric restriction prevents age-related deficits in LTP and in NMDA receptor expression. Mol Brain Res 78:154–162, 2000

Floyd RA, Hensley K: Oxidative stress in brain aging: implications for therapeutics of neurodegenerative diseases. Neurobiol Aging 23:795–807, 2002

Forster MJ, Sohal BH, Sohal RS: Reversible effects of long-term caloric restriction on protein oxidative damage. J Gerontol A Biol Sci Med Sci 55:522–529, 2000

Freude S, Plum L, Schnitker J, et al: Peripheral hyperinsulinemia promotes tau phosphorylation in vivo. Diabetes 54:3343–3348, 2005

Goodman Y, Mattson MP: Secreted forms of beta-amyloid precursor protein protect hippocampal neurons against amyloid beta-peptide-induced oxidative injury. Exp Neurol 128:1–12, 1994

Gredilla R, Barja G: Minireview: the role of oxidative stress in relation to caloric restriction and longevity. Endocrinology 146:3713–3717, 2005

Greenwood CE, Winocur G: High-fat diets, insulin resistance and declining cognitive function. Neurobiol Aging 26:S42–S45, 2005

Gustafson D, Rothenberg E, Blennow K, et al: An 18-year follow-up of overweight and risk of Alzheimer disease. Arch Intern Med 163:1524–1528, 2003

Halagappa VK, Guo Z, Pearson M, et al: Intermittent fasting and caloric restriction ameliorate age-related behavioral deficits in the triple-transgenic mouse model of Alzheimer's disease. Neurobiol Dis 26:212–220. 2007

Hemond P, Jaffe DB: Caloric restriction prevents aging-associated changes in spike-mediated Ca2+ accumulation and the slow afterhyperpolarization in hippocampal CA1 pyramidal neurons. Neuroscience 135:413–420, 2005

Ho L, Qin W, Pompl PN, et al: Diet-induced insulin resistance promotes amyloidosis in a transgenic mouse model of Alzheimer's disease. FASEB J 18:902–904, 2004

Hunt ND, Hyun DH, Allard JS, et al: Bioenergetics of aging and calorie restriction. Ageing Res Rev 5:125–143, 2006

Idrobo F, Nandy K, Mostofsky DI, et al: Dietary restriction: effects on radial maze learning and lipofuscin pigment deposition in the hippocampus and frontal cortex. Arch Gerontol Geriatr 6:355–362, 1987

Jackson-Guilford J, Leander JD, Nisenbaum LK: The effect of streptozotocin-induced diabetes on cell proliferation in the rat dentate gyrus. Neurosci Lett 293:91–94, 2000

Janson J, Laedtke T, Parisi JE, et al: Increased risk of type 2 diabetes in Alzheimer disease. Diabetes 53:474–481, 2004

Julien C, Tremblay C, Phivilay A, et al: High-fat diet aggravates amyloid-beta and tau pathologies in the 3xTg-AD mouse model. Neurobiol Aging October 14, 2008 (Epub ahead of print)

Kruman I, Bruce-Keller AJ, Bredesen D, et al: Evidence that 4-hydroxynonenal mediates oxidative stress–induced neuronal apoptosis. J Neurosci 17:5089–5100, 1997

Kruman II, Kumaravel TS, Lohani A, et al: Folic acid deficiency and homocysteine impair DNA repair in hippocampal neurons and sensitize them to amyloid toxicity in experimental models of Alzheimer's disease. J Neurosci 22:1752–1762, 2002

Larson EB, Wang L, Bowen JD, et al: Exercise is associated with reduced risk for incident dementia among persons 65 years of age and older. Ann Intern Med 144:73–81, 2006

Launer LJ: Diabetes and brain aging: epidemiologic evidence. Curr Diab Rep 5:59–63, 2005

Lazarov O, Robinson J, Tang YP, et al: Environmental enrichment reduces Abeta levels and amyloid deposition in transgenic mice. Cell 120:701–713, 2005

Le Bourg E: Delaying aging: could the study of hormesis be more helpful than that of the genetic pathway used to survive starvation? Biogerontology 4:319–324, 2003

Lee J, Duan W, Mattson MP: Evidence that brain-derived neurotrophic factor is required for basal neurogenesis and mediates, in part, the enhancement of neurogenesis by dietary restriction in the hippocampus of adult mice. J Neurochem 82:1367–1375, 2002

Lee J, Auyeung WW, Mattson MP: Interactive effects of excitotoxic injury and dietary restriction on microgliosis and neurogenesis in the hippocampus of adult mice. Neuromolecular Med 4:179–196, 2003

Li L, Cao D, Kim H, et al: Simvastatin enhances learning and memory independent of amyloid load in mice. Ann Neurol 60:729–739, 2006

Li Y, Grupe A: Genetics of late-onset Alzheimer's disease: progress and prospect. Pharmacogenomics 8:1747–1755, 2007

Lim GP, Calon F, Morihara T, et al: A diet enriched with the omega-3 fatty acid docosahexaenoic acid reduces amyloid burden in an aged Alzheimer mouse model. J Neurosci 25:3032–3040, 2005

Luchsinger JA, Tang MX, Shea S, et al: Caloric intake and the risk of Alzheimer disease. Arch Neurol 59:1258–1263, 2002

Luchsinger JA, Tang MX, Shea S, et al: Hyperinsulinemia and risk of Alzheimer disease. Neurology 63:1187–1192, 2004a

Luchsinger JA, Tang MX, Shea S, et al: Plasma homocysteine levels and risk of Alzheimer disease. Neurology 62:1972–1976, 2004b

Luth HJ, Ogunlade V, Kuhla B, et al: Age- and stage-dependent accumulation of advanced glycation end products in intracellular deposits in normal and Alzheimer's disease brains. Cereb Cortex 15:211–220, 2005

Markesbery WR: Oxidative stress hypothesis in Alzheimer's disease. Free Radic Biol Med 23:134–147, 1997

Mastrocola R, Restivo F, Vercellinatto I, et al: Oxidative and nitrosative stress in brain mitochondria of diabetic rats. J Endocrinol 187:37–44, 2005

Maswood N, Young J, Tilmont E, et al: Caloric restriction increases neurotrophic factor levels and attenuates neurochemical and behavioral deficits in a primate model of Parkinson's disease. Proc Natl Acad Sci USA 101:18171–18176, 2004

Mattson MP: Pathways towards and away from Alzheimer's disease. Nature 430:631–639, 2004

Mattson MP: Awareness of hormesis will enhance future research in basic and applied neuroscience. Crit Rev Toxicol 38:633–639. 2008

Mattson MP, Cheng A: Neurohormetic phytochemicals: low-dose toxins that induce adaptive neuronal stress responses. Trends Neurosci 29:632–639, 2006

Mattson MP, Shea TB: Folate and homocysteine metabolism in neural plasticity and neurodegenerative disorders. Trends Neurosci 26:137–146, 2003

Mattson MP, Fu W, Waeg G, et al: 4-Hydroxynonenal, a product of lipid peroxidation, inhibits dephosphorylation of the microtubule-associated protein tau. Neuroreport 8:2275–2281, 1997

Mattson MP, Maudsley S, Martin B: A neural signaling triumvirate that influences ageing and age-related disease: insulin/IGF-1, BDNF and serotonin. Ageing Res Rev 3:445–464, 2004

McCaddon A, Davies G, Hudson P, et al: Total serum homocysteine in senile dementia of Alzheimer type. Int J Geriatr Psychiatry 13:235–239, 1998

Mischoulon D, Raab MF: The role of folate in depression and dementia. J Clin Psychiatry 68 (suppl 10):28–33, 2007

Moreira PI, Santos MS, Sena C, et al: Insulin protects against amyloid beta–peptide toxicity in brain mitochondria of diabetic rats. Neurobiol Dis 18:628–637, 2005

Morris MC, Evans DA, Tangney CC, et al: Fish consumption and cognitive decline with age in a large community study. Arch Neurol 62:1849–1853, 2005

Oddo S, Caccamo A, Shepherd JD, et al: Triple-transgenic model of Alzheimer's disease with plaques and tangles: intracellular Abeta and synaptic dysfunction. Neuron 39:409–421, 2003

Oksman M, Iivonen H, Hogyes E, et al: Impact of different saturated fatty acid, polyunsaturated fatty acid and cholesterol containing diets on beta-amyloid accumulation in APP/PS1 transgenic mice. Neurobiol Dis 23:563–572, 2006

Ott A, Stolk RP, van Harskamp F, et al: Diabetes mellitus and the risk of dementia: the Rotterdam Study. Neurology 53:1937–1942, 1999

Patel NV, Gordon MN, Connor KE, et al: Caloric restriction attenuates Abeta-deposition in Alzheimer transgenic models. Neurobiol Aging 26:995–1000, 2005

Reynolds MR, Lukas TJ, Berry RW, et al: Peroxynitrite-mediated tau modifications stabilize preformed filaments and destabilize microtubules through distinct mechanisms. Biochemistry 45:4314–4326, 2006

Sarwark JF: Spina bifida. Pediatr Clin North Am 43:1151–1158, 1996

Seshadri S, Beiser A, Selhub J, et al: Plasma homocysteine as a risk factor for dementia and Alzheimer's disease. N Engl J Med 346:476–483, 2002

Sharma S, Kaur G: Neuroprotective potential of dietary restriction against kainate-induced excitotoxicity in adult male Wistar rats. Brain Res Bull 67:482–491, 2005

Shelke RR, Leeuwenburgh C: Lifelong caloric restriction increases expression of apoptosis repressor with a caspase recruitment domain (ARC) in the brain. FASEB J 17:494–496, 2003

Siegel GJ, Chauhan NB: Neurotrophic factors in Alzheimer's and Parkinson's disease brain. Brain Res Rev 33:199–227, 2000

Sinclair DA: Toward a unified theory of caloric restriction and longevity regulation. Mech Ageing Dev 126:987–1002, 2005

Sriram K, Benkovic SA, Miller DB, et al: Obesity exacerbates chemically induced neurodegeneration. Neuroscience 115:1335–1346, 2002

Steen E, Terry BM, Rivera EJ, et al: Impaired insulin and insulin-like growth factor expression and signaling mechanisms in Alzheimer's disease—is this type 3 diabetes? J Alzheimers Dis 7:63–80, 2005

Stranahan AM, Arumugam TV, Cutler RG, et al: Diabetes impairs hippocampal function through glucocorticoid-mediated effects on new and mature neurons. Nat Neurosci 11:309–317, 2008

Ubeda M, Kemp DM, Habener JF: Glucose-induced expression of the cyclin-dependent protein kinase 5 activator p35 involved in Alzheimer's disease regulates insulin gene transcription in pancreatic beta-cells. Endocrinology 145:3023–3031, 2004

Ugochukwu NH, Mukes JD, Figgers CL: Ameliorative effects of dietary caloric restriction on oxidative stress and inflammation in the brain of streptozotocin-induced diabetic rats. Clin Chim Acta 370:165–173, 2006

van Praag H, Lucero MJ, Yeo GW, et al: Plant-derived flavanol (−)epicatechin enhances angiogenesis and retention of spatial memory in mice. J Neurosci 27:5869–5878, 2007

Wan R, Camandola S, Mattson MP: Intermittent food deprivation improves cardiovascular and neuroendocrine responses to stress in rats. J Nutr 133:1921–1929, 2003

Wang J, Ho L, Qin W, et al: Caloric restriction attenuates beta-amyloid neuropathology in a mouse model of Alzheimer's disease. FASEB J 19:659–661, 2005

Xu WL, Qiu CX, Wahlin A, et al: Diabetes mellitus and risk of dementia in the Kungsholmen project: a 6-year follow-up study. Neurology 63:1181–1186, 2004

Yan SD, Chen X, Schmidt AM, et al: Glycated tau protein in Alzheimer disease: a mechanism for induction of oxidant stress. Proc Natl Acad Sci USA 91:7787–7791, 1994

Yu BP, Chung HY: Stress resistance by caloric restriction for longevity. Ann N Y Acad Sci 928:39–47, 2001

Yu ZF, Mattson MP: Dietary restriction and 2-deoxyglucose administration reduce focal ischemic brain damage and improve behavioral outcome: evidence for a preconditioning mechanism. J Neurosci Res 57:830–839, 1999

Zhu H, Guo Q, Mattson MP: Dietary restriction protects hippocampal neurons against the death-promoting action of a presenilin-1 mutation. Brain Res 842:224–229, 1999

12 Molecular Genetic Building Blocks of Successful Cognitive and Emotional Aging

Brinda K. Rana, Ph.D.

Aging is a physiological process impacting all organisms—one that is typically gradual, associated with losses and gains, and marked by reduced fecundity and increased risk of mortality and susceptibility to disease. *Successful aging* can be characterized by longevity and also by the sustained ability of individuals to perform essential physical and cognitive functions in old age. Understanding the molecular genetic bases underlying successful aging and the environmental factors that influence genetic expression can help us develop effective therapeutic and disease preventive strategies to increase the likelihood that the majority of the population will achieve successful cognitive and physical aging. In this chapter, I use the term *molecular genetics* to refer to the complex interactions among the multitude of systems within a cell, particularly emphasizing the interactions among DNA, RNA,

This work was supported, in part, by National Institute of Mental Health Grant MH080002 and by the Department of Veterans Affairs.

and protein biosynthesis, and the mechanisms governing these interactions. I describe concepts in molecular genetics that may be applied to unlock the mysteries in the biological processes leading to successful aging. Studies in this area will enable us to determine harmful genetic variants, elucidate the underlying biological systems and processes determining whether an individual ages successfully, and determine the mechanisms by which nongenetic factors (e.g., diet and lifestyle) play a role in successful aging. It is the ultimate goal of these studies to identify targets for therapeutic and lifestyle interventions that will promote successful aging and prevent age-related disease (e.g., dementia) in middle-aged populations.

Genes and Aging

It is often heard in the popular media that researchers have found *the* gene for a particular disease. Although such reports hold true for relatively rare single-gene disorders such as cystic fibrosis, identifying *the* gene governing aging is unlikely, because genes work together in gene networks through a complex interplay of DNA and environmental factors to result in the phenotypes observed in aging. Unraveling the complexity of these gene networks, the interactions among genes, and the interactions between genes and the environment that lead to the expression of phenotypes has been a daunting task.

Over the past three decades, the race for the completion of the Human Genome Project and subsequent data generated by its successor, the International HapMap Project (an international effort to develop a haplotype map of the human genome), have led to rapid development of numerous high-throughput genomic technologies that have been applied to identifying genetic determinants of traits and diseases. In addition, these projects have resulted in a massive generation of genetic data and development of new statistical methodologies to analyze these data. This progress has brought us closer to understanding the mechanisms underlying the genetic basis of common traits and disease, but genomic medicine is still a long distance away from the kind of specificity and sensitivity needed for clinical decision making.

Successful cognitive aging thus is influenced by a combination of very small effects contributed by a number of variants of genes involved in multiple biological pathways, by environmental factors to which an individual is exposed throughout her or his lifetime, and by interactions of genes with each other and the environment. The interaction of gender with genes may also impact phenotypes associated with successful aging, thereby creating an additional dimension of complexity. Interwoven with these inherited and environmental factors are the mechanisms regulating the expression of the genes.

This chapter begins with a brief description of the epidemiological and genetic studies designed to characterize successful aging and using genetic association and genomewide approaches. Genes, however, are only the first step in the flow of genetic information in our cells. For physiological processes to proceed, the DNA sequence of a gene must be transcribed into a messenger (mRNA), which is then translated into a protein, the functional unit of biological pathways. A *gene expression profile* provides a global picture of the genes that are being actively transcribed in an individual at a given time based on the DNA sequence and the interaction of the individual's genome with his or her environment—either the lifetime accumulation of events or the immediate surroundings. Cells of different tissues have different gene expression profiles at the same time point in any organism. Researchers have just begun to investigate how an individual's gene expression profile relates to the individual's aging process and can be used as a phenotypic marker for successful aging. Investigations into the mechanisms controlling how gene expression is biologically and environmentally regulated are even less abundant. A few studies have implied that the processes regulating gene expression (e.g., those involving epigenetics and microRNAs) may be therapeutically or environmentally modified and are therefore an exciting new avenue in aging research.

Defining Successful Aging Traits for Genetic Association Studies

In a genetic association study, one tests whether there is a statistically significant association between differences in genotypes at a particular genetic marker and differences in a qualitatively or quantitatively measured trait. Identifying genetic associations for complex traits is complicated by the lack of precision in many phenotypes (e.g., cognitive health), as well as the interplay between genes and the environment, and because any given gene may only impart very small quantitative effects.

Foremost to a genetic association study of complex disease and traits is clearly defining the associated phenotypes and the ability to accurately measure candidate phenotypes. Measurable phenotypes of particular value are those that show high heritability, are related to gene products or pathways involved in aging, and have minimum or at least measurable environmental influences. The most commonly examined phenotype in aging studies has been longevity. Taken together, these studies have provided evidence that longevity is heritable, with reports that 25%–50% of individual variability is attributable to genetic factors (Herskind et al. 1996; Iachine et al. 1998; McGue et al. 1993). There are many reasons to look beyond longevity. For example, variability in longevity is likely to be impacted by modern health care and technology, and survival rates in people with chronic diseases such as cancer and cardiovascular disease continue to increase. Much less work has been done in characterizing the heritability of functioning, quality of life, and adaptation (Karasik et al. 2005).

The late age at onset (*late penetrance*) of many adverse events deterring an individual from achieving successful aging adds another complexity. One way geneticists handle such obstacles is by identifying simple monogenic (or intermediate) traits that are associated with their disease or trait of interest. *Intermediate traits* often display greater heritability than the primary trait itself; are less influenced by environmental factors; can often be elicited, and therefore measured, in younger individuals; and may suggest testable candidate genes for the primary trait itself. For example, performance measures on neuropsychological tests or brain imaging may serve as intermediate traits for successful cognitive aging.

Family studies, especially those employing twins, can be a powerful approach to determining the relative influence of genetic and environmental factors on intermediate traits. These studies provide genetic researchers with valuable information on the heritability of traits associated with their primary trait of interest and potential candidate genes. Highlighted here are examples of the type of knowledge that can be gained from twin and family studies on the heritability of traits associated with successful aging:

- A study by Finkel et al. (1995) enlisted 140 monozygotic twin pairs and 97 dizygotic twin pairs and collected demographic, cognitive, physiological, personality, and behavioral data on them. This study identified major environmental factors contributing to aging and revealed that the influence of genetic and environmental factors varied for different components of functional aging. Although limited by the available age range and small sample size, this study provided researchers with candidate intermediate phenotypes for further genetic studies.
- A much larger study on twins, by Gurland et al. (2004), assessed 1,384 monozygotic and 1,337 dizygotic twin pairs in a narrower age range of the eighth decade of life and showed that 20%–25% of age-related functional impairment in this population was attributable to genes.
- In the largest family study reported thus far, Frederiksen et al. (2002) phenotyped 9,300 adult children as a function of their parents' age at death with indices including 1) physical functioning measured by hand grip strength, 2) cognitive performance as determined by established tests such as the Mini-Mental State Examination, and 3) self-reported health and diseases. Advanced parental age was significantly associated with these indices of successful aging.

The results of these and other family studies allow genetic researchers to draw some general conclusions regarding genetic and environmental contributions to successful aging. Evidence suggests that successful aging is a multifactorial trait influenced by numerous genes and environmental factors, each making a small overall contribution to the phenotype. These family studies have shown that longevity and other indicators of the *health span* (e.g., the number of years during which we can enjoy a satisfactory quality of life) have a moderate degree of heritability, warranting a continued search for contributory genes and their variants. Finally, the variance unaccounted for by genes suggests that successful aging is influenced by an environmental component or yet-to-be-investigated molecular genetic factors that interact with the environment.

Candidate Genes for Successful Aging

A sensitive approach for identifying genetic contributors with small gene effects is to employ a case-control association study in which genetic allelic markers are used to identify genomic regions enriched in a specific trait-contributing allele among the cases (i.e., successful agers) and control subjects (i.e., nonsuccessful agers). Many case-control-based studies have been published in which one or several candidate genes were examined for association with successful aging phenotypes. Readers are referred to Glatt et al. (2007) for an extensive review of case-control studies on successful aging. The authors identified 29 publications on successful aging that examined at least one other characteristic of healthy aging in addition to longevity through case-control–based association studies as well as family, twin, and linkage studies. Some of the key candidate genes implicated in successful aging and referred to in this article are highlighted in Table 12–1. The genes are organized according to the biological processes related to successful aging for which the genes were examined. Highlighted below is a subset of the candidate genes implicated in successful aging through these studies.

1. Several of the genes implicated in successful aging are involved in cardiovascular health or the ability to metabolize or transport cholesterol, lipids, and lipoproteins related to cardiovascular health. Such functions potentially influence physical activity levels. Genes in this group include those that code for proteins involved in the regulation of coagulation (e.g., *PAI1*, the gene for serpin peptidase inhibitor E1), circulation (e.g., *MTHFR*, the gene for 5,10-methylenetetrahydrofolate reductase),

TABLE 12–1. Genes and their variants that have been associated with successful aging and related traits based on genetic association studies

Gene	Variant	Association (*P* value)	Phenotype	Subjects, *n*	Reference
Cardiovascular health; cholesterol, lipid, lipoprotein metabolism and transport					
APOA1	−75P allele	Positive in men (0.0013)	≥81 years old Free of clinically overt pathologies Blood and biochemical parameters in the normal range	229 cases 571 controls	Garasto et al. 2003
APOE	E2 allele E4 allele	Positive (<0.05) Negative (<0.0001)	70–79 years old No reported disability, no more than one minor physical disability No impairment in balance or difficulty standing No impairment in mental status No impairment in verbal memory	965 cases, prospective study	Bretsky et al. 2003
APOE	E2 allele E4 allele	Positive (<0.05) Negative (<0.05)	≥90 years old No cognitive impairment	100 cases 100 controls	Zubenko et al. 2002
CETP	405Val/Val genotype	Positive (<0.001)	≥95 years old Living independently	213 cases 258 controls	Barzilai et al. 2003
KL	VS F/V genotype	Positive (<0.004)	≥95 years old Living independently	435 cases 309 controls	Arking et al. 2005

TABLE 12–1. Genes and their variants that have been associated with successful aging and related traits based on genetic association studies *(continued)*

Gene	Variant	Association (*P* value)	Phenotype	Subjects, *n*	Reference
Cardiovascular health; cholesterol, lipid, lipoprotein metabolism and transport *(continued)*					
MTHFR	677+/+ genotype	Positive (0.006)	≥75 years old No cardiovascular disease	30 cases 191 controls	Zuliani et al. 2002
PON1	–107 C/C genotype	Positive (0.01)	≥80 years old Normal electrocardiography pattern No cardiovascular disease No cognitive or functional impairment No thyroid, hepatic, or kidney disease No infectious or autoimmune disease	100 cases 200 controls	Campo et al. 2004
PON1	192R allele 192R/R genotype 55L/G alleles and genotypes	Positive (0.007) Positive (0.02) None (NS)	≥80 years old Well Mobile Living in the community	604 cases 875 controls	Rea et al. 2004
PON1	192Q allele	Negative (<0.006)	≥75 years old No cardiovascular disease	30 cases 191 controls	Zuliani et al. 2002

TABLE 12–1. Genes and their variants that have been associated with successful aging and related traits based on genetic association studies *(continued)*

Gene	Variant	Association (*P* value)	Phenotype	Subjects, *n*	Reference
Inflammation and immune responses					
HLA-B	*35 allele	Positive (<0.05)	≥65 years old No chronic physical or mental disease No acute infection in last 4 months	17 cases 105 controls	Naumova et al. 2004
HLA-DRB1	*12 allele	Positive (<0.05)	≥65 years old No chronic physical or mental disease No acute infection in last 4 months	17 cases 105 controls	Naumova et al. 2004
IL6	–174G/G genotype	Negative (0.04)	≥80 years old Living independently Mentally competent	193 cases 182 controls	Ross et al. 2003a
IL8	3470T/T genotype	Positive in men (0.05)	≥80 years old Healthy Living independently No signs of age-related disorders	182 cases 189 controls	Ross et al. 2003b
IL10	–1082A, –819C, –592C haplotype	Positive (0.039)	≥90 years old No cardiovascular disease	109 cases 495 controls	Lio et al. 2004

TABLE 12–1. Genes and their variants that have been associated with successful aging and related traits based on genetic association studies *(continued)*

Gene	Variant	Association (*P* value)	Phenotype	Subjects, *n*	Reference
Inflammation and immune responses *(continued)*					
IL10	−1082A, −819C, −592C haplotype	Positive (<0.05)	≥65 years old No chronic physical or mental disease No acute infection in last 4 months	40 cases 105 controls	Naumova et al. 2004
IL12	16974A/A genotype	Negative in men (<0.05)	≥80 years old Healthy Living independently No signs of age-related disorders	182 cases 189 controls	Ross et al. 2003b
KIR	2DS3 allele 2DL5 allele	Positive (0.02) Positive (0.03)	≥80 years old Healthy Living independently No signs of age-related disorders	93 cases 100 controls	Maxwell et al. 2004

TABLE 12–1. Genes and their variants that have been associated with successful aging and related traits based on genetic association studies (*continued*)

Gene	Variant	Association (*P* value)	Phenotype	Subjects, *n*	Reference
Cell cycling, growth, motility, and signaling					
PPARG	12Pro/Ala genotype	Positive in men (0.035)	≥86 years old No mental impairment Normal liver, kidney, and thyroid function No diabetes	222 cases 250 controls	Barbieri et al. 2004
SIRT3	Intron 5 VNTR 2/2 genotype Intron 5 VNTR 2/1 genotype	Positive in men (0.026) Positive in men (0.026)	≥90 years old Free of clinically overt pathologies Blood and biochemical parameters within normal ranges Good health: categories A and B (Franceschi et al. 2000)	242 cases 703 controls	Bellizzi et al. 2005
SIRT3	477T/T genotype 477G/T genotype	Positive (0.027) Negative (0.039)	≥90 years old Free of clinically overt pathologies Blood and biochemical parameters within normal ranges Good health: categories A and B (Franceschi et al. 2000)	120 cases 681 controls	Rose et al. 2003

TABLE 12–1. Genes and their variants that have been associated with successful aging and related traits based on genetic association studies *(continued)*

Gene	Variant	Association (*P* value)	Phenotype	Subjects, *n*	Reference
Cell cycling, growth, motility, and signaling (continued)					
TGFB[a]	915C allele	Negative (0.034)	≥100 years old	172 cases 247 controls	Carrieri et al. 2004
	915C/C genotype	Negative (0.028)	Good health: categories A and B (Franceschi et al. 2000)		
	800G, 509C, 869C, 915C haplotype	Negative (0.007)	No physical disabilities No cognitive impairment No severe diseases (e.g., cancer, ictus, liver disease)		
Drug metabolism					
GSTT1	Del allele	Positive (<0.05)	≥90 years old Good health	66 cases 150 controls	Gaspari et al. 2003
GSTT1	Del/Del genotype	Positive (0.03)	≥98 years old Good health: categories A and B (Franceschi et al. 2000)	94 cases 418 controls	Taioli et al. 2001

TABLE 12–1. Genes and their variants that have been associated with successful aging and related traits based on genetic association studies (*continued*)

Gene	Variant	Association (*P* value)	Phenotype	Subjects, *n*	Reference
Heat shock proteins					
HSP701	–110A/A genotype	Positive (<0.01)	≥80 years old Very good self-rated health	127 cases 271 controls	Singh et al. 2004
	–110C/C genotype	Positive (<0.01)			
HSP70-HOM	2437T/T genotype	Positive (<0.03)	≥80 years old Healthy Living independently No signs of age-related disorders	129 cases 100 controls	Ross et al. 2003a
Insulin/IGF-1 signaling pathway					
IGF1R	1013A allele	Positive (0.036)	≥86 years old Normal kidney, liver, and thyroid function No diabetes No major age-related diseases	218 cases 278 controls	Bonafe et al. 2003

Note. The studies cited in this table used genetic allelic markers to identify genomic regions enriched in a specific trait–contributing allele among the cases (successful agers) and control subjects (nonsuccessful agers).

IGF-1=insulin-like growth factor 1; NS=not significant.

[a]Included centenarians in good health status, defined as absence of physical disabilities, absence of severe cognitive impairment, absence of severe diseases such as cancer, ictus, and liver disease, and "intermediate health status" as defined in Franceschi et al. 2000.

Source. Data adapted from Glatt et al. 2007.

and the maintenance of cholesterol, lipid, and lipoproteins (e.g., *CETP*, the gene for plasma cholesteryl ester transfer protein; *KL*, the gene for klotho (this gene has been implicated in arteriosclerosis in animal models); *MTP*, the gene for microsomal triglyceride transfer protein; and *PON1*, the gene for paraoxonase 1).

Genes encoding the apolipoproteins that catabolize lipoproteins have been assessed for their contribution to successful aging, but only certain variants of genes encoding apolipoprotein A-I and apolipoprotein E (ApoE) have been implicated in successful aging. Although *APOE* and *APOA1* are involved in cardiovascular health, they may have substantial crossover into cognitive functions such as memory. For example, ApoE has critical functions in redistributing lipids among central nervous system cells for normal lipid homeostasis, repairing injured neurons, and maintaining synaptic connections. There is well-established evidence linking an *APOE* variant, *APOE4*, to Alzheimer disease (Mahley et al. 2006).

2. Inflammatory markers are predictors of disability and mortality in the elderly, and proinflammatory and regulatory cytokines may play a pathogenetic role in age-related diseases and may be biomarkers for other ailments that impair aspects of successful aging, such as renal and cardiovascular disorders (Brod 2000; Harris et al. 1999; Shlipak et al. 2003). Several genes encoding cytokines have been assessed, and genes encoding the interleukins and human leukocyte antigens have been shown to contribute to phenotypes related to successful aging.

3. Genes involved in cell cycling, growth, motility, and signaling impact aging by regulating *cellular senescence,* and they determine a person's susceptibility to age-related cancers. Genes identified in the Glatt et al. (2007) review of case-control studies are genes coding for transforming growth factor 1 (*TGFB*), tumor protein p53 (*p53*), and transcription factors such as peroxisome proliferative activated receptor γ (*PPARG*), and sirtuin 3 (*SIRT3*).

The candidate genes discussed above were examined in studies of *successful aging,* howsoever defined. It is evident that many of the genes studied are relevant to age-associated pathological processes (e.g., Alzheimer disease, inflammation) or affect biological pathways related to successful aging traits. Some studies have provided evidence of a gene's effect on function in aging based on animal models (Glatt et al. 2007; these are not included in Table 12–1). Of note, some genes, including *APOE, IL10, PON1,* and *SIRT3,* were found to be significantly associated with a phenotype for successful aging in two or more studies. Given that the body of literature reviewed in Glatt et al. (2007) was small, genes that were not significantly associated with successful aging traits cannot be passed over, because nonsignificant association may be a product of underpowered samples, specification of the phenotype, or the specific population studied. Conversely, those genes implicated by association studies will need validation through additional population studies or molecular approaches. Nevertheless, this literature indicates that genetic approaches can be used to identify genetic variations that may be meaningfully tied to disease processes that relate to the life span and the health span.

Whole Genome Approaches to Identifying Candidate Genes for Successful Aging

Researchers have a choice of several strategies to discover genes that influence a trait or disease. These include the following:

- Assessing gene expression differences between diseased and nondiseased tissues
- Mapping genes via crosses of inbred strains of a model organism and studying the human orthologues of those genes
- Using *linkage* (family-based) and *linkage disequilibrium* (non-family-based) mapping approaches

In addition, new genomewide approaches (systematically examining markers spanning the entire genome) are gaining popularity, and have become more accessible to researchers due to the emergence of efficient genomic technologies.

A major catalyst in the advancement of efficient genomewide technologies has been the data generated by the International HapMap Project (http://www.hapmap.org). The HapMap project has provided invaluable information on a particular type of common genetic polymorphism known as *single nucleotide polymorphisms* (SNPs, pronounced *snips*) and has created a free public database cataloguing more than 3 million common SNPs existing within and in close proximity to most known genes. SNPs, single nucleotide variations that are dispersed throughout the genome, are used in both candidate gene and genomewide association studies. In addition, the HapMap project has determined the frequencies of the SNPs in four ethnic populations of European, Asian, and African ancestry, enabling researchers to choose SNPs appropriate to their population of interest. For each of these populations, the HapMap project has determined the combinations of SNPs that are inherited together as blocks known as *haplotypes*. Haplotype information allows researchers to choose a subset of SNPs within a gene to represent other SNPs on the same haplotype block, thereby dramatically reducing the number of SNP assays and statistical tests required for genetic association studies. These data have enabled the creation of time- and cost-efficient tools for high-throughput genotyping in the form of whole genome SNP chips. Such chips allow researchers to genotype subjects on more than 600,000 SNPs within days (Mägi et al. 2007).

Genomewide association studies can be case-control based or family based. A handful of studies have utilized family-based methods in combination with genomewide methods to discover new candidate genes for successful aging. In one study, Zubenko et al. (2002) conducted a systematic survey of the genomes of 100 elders (50 men and 50 women) who had reached at least 90 years of age without evidence of cognitive impairment and 100 young (ages 18–25 years) adults. The researchers found evidence for significantly tight linkage between two markers on the Y chromosome and an as-yet-unidentified gene for successful aging, which was defined as the co-occurrence of exceptional longevity (≥90 years) and preserved cognition. In a follow-up study, Zubenko et al. (2007) identified 16 different autosomal markers (markers not on a sex chromosome) that showed evidence of influencing the ability to reach age 90 with preserved cognition. Fifteen of the 16 markers were shown to influence this trait in men or women but not both, suggesting the need to consider gene and gender interaction effects in future studies.

Two recent family-based association studies have drawn out potential genetic contributors to successful aging traits by taking advantage of whole genome chip genotyping technologies and a well-phenotyped cohort of subjects recruited from the Framingham study (Lunetta et al. 2007; Seshadri et al. 2007). The Framingham cohort was collected as part of a large epidemiological study begun in 1948 with 5,209 adult subjects from Framingham, Massachusetts, and is currently on its third generation of participants. Lunetta et al. (2007) examined 1,345 members of the 330 largest families from the Framingham cohort for five healthy aging phenotypes that could be associated with successful aging: 1) physiological function as measured by walking speed; 2) longevity as measured by age at death; 3) reaching age 65 without cardiovascular disease, dementia, or cancer; 4) age of natural menopause for women; and 5) biological age as measured by the Osseographic Scoring System (described in Karasik et al. 2005), which uses data acquired from hand radiographs for skeletal morphologies. Family-based genetic association tests identified several genes associated with a combination of these successful aging–related phenotypes: *FOXO1A, GAPDH, KL, LEPR, PON1, PSEN1, SOD2, CYP19A1,* and *WRN.* Interestingly, *KL* and *PON1* were also previously implicated by the candidate gene case-control study approach as discussed earlier (see section "Candidate Genes for Successful Aging"). It should be noted that this study falls short in whole genome coverage, leaving out several key candidate genes for successful aging.

A second study, conducted by Seshadri et al. (2007), involved 705 stroke- and dementia-free subjects of the Framingham cohort phenotyped by volumetric brain magnetic resonance imaging and cognitive tests such as the Boston Naming Test and the Wide Range Achievement Test. Statistical analysis of the data revealed 163 possible candidate genes for association with the phenotypes. The next steps for pinpointing successful aging genes is to replicate these findings in other populations, utilize whole genome chips with better coverage of the genome, expand to other ethnic populations, and conduct association studies on SNPs within candidate genes identified through whole genome approaches.

Successful Aging and Mitochondrial DNA, the Other Genome

In addition to and distinct from the genome encoded by nuclear DNA, humans possess a 16,569–base pair, maternally inherited, circular mitochondrial DNA (mtDNA) that serves as yet another source of potential genetic biomarkers for successful aging. Like nuclear DNA, mtDNA possesses inherited variants that have evolved together from common ancestors to define groups of mtDNA known as *haplogroups*. MtDNA encodes a total of 37 genes, 13 of which are for polypeptides that, together with proteins encoded by nuclear DNA, compose the respiratory chain complex crucial for supplying cells with energy in the form of adenosine 5'-triphosphate (ATP).

The *free radical theory of aging* (reviewed by Rattan [2006]) suggests that reactive oxidative species—highly reactive ions and free radicals that are formed as a consequence of ATP production by the respiratory chain in the mitochondria—contribute to the cellular aging process. Factors controlling the balance of ATP synthesis and reactive oxidative species production play a major role in oxidative mitochondrial damage and cell aging. Both somatic mutations (not inherited from parents) and inherited variants of mtDNA may alter the coupling state of the respiratory chain and thereby cause variation in ATP synthesis and reactive oxidative species production. Consistent with this theory is the vast number of reports identifying mtDNA deletions and mutations that occur with age in various human tissues (Liu et al. 1998; Michikawa et al. 1999; Wang et al. 2001). As with genetic association studies on candidate nuclear genes, existing studies on common inherited mtDNA variants have focused primarily on longevity as the primary successful aging phenotype. For example, De Benedictis et al. (1999) studied haplogroups in 212 Italian centenarians selected for their self-sufficiency, active lifestyle, and good health. Compared with 275 younger subjects (age range=20–75 years; median age=38 years) in a control group, the healthy aging centenarians were found to have an enriched haplogroup.

The possibility that certain inherited mtDNA polymorphisms may predispose certain individuals to be more resistant to age-related diseases and may promote successful cognitive and emotional aging is an attractive hypothesis that still needs to be systematically tested. Difficulties with mtDNA association studies are similar to those faced by genetic association studies, discussed earlier (see section "Defining Successful Aging Traits for Genetic Association Studies"), with the additional tendency of mtDNA association studies to be highly sensitive to population structure.

Regulating Gene Expression in Aging

The technologies and data resulting from the Human Genome Project have provided much evidence for the complex molecular networks that drive phenotypes, and have inspired researchers to look beyond simple genotype–phenotype correlations. We emphasize that the molecular genetic building blocks for successful aging will go beyond those of common genetic variations at the DNA sequence level and will reflect the interaction of genetic and environmental influences on successful aging–related traits. Examples of promising biological markers related to aging include the length of chromosomal telomeres, copy number variation, and factors regulating the pattern of expression of genes and their variants.

Many studies have described the correlation between gene expression profiles and successful aging or age-related disorders. For example, studies comparing gene expression in brains from postpartum healthy individuals versus those from subjects with dementia such as Alzheimer disease have shown significant differences in gene expression patterns (Pasinetti 2001; Ricciarelli et al. 2004). Biochemical pathways involved in cell-cell signaling, cell division, neuroplasticity, and apoptosis are upregulated during normal brain development but downregulated in normal adulthood and then aberrantly upregulated in the course of neurodegeneration (Nguyen et al. 2002). We will likely find that additional physical and cognitive disorders of aging reflect changes in gene expression. Researchers have already provided evidence in animal models such as worm and mouse models that there are differences in gene expression levels in the brains of old and young animals, but these differences can be modulated by changing their environment (Golden and Melov 2007; Sharman et al. 2007). Two emerging fields that are likely to provide exciting revelations in the near future about the processes regulating gene expression are epigenetics and the study of microRNAs.

Epigenetic Mechanisms in Successful Aging

The literal meaning of *epigenetics* is "going beyond the genes." The modern definition of epigenetics is the study of heritable (mitotically and/or meiotically) yet reversible regulation of gene functions through molecular modification of DNA or the chromatin proteins that package DNA that cannot be explained by changes in DNA sequence. Epigenetic processes are important in the understanding of developmental processes and the phenotype of an organism. They possess the features of not changing (mutating) the DNA sequence and being stable (heritable) through cell division (mitosis). In addition, epigenetic patterns may be inherited from one generation to the next. Epigenetic processes are essential in development and cell differentiation, but more relevant to successful aging is the fact that epigenetic processes occur in mature organisms, either through random change or due to the influence of the environment (see the review by Jaenisch and Bird [2003]). Although many different forms of epigenetic modifications are known, the best understood and readily assayed mechanisms are DNA methylation and histone modification.

If aging and its associated disorders are related to changes in an individual's molecular and cellular responsiveness to environmental stress, epigenetic mechanisms may be the ideal explanation of events leading to aging phenotypes. A paramount study by Fraga et al. (2005) assessed both global and locus-specific DNA methylation and histone modification differences in a large cohort of monozygotic twins to provide clear evidence that epigenetic variants accumulate during aging independently of the genetic sequence. These investigators showed that the effect of environment on gene function was associated with an epigenetic drift between siblings during aging. A comparison of gene expression profiles for pairs of 3-year-old twins with profiles for 50-year-old twins led Fraga and colleagues to hypothesize that the observed epigenetic drift causes large differences in gene expression profiles in older twins. Studies designed to reveal the history of epigenetic changes in an individual over time (longitudinal studies) rather than performing a cross-sectional assessment of epigenetic patterns in a population are warranted.

A few recent studies highlight the importance of epigenetics as an integral part of various age-related cognitive functions. Siegmund et al. (2007) assessed DNA methylation patterns at 50 genes related to central nervous system growth and development in 125 subjects ranging in age from 17 weeks of gestation to 104 years, including patients with Alzheimer disease. The study revealed that DNA methylation is dynamically regulated in the human cerebral cortex throughout the life span, involves differentiated neurons, and affects a substantial portion of genes predominantly by an age-related increase. Animal models have revealed the significance of epigenetic modification for cognitive functions such as memory function, and have demonstrated that DNA methylation and histone acetylation may be working together to regulate neuronal synaptic plasticity and long-term memory formation in the hippocampus (Levenson et al. 2004).

Epigenetic mechanisms are attractive therapeutic targets because they are, by definition, reversible, unlike an individual's inherited DNA sequence. This allows for the possibility of intervening at the intersection between the environment (e.g., nutrition, drugs, lifestyle) and the genome and modifying the effects of inherited deleterious genetic variants. However, many questions including the following still face epigenetics researchers before such interventions can be applied clinically:

- To what extent does the environment evoke an epigenetic response?
- Do environmental conditions such as diet or lifetime exposure to pollutants influence the observed methylation changes that occur with age?
- Do epigenetic alterations predispose individuals to age-related cognitive and physical decline?

Advances in programs such as the Human Epigenome Project (http://www.epigenome.org) aimed at providing researchers with comprehensive information on epigenetic patterns in individuals of different ages and in distinct tissue types will provide us with a more complete view of the connections between epigenetic modifications in the aging process.

MicroRNAs

Human phenotypes are derived from the complex interactions among the finely tuned genetic programs that are engaged during cell and tissue differentiation and maintenance. A major group of contributors to the regulation of these processes is *microRNAs*. MicroRNAs are small RNA molecules about 18–25 nucleotides in length, encoded by the genome, that are not translated into proteins. They control the expression of genes by regulating mRNA function (i.e., translation of proteins) and are enriched in human and rodent brains (Beuvink et al. 2007). MicroRNAs are now thought to play a dynamic role in many mammalian brain–related biochemical pathways (Sempere et al. 2004), including neuroplasticity, stress responses (Nelson et al. 2008), and neurodegeneration (Kim et al. 2007). However, microRNA studies are still in very early stages and many questions remain unaddressed.

Copy Number Variants

Copy number variants (CNVs) are large stretches of deletions or duplications of genomic DNA segments (>1 kilobase in length) that are found across the genome and are likely to play a major role in functional variation. Recent studies have demonstrated that as much as 12% of the human genome and thousands of genes are variable in copy number (Center for Applied Genomics 2006; Redon et al. 2006), producing an additional source of genetic diversity, beyond coding sequence, that has a potential impact on an individual's response to therapeutic drugs and components of the changing environment. CNVs may be yet another form of interindividual variation that may explain the differences in phenotypic expression and penetrance of multifactorial diseases and traits. There now is evidence that CNVs also play a central role in the pathogenesis of several neurological disorders, and animal studies have demonstrated that CNVs can be responsible for complex behavioral disorders (Lee et al. 2007). Recently, Bruder et al. (2008) explored copy number variation in 19 pairs of monozygotic twins with discordant or concordant phenotypes, demonstrating evidence for CNV involvement in discordant neurodegenerative phenotypes. Studies assessing the interaction of CNVs with environmental factors will help elucidate the contribution of CNVs to common diseases and traits such as those associated with cognitive aging.

Conclusion

Phenotypes representing successful aging are the result of the orchestra of biological processes of the cell. These processes are governed by the complex interactions among DNA, RNA, and protein biosynthesis and the mechanisms governing those interactions. Critical to identifying the molecular building blocks is the characterization of well-defined heritable traits associated with successful aging. Aging research can apply an ever-growing set of novel genomic technologies to identify candidate genes for these traits. Studies combining investigation of the genetic contribution to successful aging with investigation of processes regulating gene expression are a future direction of molecular genetic research on successful aging.

Although genomic medicine is still in its early stages, molecular genetic research has important implications for understanding the etiology of diseases that could impact successful aging. The ultimate goal is to use knowledge from molecular genetics to slow or prevent disease progression as a way to increase successful aging in the population. The molecular genetic building blocks presented in this chapter have the potential to be utilized both as therapeutic targets and as biomarkers for predicting who is resilient and who is susceptible to diseases. This knowledge should lead to refinement of individualized treatments with the predicted impact of improving health and increasing the quality of life and longevity.

KEY POINTS

■ *Molecular genetics* refers to the study of the complex interactions among the multitude of systems of a cell, particularly emphasizing the interactions among DNA, RNA, and protein biosynthesis and the mechanisms governing those interactions.

■ Molecular genetic studies can determine genetic factors (e.g., mutations at genes) that contribute to successful aging, and, just as important, they can help elucidate the extent to which nongenetic factors (e.g., diet, lifestyle, exposure to stress) play a role in successful aging.

■ Successful aging is likely influenced by many genes working together and interacting with environmental factors to which an individual has been exposed throughout her or his lifetime.

■ An immediate challenge for genetic association studies is clearly defining the phenotypes associated with successful aging and the ability to accurately measure those phenotypes.

■ Looking beyond the DNA sequence to molecular mechanisms governing the expression of genes encoded by DNA is the future direction of research for understanding heritable factors associated with aging.

References

Arking DE, Atzmon G, Arking A, et al: Association between a functional variant of the KLOTHO gene and high-density lipoprotein cholesterol, blood pressure, stroke, and longevity. Circ Res 96:412–418, 2005

Barzilai N, Atzmon G, Schechter C, et al: Unique lipoprotein phenotype and genotype associated with exceptional longevity. JAMA 290:2030–2040, 2003

Beuvink I, Kolb FA, Budach W, et al: A novel microarray approach reveals new tissue-specific signatures of known and predicted mammalian microRNAs. Nucleic Acids Res 35:e52, 2007

Bretsky P, Guralnik JM, Launer L, et al: The role of APOE-epsilon4 in longitudinal cognitive decline: MacArthur Studies of Successful Aging. Neurology 60:1077–1081, 2003

Brod SA: Unregulated inflammation shortens human functional longevity. Inflamm Res 49:561–570, 2000

Bruder CE, Piotrowski A, Gijsbers AA, et al: Phenotypically concordant and discordant monozygotic twins display different DNA copy-number-variation profiles. Am J Hum Genet 82:763–771, 2008

Center for Applied Genomics: Database of genomic variants. Toronto, ON, Department of Genetics and Genomic Biology, The Hospital for Sick Children, 2006. Available at: http://projects.tcag.ca/variation. Accessed April 6, 2009.

De Benedictis G, Rose G, Carrieri G, et al: Mitochondrial DNA inherited variants are associated with successful aging and longevity in humans. FASEB J 13:1532–1536, 1999

Finkel D, Whitfield K, McGue M: Genetic and environmental influences on functional age: a twin study. J Gerontol B Psychol Sci Soc Sci 50:P104–P113, 1995

Fraga MF, Ballestar E, Paz MF, et al: Epigenetic differences arise during the lifetime of monozygotic twins. Proc Natl Acad Sci USA 102:10604–10609, 2005

Franceschi C, Motta L, Valensin S, et al: Do men and women follow different trajectories to reach extreme longevity? Italian Multicenter Study on Centenarians (IMUSCE). Aging (Milano) 12:77–84, 2000

Frederiksen H, Gaist D, Petersen HC, et al: Hand grip strength: a phenotype suitable for identifying genetic variants affecting mid- and late-life physical functioning. Genet Epidemiol 23:110–122, 2002

Garasto S, Rose G, Derango F, et al: The study of APOA1, APOC3 and APOA4 variability in healthy ageing people reveals another paradox in the oldest old subjects. Ann Hum Genet 67:54–62, 2003

Glatt SJ, Chayavichitsilp P, Depp C, et al: Successful aging: from phenotype to genotype. Biol Psychiatry 62:282–293, 2007

Golden TR, Melov S: Gene expression changes associated with aging in C. elegans. February 12, 2007. WormBook, doi/10.1895/wormbook.1.127.2. Edited by the C. elegans research community. Available at: http://www.wormbook.org. Accessed April 2009.

Gurland BJ, Page WF, Plassman BL: A twin study of the genetic contribution to age-related functional impairment. J Gerontol A Biol Sci Med Sci 59:859–863, 2004

Harris TB, Ferrucci L, Tracy RP, et al: Associations of elevated interleukin-6 and C-reactive protein levels with mortality in the elderly. Am J Med 106:506–512, 1999

Herskind AM, McGue M, Holm NV, et al: The heritability of human longevity: a population-based study of 2872 Danish twin pairs born 1870–1900. Hum Genet 97:319–323, 1996

Iachine IA, Holm NV, Harris JR, et al: How heritable is individual susceptibility to death? The results of an analysis of survival data on Danish, Swedish and Finnish twins. Twin Res 1:196–205, 1998

Jaenisch R, Bird A: Epigenetic regulation of gene expression: how the genome integrates intrinsic and environmental signals. Nat Genet 33(suppl):245–254, 2003

Karasik D, Demissie S, Cupples LA, et al: Disentangling the genetic determinants of human aging: biological age as an alternative to the use of survival measures. J Gerontol A Biol Sci Med Sci 60:574–587, 2005

Kim J, Inoue K, Ishii J, et al: A microRNA feedback circuit in midbrain dopamine neurons. Science 317:1220–1224, 2007

Lee JA, Carvalho CM, Lupski JR: A DNA replication mechanism for generating nonrecurrent rearrangements associated with genomic disorders. Cell 131:1235–1247, 2007

Levenson JM, O'Riordan KJ, Brown KD, et al: Regulation of histone acetylation during memory formation in the hippocampus. J Biol Chem 279:40545–40559, 2004

Lio D, Candore G, Crivello A, et al: Opposite effects of interleukin 10 common gene polymorphisms in cardiovascular diseases and in successful ageing: genetic background of male centenarians is protective against coronary heart disease. J Med Genet 41:790 –794, 2004

Liu VW, Zhang C, Pang CY, et al: Independent occurrence of somatic mutations in mitochondrial DNA of human skin from subjects of various ages. Hum Mutat 11:191–196, 1998

Lunetta KL, D'Agostino RB Sr, Karasik D, et al: Genetic correlates of longevity and selected age-related phenotypes: a genome-wide association study in the Framingham study. BMC Med Genet 8 (suppl 1):S1–S13, 2007

Mägi R, Pfeufer A, Nelis M, et al: Evaluating the performance of commercial whole-genome marker sets for capturing common genetic variation. BMC Genomics 8:159, 2007

Mahley RW, Weisgraber KH, Huang Y: Apolipoprotein E4: a causative factor and therapeutic target in neuropathology, including Alzheimer's disease. Proc Natl Acad Sci USA 103:5644–5651, 2006

Maxwell LD, Ross OA, Curran MD, et al: Investigation of KIR diversity in immunosenescence and longevity within the Irish population. Exp Gerontol 39:1223–1232, 2004

McGue M, Vaupel JW, Holm N, et al: Longevity is moderately heritable in a sample of Danish twins born 1870–1880. J Gerontol 48:B237–B244, 1993

Michikawa Y, Mazzucchelli F, Bresolin N, et al: Aging-dependent large accumulation of point mutations in the human mtDNA control region for replication. Science 286:774–779, 1999

Naumova E, Mihaylova A, Ivanova M, et al: Immunological markers contributing to successful aging in Bulgarians. Exp Gerontol 39:637– 644, 2004

Nelson PT, Wang WX, Rajeev BW: MicroRNAs (miRNAs) in neurodegenerative diseases. Brain Pathol 18:130–138, 2008

Nguyen MD, Mushynski WE, Julien JP: Cycling at the interface between neurodevelopment and neurodegeneration. Cell Death Differ 9:1294–1306, 2002

Pasinetti GM: Use of cDNA microarray in the search for molecular markers involved in the onset of Alzheimer's disease dementia. J Neurosci Res 65:471–476, 2001

Rattan SI: Theories of biological aging: genes, proteins, and free radicals. Free Radic Res 40:1230–1238, 2006

Redon R, Ishikawa S, Fitch KR, et al: Global variation in copy number in the human genome. Nature 444:444–454, 2006

Reiner AP, Diehr P, Browner WS, et al: Common promoter polymorphisms of inflammation and thrombosis genes and longevity in older adults: the Cardiovascular Health Study. Atherosclerosis 181:175–183, 2005

Ricciarelli R, d'Abramo C, Massone S, et al: Microarray analysis in Alzheimer's disease and normal aging. IUBMB Life 56:349–354, 2004

Ross OA, Curran MD, Crum KA, et al: Increased frequency of the 2437T allele of the heat shock protein 70-Hom gene in an aged Irish population. Exp Gerontol 38:561–565, 2003a

Ross OA, Curran MD, Meenagh A, et al: Study of age-association with cytokine gene polymorphisms in an aged Irish population. Mech Ageing Dev 124:199–206, 2003b

Sempere LF, Freemantle S, Pitha-Rowe I, et al: Expression profiling of mammalian microRNAs uncovers a subset of brain-expressed microRNAs with possible roles in murine and human neuronal differentiation. Genome Biol 5:R13, 2004

Seshadri S, DeStefano AL, Au R, et al: Genetic correlates of brain aging on MRI and cognitive test measures: a genome-wide association and linkage analysis in the Framingham study. BMC Med Genet 8 (suppl 1):S1–S15, 2007

Sharman EH, Bondy SC, Sharman KG, et al: Effects of melatonin and age on gene expression in mouse CNS using microarray analysis. Neurochem Int 50:336–344, 2007

Shlipak MG, Fried LF, Crump C, et al: Elevations of inflammatory and procoagulant biomarkers in elderly persons with renal insufficiency. Circulation 107:87–92, 2003

Siegmund KD, Connor CM, Campan M, et al: DNA methylation in the human cerebral cortex is dynamically regulated throughout the life span and involves differentiated neurons. PLoS ONE 2:e895, 2007

Wang Y, Michikawa Y, Mallidis C, et al: Muscle-specific mutations accumulate with aging in critical human mtDNA control sites for replication. Proc Natl Acad Sci USA 98:4022–4027, 2001

Zubenko GS, Stiffler JS, Hughes HB 3rd, et al: Genome survey for loci that influence successful aging: sample characterization, method validation, and initial results for the Y chromosome. Am J Geriatr Psychiatry 10:619–630, 2002

Zubenko GS, Hughes HB 3rd, Zubenko WN, et al: Genome survey for loci that influence successful aging: results at 10-cM resolution. Am J Geriatr Psychiatry 15:184–193, 2007

Zuliani G, Cherubini A, Volpato S, et al: Genetic factors associated with the absence of atherosclerosis in octogenarians. J Gerontol A Biol Sci Med Sci 57:M611–M615, 2002

Recommended Readings and Web Sites

Glatt SJ, Chayavichitsilp P, Depp C, et al: Successful aging: from phenotype to genotype. Biol Psychiatry 62:282–293, 2007

Liu L, van Groen T, Kadish I, et al: DNA methylation impacts on learning and memory in aging. Neurobiol Aging 30:549–560, 2009

Sethupathy P, Collins FS: MicroRNA target site polymorphisms and human disease. Trends Genet 24:489–497, 2008

WikiGenetics (encyclopedia on human genetics). Available at: http://www.wikigenetics.org/index.php/Main_Page.

13 Animal Models of Successful Cognitive Aging

Jared W. Young, Ph.D.
Victoria Risbrough, Ph.D.

Since the time of Aristotle and Socrates, researchers have been using animal experimentation as a means to further our knowledge of the world in which we live. In fact, the majority of medical advancements have occurred as a direct result of animal experimentation. In this chapter we 1) introduce readers to common behavioral tasks in rodents relevant to the study of cognitive aging and 2) highlight recent examples of important findings from animal models of healthy aging. We begin the chapter by reviewing animal research from a historical perspective, and how it relates to investigating successful cognitive aging. Then, in each section, we highlight a recent finding in preclinical, animal models of cognitive aging, discussing the pros and cons of the methods used and the impact of the findings on aging research.

Introduction to Animal Research: A Historical Perspective

Animal experimentation in the aid of scientific research has been conducted for more than two millennia. Aristotle (384–322 B.C.E.), one of the founders of Western philosophy and science, was also one of the first recorded animal experimentalists, followed by Erasistratus (304–258 B.C.E.). Following church doctrine that banned the use of human cadavers for research, Galen (129–

200 C.E.) performed numerous animal experiments, and his approach to rational and systematic experiments led him to be dubbed the "father of vivisection." Although the knowledge and techniques developed by Galen proved useful to physicians throughout history, with translations of his work during the medieval period, little experimentation was conducted to further his research. In 1859, Charles Darwin's theory of evolution provided a scientific rationale for the use of animals to learn about humans. Given the kinship evident among animals—especially mammalian species—it was thought that animal experimental data could further the understanding of human biology and behavior. This, kinship however, also provided arguments for animal research to be humane, culminating in the British 1876 Cruelty to Animals Act, the first of many laws passed throughout the world that recognize not only the need for animal experimentation in science but also the necessity for proper treatment of and respect for the animals.

It was not until the late nineteenth century that the true worth of animal experimentation for scientific research into human diseases was realized. Despite the popular misconception among physicians at the time that diseases were caused by internal derangements, in the 1880s the French chemist Louis Pasteur demonstrated that cholera was in fact caused by a microorganism. By isolating bacteria from infected chickens, growing the culture, then administering it to healthy chickens and observing that the chickens subsequently fell ill, he demonstrated the external causation of the disease through animal research. Subsequent experiments with anthrax demonstrated similar findings, leading Pasteur to develop an anthrax vaccine. Since the introduction of the vaccine, reports of anthrax infection have become rare in many areas of the world. Vaccines for diphtheria, tetanus, rabies, whooping cough, tuberculosis, measles, mumps, and rubella have all since been developed with the aid of animal experimentation.

The necessity of *in vivo* research (in live animals), as opposed to *in vitro* research (in a test tube or culture dish), was demonstrated by Gerhard Domagk's group in Germany. Domagk insisted on assessing antibacterial agents in infected mice as opposed to bacteria in vitro, which was fortunate because sulfanilamide proved to be an effective antibacterial agent in mice but not in in vitro experiments (Botting and Morrison 1997). Through this demonstrable efficacy in animals, deaths caused by infections have been dramatically reduced, and Domagk won the Nobel Prize in 1939. The development of insulin, the treatment of meningitis, organ transplantation, open heart surgery—there are numerous examples of achievements in modern medicine that would not have occurred had it not been for animal experimentation.

Use of Animal Research in Studies of Cognitive Aging

Although most of the medical breakthroughs that we have mentioned thus far have been in physiological medicine, therapeutics for neuropsychiatric diseases with cognitive and emotional symptoms have also been developed through animal research. Memantine is the most recently approved therapeutic agent to treat cognitive dysfunction in Alzheimer disease (approved in the European Union and the United States in 2002 and 2003, respectively), with animal research conducted prior to clinical testing supporting its cognitive therapeutic efficacy (for review, see Parsons et al. 2007). Numerous antianxiety drugs have also been developed following assessment of the compounds in animal models (Millan 2003).

The benefits of using animals in research on successful cognitive aging are threefold:

1. Ensures scientific value, in that investigators are able to control the animal's environment, ensuring that experimental effects observed are a result of the intervention being tested and are not due to an unknown variable.
2. Provides opportunities to use experimental therapeutics, compounds that are selective for specific brain regions or receptors, and genetic manipulations that cannot be conducted in humans.
3. Has practical implications in reducing the time frame of aging research. Aging research is most rigorously assessed using longitudinal measures. In humans, a single study from early adulthood to old age may span 80 years. In rodents, however, this time frame would be closer to 2 years; in flies, closer to 1 month.

Because animal studies afford greater control of variables, and thus greater experimental manipulation of those variables, and investigators can thereby conduct far more studies, these studies remain an attractive option in research on successful cognitive and emotional aging research. In this chapter we focus on the examination of central nervous system aging, using animal models, in particular methods to identify biological mechanisms that incur resilience to the effects of age on mental processes. Hence, we will discuss multiple phenotypes relevant to cognition and emotional functions that can be modeled successfully in animals.

Gene Expression Analysis Using Microarray Studies

Several approaches exist that allow the identification of systems contributing to aging. One method is to examine biological "signatures" of aging using microarray gene expression patterns. Microarray studies, which can quantify the expression levels of up to 30,000 genes, allow a systemwide approach to identifying trajectories of gene expression levels with age. This technique can be used to identify clusters of interacting genes, genes that have correlated expression patterns during the aging process, with the aim of revealing critical pathways contributing to aging's effects. Clearly, many genes and systems interact to contribute to such a heterogeneous phenotype as cognitive aging. This multigene approach may aid in identifying systems that play a significant role in either accelerating or compensating for aging's effects on neural plasticity, and consequently cognition. In general, this approach can be used to identify age-related changes in gene expression patterns across a wide variety of tissues, in order to examine the effects of aging on multiple phenotypes, including neurological integrity, cardiovascular functioning, and bone density.

Conservation of Biological Systems Between Species

A number of studies have investigated what biological systems appear to be conserved in their sensitivity to age across model organisms, and the evolutionary scientific rationale put forth by Darwin for using lower-order animals to learn about humans has been supported by early microarray studies. Gene expression studies in highly divergent species, *Drosophila melanogaster* (fruit fly) and *Caenorhabditis elegans* (roundworm), indicate that a large number of genes are similarly upregulated or downregulated with age (McCarroll et al. 2004). These findings have since been extended to rodents and humans. A recent study across species—flies, worms, mice, and humans—indicated that mitochondrial genes involved in cellular respiration are most highly correlated with age in these species (Zahn and Kim 2007). These studies, among others, demonstrate conserved processes that occur with aging across species, supporting the utility of animal models of aging. In general, however, the use of higher-order animals is preferable to examine aging's effects on cognitive phenotypes, to increase the predictive potency of the results for humans. This idea is based on the need for increased homology between neural circuits (e.g., in the frontal cortex) as well as homologous behavioral phenotypes (e.g., working memory) between the animal model and the human aging phenotype.

Cognitive Function in Aging Rats

Many laboratories have reported that older rats exhibit significant variance in spatial memory, just as is seen in humans (Blalock et al. 2005; Gallagher and Nicolle 1993; Markowska et al. 1989). Spatial memory in rats is most often examined using the *Morris water maze*, a test that requires hippocampal integrity. The Morris water maze is one of the most commonly used tools to assess cognition in preclinical behavioral neuroscience, in part due to its simple and elegant design (Figure 13–1). First developed by Morris (1981) to assess spatial learning and memory in rats, the water maze is a circular pool, approximately 1.3 m in diameter, containing a submerged platform. The water is made opaque so that the platform is no longer visible. Testing involves placing the test animals in the water, around which spatial cues are used to locate the submerged platform. Time taken to locate the platform is assessed over several sessions within a day and between days as a measure of learning and memory. Whether assessing learning or short- or long-term memory, the hippocampus is predominantly required for performance of the task, as it is for all spatial memory tasks. Importantly, recently created human versions of this task using virtual reality or video game approaches have indicated that similar neural substrates and circuitry are required for performance of this spatial navigation task (Sorkin et al. 2006). Microarray analyses may identify systems linked to aging's effects on spatial memory in performing this task.

As rodents age, there is increased variability in performance of the water maze across individual animals; some old rats exhibit little difference in performance compared with young animals (and are referred to as *age-unimpaired*, or AU, rats) whereas others exhibit significantly reduced spatial memory (*age-impaired*, or AI, rats). Thus AU rats are a model of cognitive health and AI rats are a model of cognitive impairment. Researchers are beginning to exploit this variability in cognitive performance to examine biological mechanisms that are altered in both AU and AI brains, specifically in the hippocampus (for review, see Lund et al. 2004).

Rowe and colleagues (2007) recently completed an exhaustive microarray study of hippocampal gene expression patterns correlated to water maze performance across young, AI, and AU groups of rats. Although the predominant focus of the study was to identify genes linked to cognitive decline in the AI rats, the researchers also described a subset of genes upregulated only

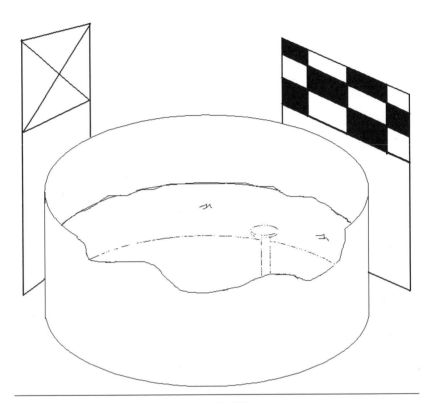

FIGURE 13–1. Cutaway drawing of a Morris water maze.

The Morris water maze consists of a circular pool, approximately 1.3 m in diameter, with a submerged platform. The water is made opaque so that the platform is no longer visible. The rodent is placed in the water and must learn where the platform is by using the spatial cues located outside of the pool. Within a few trials, the rodent will have learned where the platform is located in relation to these visual cues, and its latency to find the platform will be significantly faster than the first trial. Whether learning or short- or long-term memory is being assessed, the hippocampus is predominantly required for performance in the task, as it is for all spatial memory tasks. Importantly, recently created human versions of this task using virtual reality or video game approaches have indicated that similar neural substrates and circuitry are required for performance of this spatial navigation task. Microarray analyses may identify systems linked to age effects on spatial memory in this task.

in the AU group, suggesting that systems regulated by these genes may play a role in compensation to maintain intact cognitive functions. Included were genes for second-messenger signaling transduction factors and membrane receptors (*Adra2c, Adrbk1, Calm1, Camk2d, Gpr26, Gpr83, Grm2, Itpkb, Mtap2, Mtap6, Nrg1, Pik3c2g*)—genes that may play a role in boosting neuronal signaling. This study points to an interesting distinction between two possible mechanisms supporting successful aging: 1) the resilience of a pathway to maintain normal activity during aging (i.e., no change; in this case, expression patterns that were altered only in the AI group and not in the young and AU groups), *or* 2) the ability to correct or compensate for normal aging-induced dysfunction with modulation of other systems (genes that were expressed differently only in the AU group). Further analysis via pharmacological manipulations of these systems or genetic manipulations (overexpression and knockout of identified genes) is required to test the preliminary models supported by microarray data.

Using this strategy of identifying individual variability in spatial memory performance with age, researchers have begun to identify specific mechanisms for successful cognitive aging. Lee and colleagues (2005) reported that AU rats have different mechanisms for long-term depression (LTD; a marker of synaptic plasticity linked to memory) compared with AI and young rats, implying that with age, "normal" N-methyl-D-aspartate (NMDA) receptor–dependent LTD is disrupted; however, some animals show compensation via a switch to NMDA receptor–independent LTD. This animal model of successful hippocampal aging may identify systems that compensate for the effects of aging, and thus allow for examination of novel therapeutics that may boost these compensatory mechanisms.

Identification of Preventive Therapies for Resilience to Cognitive Aging: Enhancement of Hippocampal Neurogenesis

Many studies have been performed to examine both behavioral and pharmacological therapies that may confer resilience to cognitive aging. The use of physical exercise to promote successful cognitive aging in humans has been discussed in detail elsewhere (see Chapter 14, "Creating Environments to Encourage Physical Activity"). Studies have also been performed in animals to investigate the mechanisms underlying the positive effects of physical exercise on successful cognitive aging. Van Pragg and colleagues (2005) examined the effects of voluntary physical exercise (running wheel activity) on the spatial learning and memory of older mice in the Morris water maze test. Older mice that were given access to running wheels ascertained the location of the platform significantly faster than older mice without access to running wheels (controls). In fact, the spatial learning performance of these AU mice was equal to that of both active and sedentary young mice. van

Praag and colleagues (2005) demonstrated that this improvement coincided with a slowed decline in hippocampal neurogenesis in the exercising mice compared with controls. Thus, one mechanism for the effects of physical exercise (as well as mental exercise, which appears to produce similar results) on cognition may be to sustain neurogenesis. Hippocampal neurogenesis has been hypothesized to be critical both for the compensatory potential of the brain in the face of age- or disease-related disruptions and for the ability to maintain complex and adaptable neural networks (Kemperman 2008).

A recent example of testing pharmacological treatments that may help maintain hippocampal integrity and neural plasticity during aging is the study of retinoic acid's effects on spatial memory loss during aging (Mingaud et al. 2008). Retinoic acid is the predominant vitamin A metabolite that is critical to neuronal development, has antiapoptotic and antioxidative activity, and has recently been shown to promote neural plasticity in the adult hippocampus (McCaffery et al. 2006; Mingaud et al. 2008). Mingaud and colleagues (2008) assessed the putative procognitive effects of retinoic acid treatment on spatial memory in older mice using the *radial arm maze,* one of the oldest tests of spatial memory in rodents (Olton and Samuelson 1976). The radial arm maze consists of an octagonal central hub with eight protruding arms. The end of each arm is baited with food, and the rat must enter each arm sequentially to obtain the food (Figure 13–2). Performance is measured by the number of arms entered prior to repeating entry into an already visited arm (thus, the maximum number obtainable is 8). Access to each arm can be controlled by guillotine doors, so that delays in access to the arms after each trial can be controlled by the experimenter, increasing the difficulty of the task. The task is mediated by both frontal cortex (without delays) and the hippocampus (with delays) and provides an opportunity to assess the neural substrates contributing to successful cognitive aging in the spatial working memory domain. Some mazes now have 16 arms, which makes the task more difficult to complete without making a mistake (reentering a previously visited arm), thus increasing the sensitivity of the task to detect group differences in memory performance. The task can also be used to test short- and long-term spatial memory, by allowing the animal to visit one arm to collect the food reward, then, after a short or long delay, giving the animal a choice between entering the previously visited arm or a new arm. Performance can be measured simply by the number of arms visited before the animal repeats entry into a previously visited arm.

Mingaud and colleagues (2008) utilized the radial arm maze to assess the contribution of retinoic acid to both short- and long-term spatial memory performance in young (age 2 months), middle-aged (age 11–12 months), and older (age 23–24 months) mice. The authors demonstrated age-related reductions in performance in both the short- and long-term memory tasks,

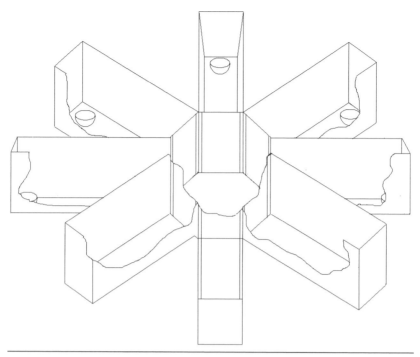

FIGURE 13–2. **Cutaway drawing of the radial arm maze apparatus.**

The radial arm maze consists of an octagonal central hub, with eight arms protruding from each side. The end of each arm is baited with food, and the rat must enter each arm sequentially to obtain the food. Performance is measured by the number of arms entered prior to repeating entry into an already visited arm (thus, the maximum is eight). Access to each arm can be controlled by guillotine doors, so that delays in access to the arms after each trial can be controlled by the experimenter, increasing the difficulty of the task. The task is mediated by both frontal cortex (without delays) and the hippocampus (with delays) and provides an opportunity to assess the neural substrates contributing to successful cognitive aging in the spatial working memory/short-term memory domain.

reductions that were not seen in mice raised on a diet enriched with retinoic acid (mice were maintained on the diet from 2 months of age until testing). The researchers further demonstrated that with age, retinoic acid expression is reduced in the hippocampus, and that the expression levels correlate with cognitive performance in older animals. Older mice exhibited a reduced hippocampal messenger RNA expression of *GAP43* (a gene related to synaptic plasticity) and a functional indicator of retinoid signaling. Mice that were fed the diet enriched in retinoic acid, however, did not exhibit reduced *GAP43* expression. The improved performance of older mice with retinoic acid enrichment was also linked to measures of increased activation in CA1–

CA3 and dentate gyrus regions of the hippocampus, as well as in the prefrontal cortex.

This study provides possible targets within retinoic acid signaling pathways, and paves the way for studies investigating genes that may contribute to successful cognitive aging as well as pointing toward potential nutritional additives that could be beneficial. As with most nutritional supplements, however, too much can also be a bad thing, and high doses of retinoic acid have been correlated with disruption of spatial memory in adults (Crandall et al. 2004). Thus, further study is required to determine the efficacy and safety of retinoic acid supplements.

Role of the Frontal Cortex in Successful Aging: Predictive Tasks in Rodents

Preclinical research in cognitive aging has thus far predominantly focused on hippocampal tissue and memory tasks, in part due to the focus on Alzheimer disease–related cognitive disruption (e.g., impaired short-term memory and memory consolidation). Reports in older humans, however, indicate that prefrontal and parietal circuitry are crucial to many cognitive domains that are affected by aging, including working memory, processing speed, executive function, and inhibitory control (Rajah and D'Esposito 2005). This circuitry may also facilitate utilization of alternative strategies and skills that are part of normal compensation associated with aging-related declines; thus intact frontal cortex function may be critical to successful aging in terms of global functioning. Below we highlight the current animal models of cognitive domains relevant to tasks affected by aging that are controlled by the frontal cortex. Such tasks will move the field forward in assessing animal models of successful cognitive aging to identify biological systems that support successful function in these domains.

Role of Cholinergic Systems in Aging's Effects on Sustained Attention

The *five-choice serial reaction-time task* (5CSRTT) is a rodent test of sustained attention (Carli et al. 1983), modeled on Leonard's five-choice test of serial reactions that was devised to assess the attention of enlisted men (Wilkinson 1963). The rodent 5CSRTT is a frontal cortex–mediated operant-based task (Robbins 2002), widely used in rats and mice, conducted in a metal testing chamber with a curved wall that contains five apertures, each facing the location where food rewards are delivered (the magazine; see Figure 13–3). In each trial, one of the five apertures is illuminated very briefly (0.5–1 second) and the rodent must poke its nose into the lit aperture. For every successful nose poke, the rodent is rewarded with food. For incorrect responses or failures to respond (e.g., having missed which aperture was lit), the rodent is punished with a time-out period of several seconds in which there is no opportunity to earn a reward. The rewards and punishments encourage consistent responding, and the rodent must attend to the apertures for 100–400 trials over a period of 30–60 minutes.

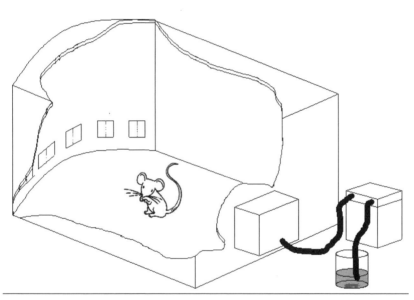

FIGURE 13–3.   **Cutaway drawing of the five-choice serial reaction-time task (5CSRTT) apparatus.**

The 5CSRTT is performed in a five-hole operant chamber. An array of five apertures is located at the rear of the chamber, facing the location of food reward delivery area (magazine). Cue lights are present in each aperture and the magazine, and entry to each of these is monitored by infra-red beams. Each trial begins with a nose-poke in the magazine. Following a predetermined duration during which the rodent must scan the array, one of the five apertures is lit and the rodent must nose-poke into the lit aperture. A reward is delivered into the magazine if the rodent is correct, and if the rodent is incorrect, a 'time-out' period ensues where all apertures are unresponsive (typically for 5 seconds). The rodent continues to perform the task for 100–400 trials, or until 30–60 minutes have elapsed. Multivariate assessment of performance allows the attention and impulsivity to be measured in rodents, with observations of age-related impairment in performance providing the opportunity to assess the genetic contribution to successful cognitive aging within the domain of attention.

Multivariate assessment of performance allows the rodent's attention and impulsivity to be measured, with observations of age-related impairment in performance providing the opportunity to assess the genetic contribution to successful cognitive aging within the domain of attention.

Jones and colleagues (1995) studied young (age 3 months), middle-aged (age 15 months), and older (age 22 months) rats' performance on the 5CSRTT. Although processing speed as measured by reaction time was slow in both middle-aged and older rats, there was also a subset of older rats that exhibited significantly worse attentional performance in the standard task. When the task was made more difficult by lowering and varying the duration the cue light was on, however, both middle-aged and older rats exhibited poorer performance than young rats. Jones et al. (1995) elegantly demonstrated that the poorer performance of middle-aged and older rats in the task was attentionally mediated, because no deficits were observed in these rats when similarly challenged in a simple reaction-time task. However, the fact that several older rats displayed poorer performance on the standard task, whereas other older rats exhibited performance comparable to that of middle-aged rats, suggests that this task may be useful in delineating the possible genetic contributions to trajectories of cognitive aging (as spatial memory tasks can; see sections "Cognitive Function in Aging Rats" and "Identification of Preventive Therapies for Resilience to Cognitive Aging" earlier in this chapter).

Consistent with theories of the degradation of cholinergic control of attention with age, older rat performance was more sensitive to manipulations of cholinergic signaling. Specifically, older rats were more sensitive to performance disruption when they were administered the cholinergic antagonist scopolamine, whereas performance was enhanced by treatment with the acetylcholinesterase inhibitor tacrine (Jones et al. 1995). One possible mechanism for successful cognitive aging may be the maintenance of signaling of the α_7 nicotinic acetylcholine receptor. Reduction in expression of this receptor has been observed in the hippocampi of Alzheimer disease patients (Guan et al. 2000). Preclinical evidence also suggests that the α_7 receptor is required specifically for attention, with mice lacking the receptor exhibiting significantly poorer attention in the 5CSRTT compared with their wild-type littermates (Young et al. 2004). Thus α_7-selective agonists are being developed by numerous pharmaceutical companies including NeuroSearch, GlaxoSmithKline, Mitsubishi, AstraZeneca, EnVivo, CoMentis, Pfizer, Targacept, and Memory Pharmaceuticals, for potential utility in treating aging-related cognitive decline.

Processing Speed: Lateralized Reaction-Time Task

Processing speed reflects the speed at which a subject solves a problem, and it appears to be among the first cognitive functions to decline with age (Hedden and Gabrieli 2004). The assessment of processing speed in humans is conducted using many different types of tasks, from the more complex solving of mazes using pen and paper, to the most basic reaction-time tasks (e.g., a task in which the subject must release the button of a computer mouse following a cue stimulus). Although mazes are used in animal behavior studies, they are rarely used to assess processing speed because of possible motoric confounding factors. In other words, if an older mouse takes longer to solve the maze, it is difficult to determine whether this is due to reduced processing speed or simply slower movement. Operant-based tasks using levers are less confounded by aging's effects on motor ability.

In one such task, rats are trained to depress a single lever, and to release the lever following the presentation of a cue stimulus (e.g., light). The reaction time is measured as time between stimulus presentation and release of the lever. Burwell and colleagues (1995) demonstrated an age-related increase in reaction time in rats from 14.5 to 25 months of age. As with the spatial memory tasks discussed above, researchers observed increased variability in reaction time in older rats, such that the reaction times of some older rats (the AU rats) were equivalent to those of younger rats, whereas other rats (the AI rats) were significantly slower. The differences between reaction times in AU and AI rats were linked to an overall decrease in dopamine levels, and an increase in dopamine type 1 receptor binding, in AU rats. These findings indicate that disruptions in dopamine neurotransmission may separate successful from unsuccessful cognitive aging in terms of processing speed. These findings are not a surprise, because across species dopamine neural circuits are very sensitive to aging, with alterations in dopamine receptor binding, dopamine synthesis, and other biomarkers of nigrostriatal viability (Stark and Pakkenberg 2004). Thus, maintenance of dopamine networks may be critical to reducing aging's effects on processing speed. A drawback to this interpretation, however, is that the lever depression and release task that Burwell and colleagues (1995) used does not provide much of a cognitive challenge, as it is a very simple one-stimulus/ one-response task. Other tasks that require more complex choices before responding (e.g., between alternate signal types or between alternate response types) can provide a more comprehensive probe of the changes in cognitive processing speed that occur with age during active problem solving.

The *lateralized reaction-time* (LRT) task provides an opportunity to assess reaction time associated with more difficult cognitive challenges than the simple reaction-time task discussed above. The LRT task was developed using the same testing chambers as the 5CSRTT (see "Role of Cholinergic Systems in Aging's Effects on Sustained Attention"), although it utilizes only three apertures (the central aperture and two extreme apertures) (Carli et al. 1985). Each trial begins with the rodent poking its nose into the central aperture and keeping it there while continuously scanning the two extreme apertures. After a variable period of time, one of the two extreme apertures illuminates, following which the rodent must remove itself from the central aperture and poke its nose into the lit aperture. To perform the task as quickly as possible, the rat must divide its attentional resources between the two extreme apertures and decide which way to move following the presentation of a stimulus. Another major benefit of the LRT task in assessing processing speed is that reaction time can be differentiated from motor speed, because reaction time is measured only as the length of time it takes the rodent to remove its head from the central aperture following the appearance of the light stimulus. Movement time is assessed as a measure of motor speed, calculated from the time the animal removes its head from the central aperture to the time the animal pokes its nose into one of the extreme apertures. This separation of reaction time and motor speed provides greater specificity in the assessment of processing speed in rodents, especially in cognitive tasks that have motoric components to performance (e.g., the 5CSRTT). To our knowledge, this task has not been employed in aging research, but certainly could be.

Executive Functioning: Attentional Set-Shifting Task

The frontal cortex is also required when performing problem-solving or executive functioning tasks. A common test of executive functioning in humans is the Wisconsin Card Sorting Test (WCST), in which the subject must sort cards based on stimuli provided on the cards—dimensions of color, shape, or number. An analogue of this test has been created for use with rodents (Eling et al. 2008), demonstrating remarkable homology to the WCST, in which animals must select bowls using stimuli based on dimensions of odor or digging medium within the bowls, or the texture of the bowls. As with humans performing the WCST, performance of animals in this *attentional set-shifting task* deteriorates with age (Nicolle and Baxter 2003), a phenomenon that varies across individual animals. In their study of rats performing this task, Nicolle and Baxter (2003) observed lower glutamatergic (kainite) receptor binding in the frontal cortices of older animals, with poorer performance related specifically to lower levels in the cingulate cortex. Interestingly, increased NMDA receptor binding in the striatum correlated negatively with performance, which may indicate that activation of basal ganglia can interfere with some executive function tasks (Nicolle and Baxter 2003). Activation of the striatum is linked to perseverative behaviors, which tend to increase with age across species. Thus, some executive function tasks may require maintenance of glutamate signaling in both the frontal cortex and the striatum. As with the LRT task described above, this task would seem to be a promising candidate for use in aging research.

Working Memory Capacity: Odor Span Task

The *odor span task* is a nonspatial task that may provide the most accurate measurement of working memory capacity in rodents (see Figure 13–4). Following training, at span 0 when no memory is required, the rodent must dig in a bowl containing material of a particular odor (odor A) to retrieve a food reward. That bowl is then relocated, to avoid the use of spatial cues, and a second bowl is placed on the table (or floor, if the task is performed on the floor), filled with material of a different odor (odor B). This is referred to as *span 1* because the rodent has one odor to remember in order to complete this span (i.e., to choose a bowl of a different odor). The previously encountered odor (A) must be remembered because it is no longer baited, whereas the bowl with the novel odor (B) is baited. If the task is performed successfully, the rodent moves to span 2, with three bowls containing different odors placed in novel locations, and it must remember odors A and B in order to select bowl C as the one containing the novel odor and therefore the food reward. This continues up to span 11 in the standard task, or span 23 in the extended challenge task. Thus, the task is simple in design, requiring rodents to remember increasing numbers of odor stimuli in order to identify the novel odor that is presented in each new span.

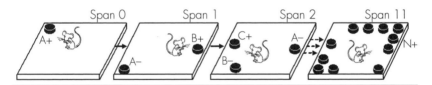

FIGURE 13–4. Schematic of the odor span task.

The odor span task measures the capacity of working memory for nonspatial, olfactory information. Following training, at span 0 when no memory span is required, the rodent must dig in a bowl containing a particular odor (A) to retrieve a food reward. That bowl is then relocated (to avoid the use of spatial cues), and a second bowl is placed on the table, filled with a different odor (B). This is referred to as *span 1* as the rodent has 1 odor to remember in order to complete this span. The previously encountered odor (A) must be remembered, as it is not baited, while the novel odor (B) is baited. If the task is performed successfully, the rodent moves to span 2, with three odors placed in novel locations, and it must remember odors A and B in order to select bowl C as the novel odor. This continues up to span 11 in the standard task, or span 23 in the extended challenge task. Increased variability on performance of mice in this task has been demonstrated with increased aging, suggesting that some aged mice may perform the task as well as young comparison mice, while others may not, providing an opportunity to assess the genetic contribution to successful cognitive aging for working memory span capacity.

Given the preference for the olfactory modality in rats and mice, it is unsurprising that they display a high level of performance, although several studies have now identified factors that contribute to performance in this task (Young et al. 2009). For more than a decade, caspases, a group of proteases integral to cell death and the apoptotic pathway, have been linked to aging and neurodegenerative diseases (McLaughlin 2004). Recent data suggest that these enzymes may be involved in synaptic plasticity and network remodeling. Mice overexpressing caspase-3, a caspase that is essential for apoptotic pathway–mediated cell death and that may be involved in synaptic plasticity, exhibited impaired performance in the odor span task irrespective of their age group (6, 12, or 18 months old) (Young et al. 2007). Overall, the data from this study indicate that increased caspase-3 activity, which is also found in some tissues with increased age, may interfere with working memory processes. Because the olfactory cortex, a region of high caspase-3 expression, is likely to interact with the frontal cortex to code for the olfactory working memory capacity, caspase-3 may be important for maintaining information held for working memory. Overall, the main effect of age on performance of this task in wild-type mice was on reaction latency, not accuracy; this may indicate that older mice exhibit slower processing speed while retaining accuracy (a speed-accuracy trade-off), or it could simply reflect slowed locomotor activity. The variability of older wild-type mice in performing this task increased with increasing task difficulty, however, suggesting that with larger groups of mice than those used in the Young et al. (2007) study, the animals could be identified as AU and AI performers for use in studies examining the mechanism of successful aging versus aging-related working memory decline.

Conclusion

Specific models of cognitive aging in rodents, though in their infancy, offer promise in providing a better understanding of mechanisms supporting successful aging. Hippocampus-dependent tasks are being used by a number of groups to identify the genetic and neural attributes of animals with reduced sensitivity to aging's effects on cognition (Blalock et al. 2005; Gallagher and Nicolle 1993; Markowska et al. 1989). Their findings indicate that at least one possible mechanism involved in maintenance of cognitive function in aging may be preservation of glutamate signaling, either via boosting receptor or second messenger expression levels or via activation of compensatory mechanisms (e.g., NMDA-independent neural plasticity). A second mechanism may be the supporting processes involved in neural plasticity of the hippocampus, including neurogenesis and retinoic acid signaling. Evidence certainly supports the notion that there may be very disparate underlying pathologies and hence different treatment strategies for successful cognitive aging involving hippocampal and frontal cortex neural circuits (Baxter 2003). Our understanding of biological mechanisms supporting frontal cortex–dependent tasks is somewhat farther behind, but with the recent development of more sophisticated animal models such as the odor span and attentional set-shifting tasks, genetic and pharmacological strategies similar to those used with hippocampus-dependent tasks (e.g., based on individual variation in performance) can be applied to identify mechanisms maintaining intact working memory and executive functioning with age. In conclusion, animal experimentation provides an invaluable resource to identify the biological systems underlying successful cognitive aging.

KEY POINTS

❚ Animal research in neuroscience has a long history and, as a result of the conservation of basic physiological attributes between species, has made major contributions to our understanding of the human brain. Progress in this area has included greater attention to ethical aspects of animal research.

❚ A number of rodent tasks assess similar cognitive domains assessed in humans, including tests for attention, working memory, and executive functioning.

❚ Performance on these tasks can be used to identify phenotypes that help us understand genetic contributions to cognition, and also to identify the biological processes associated with neurogenesis in interventional experiments (e.g., physical activities, pharmacotherapy).

❚ The use of animal models in studying cognitive aging is in its infancy, yet with proper controls for sensory and motor changes, animal models can provide many potential windows to understanding and enhancing function in the aging human brain.

References

Baxter MG: Age-related memory impairment: is the cure worse than the disease? Neuron 40:669–670, 2003

Blalock EM, Chen KC, Stromberg AJ, et al: Harnessing the power of gene microarrays for the study of brain aging and Alzheimer's disease: statistical reliability and functional correlation. Ageing Res Rev 4:481–512, 2005

Botting JH, Morrison AR: Animal research is vital to medicine. Sci Am 276(2):83–86, 1997

Burwell RD, Lawler CP, Gallagher M: Mesostriatal dopamine markers in aged Long-Evans rats with sensorimotor impairment. Neurobiol Aging 16:175–186, 1995

Carli M, Robbins TW, Evenden JL, et al: Effects of lesions to ascending noradrenergic neurones on performance of a 5-choice serial reaction task in rats: implications for theories of dorsal noradrenergic bundle function based on selective attention and arousal. Behav Brain Res 9:361–380, 1983

Carli M, Evenden JL, Robbins TW: Depletion of unilateral striatal dopamine impairs initiation of contralateral actions and not sensory attention. Nature 313:679–682, 1985

Crandall J, Sakai Y, Zhang J, et al: 13-cis-retinoic acid suppresses hippocampal cell division and hippocampal-dependent learning in mice. Proc Natl Acad Sci USA 101:5111–5116, 2004

Eling P, Derckx K, Maes R: On the historical and conceptual background of the Wisconsin Card Sorting Test. Brain Cogn 67:247–253, 2008

Gallagher M, Nicolle MM: Animal models of normal aging: relationship between cognitive decline and markers in hippocampal circuitry. Behav Brain Res 57:155–162, 1993

Guan ZZ, Zhang X, Ravid R, et al: Decreased protein levels of nicotinic receptor subunits in the hippocampus and temporal cortex of patients with Alzheimer's disease. J Neurochem 74:237–243, 2000

Hedden T, Gabrieli JD: Insights into the ageing mind: a view from cognitive neuroscience. Nat Rev Neurosci 5:87–96, 2004

Jones DN, Barnes JC, Kirkby DL, et al: Age-associated impairments in a test of attention: evidence for involvement of cholinergic systems. J Neurosci 15:7282–7292, 1995

Kemperman G: The neurogenic reserve hypothesis. Trends in Neurosciences 31:163–169, 2008

Lee HK, Min SS, Gallagher M, et al: NMDA receptor–independent long-term depression correlates with successful aging in rats. Nat Neurosci 8:1657–1659, 2005

Lund PK, Hoyt EC, Bizon J, et al: Transcriptional mechanisms of hippocampal aging. Exp Gerontol 39:1613–1622, 2004

Markowska AL, Stone WS, Ingram DK, et al: Individual differences in aging: behavioral and neurobiological correlates. Neurobiol Aging 10:31–43, 1989

McCaffery P, Zhang J, Crandall JE: Retinoic acid signaling and function in the adult hippocampus. J Neurobiol 66:780–791, 2006

McCarroll SA, Murphy CT, Zou S, et al: Comparing genomic expression patterns across species identifies shared transcriptional profile in aging. Nat Genet 36:197–204, 2004

McLaughlin B: The kinder side of killer proteases: caspase activation contributes to neuroprotection and CNS remodeling. Apoptosis 9:111–121, 2004

Millan MJ: The neurobiology and control of anxious states. Prog Neurobiol 70:83–244, 2003

Mingaud F, Mormede C, Etchamendy N, et al: Retinoid hyposignaling contributes to aging-related decline in hippocampal function in short-term/working memory organization and long-term declarative memory encoding in mice. J Neurosci 28:279–291, 2008

Morris RGM: Spatial localization does not require the presence of local cues. Learn Motiv 12:239–260, 1981

Nicolle MM, Baxter MG: Glutamate receptor binding in the frontal cortex and dorsal striatum of aged rats with impaired attentional set-shifting. Eur J Neurosci 18:3335–3342, 2003

Olton DS, Samuelson RJ: Remembrance of places passed: spatial memory in rats. J Exp Psychol Anim Behav Process 2:97–116, 1976

Parsons CG, Stöffler A, Danysz W: Memantine: a NMDA receptor antagonist that improves memory by restoration of homeostasis in the glutamatergic system—too little activation is bad, too much is even worse. Neuropharmacology 53:699–723, 2007

Rajah MN, D'Esposito M: Region-specific changes in prefrontal function with age: a review of PET and fMRI studies on working and episodic memory. Brain 128:1964–1983, 2005

Robbins TW: The 5-choice serial reaction time task: behavioural pharmacology and functional neurochemistry. Psychopharmacology (Berl) 163:362–380, 2002

Rowe WB, Blalock EM, Chen KC, et al: Hippocampal expression analyses reveal selective association of immediate-early, neuroenergetic, and myelinogenic pathways with cognitive impairment in aged rats. J Neurosci 27:3098–3110, 2007

Sorkin A, Weinshall D, Modai I, et al: Improving the accuracy of the diagnosis of schizophrenia by means of virtual reality. Am J Psychiatry 163:512–520, 2006

Stark AK, Pakkenberg B: Histological changes of the dopaminergic nigrostriatal system in aging. Cell Tissue Res 318:81–92, 2004

van Praag H, Shubert T, Zhao C, et al: Exercise enhances learning and hippocampal neurogenesis in aged mice. J Neurosci 25:8680–8685, 2005

Wilkinson RT: Interaction of noise with knowledge of results and sleep deprivation. J Exp Psychol 66:332–337, 1963

Young JW, Finlayson K, Spratt C, et al: Nicotine improves sustained attention in mice: evidence for involvement of the alpha7 nicotinic acetylcholine receptor. Neuropsychopharmacology 29:891–900, 2004

Young JW, Kerr LE, Kelly JS, et al: The odour span task: a novel paradigm for assessing working memory in mice. Neuropharmacology 52:634–645, 2007

Young JW, Powell SB, Risbrough V, et al: Using the MATRICS to guide development of a preclinical cognitive test battery for research in schizophrenia. Pharmacol Ther 122:150–202, 2009

Zahn JM, Kim SK: Systems biology of aging in four species. Curr Opin Biotechnol 18:355–359, 2007

Recommended Readings

Lund PK, Hoyt EC, Bizon J, et al: Transcriptional mechanisms of hippocampal aging. Exp Gerontol 39:1613–1622, 2004

Nicolle MM, Baxter MG: Glutamate receptor binding in the frontal cortex and dorsal striatum of aged rats with impaired attentional set-shifting. Eur J Neurosci 18:3335–3342, 2003

Robbins TW: The 5-choice serial reaction time task: behavioural pharmacology and functional neurochemistry. Psychopharmacology (Berl) 163:362–380, 2002

Rowe WB, Blalock EM, Chen KC, et al: Hippocampal expression analyses reveal selective association of immediate-early, neuroenergetic, and myelinogenic pathways with cognitive impairment in aged rats. J Neurosci 27:3098–3110, 2007

PART III

Prevention and Intervention Strategies

14

Creating Environments to Encourage Physical Activity

Jacqueline Kerr, Ph.D.
Dori Rosenberg, M.P.H., M.S.
Kevin Patrick, M.D., M.S.

Physical activity offers many health benefits for older adults (for the purposes of this chapter, those 65 years and older). The barriers to being more physically active, however, are large in this population. Older adults are the least active population group, with one-third of those over age 65 engaging in no leisure time physical activity (Centers for Disease Control and Prevention 2004). A further challenge is that although some interventions appear effective in increasing physical activity, participants are often unable to maintain improvements once the support and encouragement provided by the intervention end. Thus, interventions that are community based and seek to make permanent changes in the physical environment to support activity may be necessary. Furthermore, given the detrimental health consequences of inactivity, it is important that physicians and other health care professionals promote regular exercise for their elderly patients and engage with others in efforts to create environments that are activity-friendly for seniors. This chapter addresses the importance of physical activity for older adults and discusses the interrelated nature of psychosocial and environmental factors in promoting improvements in physical activity behaviors in this population. We first describe the benefits of and barriers to participation in physical activity among older adults. The effectiveness of exercise interventions in older adult populations is briefly reviewed. We then present research on the creation of environments that support physical activity. Finally, we provide recommendations for the role that clinicians can play in promoting physical activity among older adults.

Physical Activity and Aging

As we age our physical capacity declines; every decade after age 30, maximum oxygen uptake falls by about 8%–16% and muscle strength by about 10%–15%, and risk for falls increases (Paterson et al. 2007). In the midst of these declines, physical activity appears to positively alter trajectories in physical, cognitive, and emotional health. Longitudinal epidemiological studies have shown that physical activity is related to reduced morbidity and mortality (Paterson et al. 2007). Physical activity is a central component in the prevention and treatment of a range of health conditions, including obesity, type 2 diabetes, cardiovascular disease, osteoporosis, some forms of chronic pain, chronic obstructive pulmonary disease, high cholesterol, high blood pressure, and some cancers (Nelson et al. 2007). Physical activity is associated with a decreased risk of falls and can help older adults recover from functional limitations, serving to assist older adults in living independently (Lee and Park 2006).

Regarding cognitive health, abundant evidence from animal studies demonstrates that physical activity increases the amounts of several neurotrophic factors, including brain-derived neurotrophic factor, which are important in the creation of new neurons in the hippocampus (Cotman et al. 2007). In humans, physically active lifestyles have been related to decreased risk of dementia in longitudinal studies (Ravaglia et al. 2008). Meta-analyses of physical activity interventions have shown improvements in performance of cognitive tasks, particularly tasks related to executive function (Colcombe and Kramer 2003).

Physical activity also benefits emotional health. More active individuals are less depressed and anxious and have higher ratings of quality of life (Nelson et al. 2007). The National Institutes of Health's Cognitive and Emotional Health Project found that physical activity was related to reduced depression (Hendrie et al. 2006). A recent review (Sjösten and Kivelä 2006) also found that exercise may reduce the incidence of clinical depression and depressive symptoms in older people. A review of quality of life and independent living in older adults (Spirduso and Cronin 2001) found that although physically

TABLE 14–1. Possible weekly exercise schedule to meet American College of Sports Medicine and American Heart Association recommendations: how many older adults could exercise this often in a week?

Mon	Tues	Wed	Thurs	Fri	Sat	Sun
Aerobic		Aerobic	Aerobic	Aerobic		Aerobic
	Strength				Strength	
		Flexibility		Flexibility		
	Balance		Balance		Balance	

active older adults report higher levels of well-being and physical function, exercise participation does not show a dose–response relationship. The most consistent result was that long-term physical activity is related to postponed disability and longer independent living in the oldest of old individuals.

In 2007, the first recommendations on the amount and type of physical activity needed for health in older adults were issued by the American College of Sports Medicine and the American Heart Association (Nelson et al. 2007). The recommendations included the following:

- 30 minutes of moderate-intensity aerobic activity at least 5 days a week or 20 minutes of vigorous exercise 3 days a week
- Eight to ten strength-training exercises at least twice a week, with 10–15 repetitions for each exercise
- 10 minutes of flexibility work twice a week
- For those at risk for falls, balance training 3 days a week

These recommendations stem from individual research studies on the benefits of different types of activities; however, there has been little research on the impact of multimodal exercise programs (Baker et al. 2007). As the weekly activity chart in Table 14–1 shows, incorporating these four exercise prescriptions into daily life may be challenging. Lifestyle activities that incorporate aerobic exercise and exercise that increases strength and balance, such as walking, carrying bags of groceries, doing housework, and climbing stairs, may help contribute to achieving weekly activity goals.

Barriers to Participation in Physical Activity

Although the benefits of physical activity in older adults are convincing, older adults are one of the most inactive segments of the population. Less

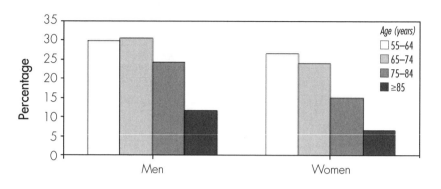

FIGURE 14–1.   Percentage of men and women who are active.[a]

Based on nationally representative data from the National Health Interview Survey, a population-based survey conducted in the United States. Statistics for adults older than age 65 reported separately from those of other age groups.

[a]Participation in light to moderate activity at least five times a week for 30 minutes or more.

Source.   Schoenborn et al. 2000–2003.

than 10% of individuals over age 85 participate in light to moderate activity at least five times a week for 30 minutes or more (Schoenborn et al. 2003) (see Figure 14–1). Less than 15% of those over age 65 perform strength-training exercises two or more times a week (Schoenborn et al. 2003). In particular, retirement often introduces a reduction in physical activity from work-related activities that is not compensated for by an increase in sports participation or leisure time physical activity (Slingerland et al. 2007).

Several barriers to physical activity prevent many elders from participating in regular physical activity (Brawley et al. 2003; Schutzer and Graves 2004). Older adults encounter barriers common to other populations such as the lack of time, motivation, someone to exercise with, energy, or skill (Brawley et al. 2003). However, there are aspects to these common impediments to physical activity that are unique to older adults, as well as additional barriers. For example, time and logistical constraints can be exaggerated in older adults if they rely on public transportation to reach an exercise destination. Older adults may view physical activity as manual labor or as a recreational pursuit, without considering it in a health context. And they may consider the labored breathing and muscle soreness that sometimes accompany physical activity as unpleasant sensations to be avoided (Brawley et al. 2003; Schutzer and Graves 2004).

In contrast to younger adults, older adults more often cite poor health, particularly illness and injury, as the main reason they do not engage in physical activity (Schutzer and Graves 2004). Lack of family support has also been identified as a key barrier to walking (Dunn 2008). Fear of falling is a major barrier to physical activity participation among older adults, particularly outdoor activities like bicycling and walking, and leads many older adults to reduce their physical activity levels (Bertera and Bertera 2008).

Another major barrier to exercise among older adults is pain, often caused by osteoarthritis, the most prevalent chronic condition among older adults. A misperception among those with pain is that they should not exercise because it will worsen the underlying condition and cause more pain. However, trials of physical activity among those with osteoarthritis suggest that physical activity does not worsen arthritis or pain and can improve physical functioning (American Geriatrics Society 2001).

Older adults also report environmental barriers to physical activity (Brawley et al. 2003; Schutzer and Graves 2004). In focus groups, seniors indicated that barriers include traffic hazards and poorly maintained or missing sidewalks, which can cause falls (Michael et al. 2006). For example, a cracked or uneven sidewalk is difficult to negotiate with an assistive device such as a walker (Lockett et al. 2005). Having lights with insufficient crossing time at intersections was an example of a traffic hazard that made it hard to be active. Poor pedestrian access to shopping venues was also a concern because access to services is important for older adults so that they can walk and take care of daily activities (Michael et al. 2006). Gardens and interesting things to see were noted to add to walking enjoyment, safety, and attractiveness and seemed more important than the distance required to walk to destinations. Interviewees in one study indicated that their choice of walking routes was influenced by the length of the route, sidewalk quality, people along the route, traffic, the presence of signaled crosswalks, safety from crime, and scenery (Kealey et al. 2005). Participants in a focus group of older ethnic minority women particularly highlighted the need for more facilities for activity (Lees et al. 2007).

Physical Activity Interventions for Older Adults

Physical activity interventions to date have dealt primarily with changing behaviors in individuals or groups (Brawley et al. 2003). Individually tailored physical activity interventions aim to address individual differences and attempt to increase physical activity. Such interventions are tailored to the individual's preferences, readiness for change, and interests by teaching behavioral skills from models such as Social Cognitive Theory and the Transtheoretical Model of behavior change (Brawley et al. 2003). Commonly used strategies include goal setting, self-monitoring, improving social support, providing feedback, using rewards and positive self-talk, problem solving, improving self-efficacy, and relapse prevention (Brawley et al. 2003; Cress et al. 2005). Interventions can be delivered individually; in groups; by mail, telephone, or other media; or in person (Kahn et al. 2002). With improvements in technology, tailored interventions are now increasingly conducted using the World Wide Web and/or over the telephone (Vandelanotte et al. 2007).

An expert panel convened by the American College of Sports Medicine summarized effective components of physical activity programs for older adults (Cress et al. 2005). These included the following:

- Social support from family, peers or friends, and professionals
- Self-efficacy improvement
- Tailored programs with choices for whether to engage in a group program or an individual activity program
- Health contracts
- Safety education
- Self-monitoring
- Feedback on performance
- Positive reinforcement

The authors stated that coupling these components with routine activities that are a normal part of daily life, often described as a lifestyle approach, may help improve maintenance of physical activity.

In a review of physical activity interventions for older adults, A.C. King et al. (1998) concluded that supervised home-based programs or a combination of group and home-based programs outperformed class or group-based exercise formats alone. The most common format for physical activity interventions for older adults is a group format—center-based, structured sessions led by an instructor (Brawley et al. 2003). Yet many older adults prefer programs that they can do on their own (Brawley et al. 2003; Prohaska et al. 2006). Home- and center-based physical activity programs for older adults have been compared in a Cochrane review (Ashworth et al. 2005): center-based programs provided better physical activity outcomes, whereas home-based programs had superior adherence. The Cochrane review supports A.C. King and colleagues' (1998) conclusion that combinations of center- and home-based programs may be most effective for older adults. Thus, offering a lifestyle approach or structured activities (in the home or in groups), with individualized counseling if needed, and behavior-changing strategies targeted to the individual's stage of change and motivation level may be optimal.

In terms of the specific kind of physical activity to be encouraged, two forms of physical activity for seniors have been subjected to considerable study: walking and tai chi.

Walking

Walking is an excellent form of physical activity for older adults. It is the most preferred physical activity for older adults, inexpensive, and gentle on the body, and can be performed almost anywhere (Belza et al. 2004). Walking is an activity that can be done on one's own (which many older adults prefer) or as part of an organized approach (Brawley et al. 2003). Walking may also serve as a gateway activity to engagement in other types of physical activity, because it can improve fitness and confidence.

A recent review of walking interventions in various age groups and countries (Ogilvie et al. 2007) concluded that there is not one specific strategy that improves walking levels uniformly. Rather, the evidence supports targeting motivated individuals, tailoring interventions to participants' needs via individualized counseling or materials, and acknowledging that certain types of interventions may work best for certain types of individuals.

Pedometers have been used as a simple means to increase physical activity and promote walking among older adults (Sarkisian et al. 2007). Although 10,000 steps a day is the general goal for adults to meet physical activity recommendations, older adults may require fewer steps to achieve health gains or maintain health. To date there is no consensus on recommended step counts for older adults. Tudor-Locke and Myers (2001) suggest that a reasonable goal for step counts would be 6,000–8,500 for healthy older adults and 3,500–5,500 for older adults with disabilities and/or chronic illnesses. Other researchers have suggested that patients with cardiac disease should attain 6,500–8,500 steps per day (Ayabe et al. 2008).

A recent review explicitly examined the use of pedometers to increase physical activity and improve health in a variety of populations and age groups (Bravata et al. 2007). Twenty-six studies were reviewed, and evidence that using pedometers increased physical activity appeared strong. An important finding was that studies requiring a specific step count goal led to increased physical activity whereas those that did not have step count goals showed no significant effects. Also, studies that required participants to keep a self-monitoring log or diary showed significant increases in physical activity whereas those without this requirement did not. Pedometer use resulted in an increase of approximately 2,000 steps per day, almost a mile. In a meta-analysis of pedometer-based walking programs, pedometers were also shown to reduce weight by about 1 kg (Richardson et al. 2008). However, these gains did not appear to be sustained in the long term (Ogilvie et al. 2007).

Reports of pedometer-based interventions for older adults are less common. One study conducted an unsupervised walking program, using pedometers and self-monitoring, in middle-aged and older adults (Tully et al. 2007). The study resulted in increased walking distance in the intervention group compared with control group participants (who did not take part in the walking program), as well as health benefits, including decreased weight, body mass index, waist and hip circumference, cholesterol levels, and blood pressure, for those walking 3 days per week, and decreased waist and hip circumference and blood pressure in those who walked 5 days per week. Other studies have found increased step counts using group-based education (Sarkisian et al. 2007), pedometers only (Engel and Lindner 2006), and behavioral strategies such as self-monitoring and goal setting (Croteau et al. 2007). Pedometers have shown efficacy in improving activity levels in clinical populations such as older adults with diabetes (Tudor-Locke and Bassett 2004) or arthritis (Talbot et al. 2003), but other studies have shown mixed results (Croteau et al. 2004).

Our research group has conducted two studies using pedometers to increase walking in older adults (mean age=84.1 years; range=69–98 years) (Rosenberg et al. 2008, 2009). Pedometers seem to be an acceptable motivational tool for this population, especially if they have a large readable display. However, in individuals with gait problems, such as those who walk very slowly or use a walker, the pedometer appears to underreport step counts. This can be frustrating for participants who are trying to be more active but find that their pedometer does not count many of the steps taken. Also, some pedometers can be hard to use for individuals with arthritic or weak fingers. In one study that used clamshell pedometers (pedometers that needed to be opened to be read), researchers had to alter the opening clasp (by filing it down) to make the pedometer easier to open. Once this was accomplished participants could use the pedometer and saw it as a useful tool.

Tai Chi

Tai chi is a gentle "mind-body" exercise that is appropriate for persons with impairments and functional limitations (Fontana et al. 2000). Several reviews of the benefits of tai chi have been conducted (Adler and Roberts 2006; Verhagen et al. 2004; Wang et al. 2004; Wu 2002). Benefits have been found in cardiovascular and respiratory function in healthy subjects and in patients who have undergone coronary artery bypass surgery as well as in patients with heart failure, hypertension, myocardial infarction, arthritis, or multiple sclerosis (Adler and Roberts 2006). Benefits have also been found in improving balance, strength, and flexibility in older subjects; reducing falls in frail elderly subjects; and reducing pain, stress, and anxiety in healthy subjects (Adler and Roberts 2006). Overall, tai chi has physiological and psychosocial benefits and has been shown to be safe and effective in promoting balance control, flexibility, and cardiovascular fitness for older adults with chronic conditions (Wang et al. 2004). However, there have been only a few randomized, controlled trials of tai chi, most of which were only 8–16 weeks long and did not have long-term follow-up. A review of studies assessing tai chi's effects on balance and reducing the risk of falling found inconsistent study methods and infrequent and nonstandardized measurement of falls (Wu 2002). A review of a specific but common style of tai chi, tai chi chuan, concluded that there is limited evidence that it is effective in reducing falls and blood pressure in the elderly, due to the lack of randomized, controlled trials (Verhagen et al. 2004).

Finally, studies have seldom compared tai chi to other forms of exercise. One study in Japan found that tai chi, resistance exercises, and balance exercises had similar effects on balance but that the resistance and balance exercises had greater effects on strength and functional reach (Takeshima et al. 2007). Studies on the effects of tai chi on cognitive and emotional functioning are currently lacking. Overall, tai chi holds promise as an exercise option for older adults, especially if it is supplemented by aerobic activity.

Creating Environments to Encourage Physical Activity

Much of the research on the clinical and health benefits of physical activity has been performed in laboratory settings using strict exercise prescriptions. The physical activity recommendations for public health are based, in part, on such studies, but these types of programs are not likely to be sustainable in the population at large. Granted, there are some successful individual-based interventions, but these may also have limited effects in the long term. To increase physical activity levels in the general population, it is important to create social and physical (built) environments that support daily physical activity. This may involve changing societal expectations about aging and physical activity—for example, dispelling the notion that retirement should focus on relaxation and passive leisure.

Changes in the built environment may facilitate, promote, and encourage regular physical activity in the course of usual activities of living. If these environmental supports are in place, physical activity can be better promoted to older adults by respected and influential information gatekeepers such as physicians and the media. At a population level, the more individuals who are active, especially in public locations, the more physical activity becomes an expected part of daily living.

Building Supportive Physical Environments

Because of the barriers to physical activity in all populations, researchers are investigating ways to engineer physical activity into our daily lives. The built environment can directly and indirectly shape participation in physical activity, and making changes to the design of communities and living spaces may increase activity levels. The advantage of such changes is that they are essentially permanent and thus can have a long-term impact and reach large numbers of people.

Several reviews of built environment characteristics that are associated with physical activity include studies on older adults (Cunningham and Michael 2004; Sallis and Kerr 2006). The evidence suggests that streets with short block lengths, multiple route choices, and many destinations encourage walking for transportation. The presence of parks and recreation facilities, sidewalks, and pleasant landscaping promotes walking for leisure. A few quantitative studies illustrate the potential for the built environment to support older adults' physical activity. In a Canadian study, physical activity was related to the presence of hills, biking and walking trails, streetlights, recreation facilities, seeing other people, and unattended dogs (Chad et al. 2005). Li and colleagues (2005) found density, street connectivity, and safety were related to walking. Patterson and Chapman (2004) reported more walking in women over age 70 who lived in neighborhoods with mixed services and good pedestrian access to services. Studies using pedometers as objective measures of physical activity provide more convincing results. Older women living within a 20-minute walk of a park, trail, or store had more total walking than those with no destinations, and there was a direct relation between number of nearby destinations and walking (W. C. King et al. 2003). In older overweight women, the predominance of older homes (representing more pedestrian-friendly neighborhoods) and access to destinations were related to more walking (W. C. King et al. 2005). In particular, proximity to parks was related to duration of park use, physical activity levels, and health in 1,515 older adults in Ohio (Mowen et al. 2007). In one study comparing those younger than age 50 to those age 50 years and older, the older adults were more influenced by environmental characteristics, particularly pleasant scenery, hills, and residential neighborhoods, than the younger adults (Sallis et al. 2007).

Older adults who live in neighborhoods with more incivilities such as heavy traffic, noise, trash, and poor lighting have been shown to have worse physical function than older adults living in neighborhoods without these characteristics (Prohaska et al. 2006). Lower function could be due to fewer opportunities for physical activity, given what we know about the causes of decline in things such as strength and flexibility.

Physical Activity and Retirement Communities

The environmental characteristics of facilities where older adults live, such as continuing care retirement communities (CCRCs), which offer a continuum of care ranging from independent living to assisted living and skilled nursing, also play a role in shaping activity levels of residents. Few studies have examined the activity environments of CCRCs, but there is increasing interest in this field. Joseph and Zimring (2007) explored relationships between recreational walking and environment characteristics among older adults living in CCRCs in Atlanta. Walking was related to having outdoor and longer walking paths rather than indoor and shorter paths, although many older adults used indoor corridors for walking, especially in inclement weather. Residents were more likely to use paths without stairs. Highly connected paths were more likely to be used, as were paths with more attractive scenery. Path segments with more connections to central destinations related to activity, administration, or residences were used more for utilitarian walking.

A survey of administrators from 400 CCRCs across the United States asked about indoor and outdoor physical activity resources and resident participation in physical activity (Joseph et al. 2005). Findings suggest that independent-living residents walk more when CCRCs have walking paths, gardens, or outdoor recreation areas such as an area for lawn bowling. CCRCs with multipurpose activity rooms have more residents who participate in aerobics, as do CCRCs with indoor pools.

Intervening at the Level of the Environment

At present there are few studies assessing the influence of changes to the built environment on subsequent changes in physical activity. Changes to the built environment are often costly and impractical for most research studies. However, a recent review of studies on initiatives to promote physical activity conducted by Britain's National Institute for Health and Clinical Excellence (NICE) concluded that when trails, traffic-calming initiatives, cycling infrastructure, road restrictions, and charging for road use are introduced into communities, levels of physical activity increase (National Institute for Health and Clinical Excellence 2006). These studies did not focus particularly on older adults' physical activity levels.

The U.S. Environmental Protection Agency has a policy approach to reward excellence in building healthy communities for active aging (http://www.epa.gov/aging/bhc). Case studies from this program include affordable senior housing near stores and public transportation in Seattle, building sidewalks in Naples, Florida, and developing a new senior-friendly village center in Barrington, New Hampshire. Studies of subtle changes such as point-of-choice prompts to increase stair use demonstrate that these relatively simple interventions in specific locations can be effective in increasing physical activity in older adults and that these changes can last several months (Kerr et al. 2001).

The design of the environment for older adults must accommodate the declining acuity of senses such as vision, hearing, and balance (Crews 2005). Impaired hearing and vision need to be compensated for by louder crossing signals and increased lighting. Changes in gait and balance mean that hazards such as uneven sidewalks and high curbs need to be eliminated. Diminution of stamina suggests that more resting places are required. Even if better environments are built, individual and motivational barriers to using them may still need to be addressed. Examples of this can be seen in supportive environments already in existence that are not fully used by older adults. One barrier, awareness, can be addressed via educational tools such as walking route maps (Rosenberg et al. 2009) and/or maps of local recreational amenities (Reed et al. 2008). Participants can also be taught strategies for walking safely. For example, researchers explored adding an environmentally tailored component to an individually tailored walking program targeting older adults in a retirement community (Rosenberg et al. 2009). Participants took part in a weekly group session and received printed materials, pedometers, and walking route maps aimed at improving awareness of places to walk both on site and in the nearby neighborhood. Over a period of 3 weeks, participants significantly increased their step counts. Although this was only a small feasibility study, acceptability was high, suggesting the promise of this approach.

Capitalizing on Community Networks

One walking intervention has attempted to improve both motivation and environments for walking through the creation of walking groups in neighborhoods led by a designated leader (Fisher and Li 2004). The study showed significantly increased walking behavior in the intervention group compared with control subjects. Another study evaluated a resident-run walking club in an assisted-living facility (Taylor et al. 2003). Although walking behavior was not examined, over the course of 9 weeks participants had improvements in balance, gait, and ability to reach. An intervention incorporating the use of pedometers and a street-sign social marketing campaign for a "10,000 Step Challenge" was found to be particularly effective in individuals age 45 and older (Eakin et al. 2007). And education and counseling can result in reduced environmental hazards in the home, such as poor lighting (Wyman et al. 2007). Overall, environmental approaches to promote physical activity in older adults appear promising, in particular multilevel approaches that also include individualized counseling and social elements (Prohaska et al. 2006).

Community-Based Programs

Several community-based programs that target older adults are summarized in Table 14–2: Enhance Fitness (Belza et al. 2006), Fit and Strong! (Hughes et al. 2006), Active Choices (Wilcox et al. 2006), Active Living Every Day (Wilcox et al. 2006, 2008), and the Community Healthy Activities Model Program for Seniors (Stewart et al. 2001). Each of these programs has been associated with positive effects on indicators of functioning and/or physical activity. The monograph "Moving Ahead: Strategies and Tools to Plan, Conduct and Maintain Effective Community-Based Physical Activity Programs for Older Adults" (http://www.cdc.gov/Aging/pdf/Community-Based_Physical_Activity_Programs_For_Older_Adults.pdf) is a useful document summarizing best practices in community-based programs.

One drawback for seniors' participation in community-based programs is that access and transportation may need to be provided (Tannenbaum and Shatenstein 2007). Fixed schedules and limited open hours may dissuade some from participating in exercise classes, and fear of injury may prevent others. If older adults have been sedentary for extended periods of time, starting them on a very modest walking program may be more acceptable than an exercise class and it can lead to the self-efficacy and confidence to continue to be active. The Center for Healthy Aging has seven documents ("issue briefs") (Table 14–3) that address the difficulties of motivating, recruiting, and reengaging older adults in community-based physical activity programs (http://www.healthyagingprograms.com/content.asp?sectionid=73). Suggestions include the following:

- Offering a range of classes
- Offering classes that include one-on-one monitoring and individual adaptations
- Enlisting older adults to help design classes
- Having appropriate exercise leaders and peer mentors
- Having tracking systems with follow-up contact to check with participants who disengage from a program
- Offering incentives and celebrating achievement milestones

There are other resources available on-line to help community groups develop physical activity programs for older adults (see "Recommended Web Sites" at end of chapter).

Recommendations for Practitioners and Clinicians

Physicians and other health care providers can be a key source of information on physical activity for older adults. This is because older adults are more likely to respect and trust medical advice, and older people make more visits

TABLE 14–2. Community-based physical activity programs for older adults

Program	Study	N	Sessions	Type of exercise/goal	Outcomes
Active Choices	Wilcox et al. 2006	275	One face-to-face meeting with health educator, biweekly and monthly counseling by telephone tailored to stage of change	Learn behavior-changing skills	Increases in physical activity by 2–3 hours/week
Active Living Every Day	Wilcox et al. 2006	333	20-week group program at a variety of community locations; groups met for 1 hour per week	Learn behavior-changing skills and gain social support	Increases in physical activity by 2–3 hours/week
Community Healthy Activities Model Program for Seniors (CHAMPS)	Stewart et al. 2001	81 (I) 83 (C)	Telephone support and one personal planning session, 10 group workshops, newsletters, activity logs	Acquire tailored behavior-changing skills	Significant increases in physical activity after 1 year compared with wait-list control group
Enhance Fitness	Belza et al. 2006	2,889	1-hour exercise classes three times per week at a variety of community locations (e.g., YMCAs)	Aerobic, strengthening, flexibility, balance	Improvements on several measures of physical functioning from the Functional Fitness Test (i.e., arm curls, eight foot up and go, and chair stands)

TABLE 14–2. Community-based physical activity programs for older adults *(continued)*

Program	Study	*N*	Sessions	Type of exercise/goal	Outcomes
Fit and Strong!	Hughes et al. 2006	115 (I) 100 (C)	90-minute sessions three times per week for 8 weeks in senior centers and senior housing residencies	Flexibility, walking, resistance training, discussion/education	Increases in exercise by 100 minutes/week compared with wait-list control group given a list of exercise programs in the community

Note. Physical activity is "any bodily movement produced by the contraction of skeletal muscle that increases energy expenditure above a basal level." Exercise is "a subcategory of physical activity that is planned, structured, repetitive, and purposive in the sense that the improvement or maintenance of one or more components of physical fitness is the objective. 'Exercise' …generally refer[s] to physical activity performed during leisure time with the primary purpose of improving or maintaining physical fitness, physical performance, or health" (Centers for Disease Control and Prevention; http://www.cdc.gov/physicalactivity/everyone/glossary/index.html).

TABLE 14–3.   Center for Healthy Aging resources: issue briefs and physical activity series

Best Practices in Physical Activity

Designing Safe and Effective Physical Activity Programs

Keeping Current on Research and Practice in Physical Activity for Older Adults

Maintaining Participation of Older Adults in Community-Based Physical Activity Programs

Motivating Participants to Be More Physically Active

Recruiting and Retaining Effective Instructors for Physical Activity Programs

Recruiting Older Adults Into Your Physical Activity Programs

Source.   http://www.healthyagingprograms.com/content.asp?sectionid=73.

to physicians than do younger individuals, thus providing more opportunities. A Scandinavian study found that older patients whose physicians had advised them to exercise were five to six times more likely to participate in supervised exercise classes (Hirvensalo et al. 2003). In the United Kingdom, practitioners referred frail elderly patients to weekly group sessions with specialist exercise instructors within their clinic, leading to improvements in measures of physical function related to movement and walking (Dinan et al. 2006). In New Zealand, doctors and nurses delivered brief activity counseling and exercise specialists provided telephone support for 3 months. This exercise prescription led to improved activity, energy expenditure, and quality of life, and reduced hospitalizations (Kerse et al. 2005), and the effects were maintained at 12 months postbaseline (Kolt et al. 2007). In the United States, however, few older adults receive exercise advice from their primary care physician (Figure 14–2). There may also be additional unknown barriers to participation in such programs. For example, one study attempted to translate a motivational support program for physical activity, Active Choices, for use by a group of diverse, low-income, community-dwelling elders with diabetes and found that only 21% of those offered referral enrolled in the program (Batik et al. 2008).

A successful exercise prescription is "succinct, measurable, patient-appropriate and in a form that allows the physician to address compliance expectations and barriers" (McDermott and Mernitz 2006, p. 439). Physicians should be aware that the physical activity recommendations include aerobic, strength, flexibility, and balance exercises, but understand that older adults may need to start with lifestyle modifications such as watching television less, walking more (even in short bouts or indoors), and taking the

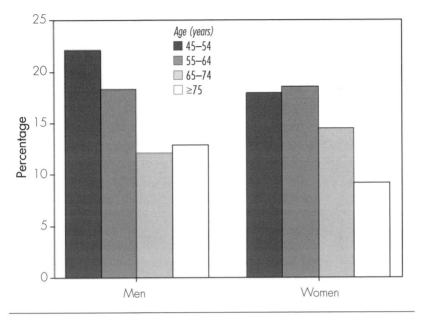

FIGURE 14–2.   **Estimated percentage of patients 45 years and older who received exercise counseling from their primary care physician, by sex and age group, United States.**

Exercise counseling defined as "any topics related to the patient's physical conditioning or fitness" (e.g., "information aimed at general health promotion and disease prevention"). Patient's primary-care physician or provider defined by "survey respondents in physician offices and hospital outpatient departments who responded 'yes' to the question 'Are you the patient's primary-care physician?'" Visit data were reweighted to provide estimates of patients receiving counseling during any visit within the preceding 12 months."

Source.   National Ambulatory Medical Care Survey and National Hospital Ambulatory Medical Care Survey, United States, 2003–2005.

stairs. Physicians can improve their communication and achievement of exercise goals by using the five *A*'s model: assessing, providing advice, gaining agreement, assisting, and arranging services for their patient to be more active (McDermott and Mernitz 2006). Special consideration is needed for patients with particular comorbidities. For example, those with arthritis may need to avoid exercising in the morning and limit repetition and stretching of joints; obese and diabetic patients may need to include low-intensity exercise for longer durations; hypertensive patients may need focus on aerobic activities rather than resistance training; and osteoporosis patients may need to include more weight-bearing activities (McDermott and Mernitz 2006).

KEY POINTS: SUGGESTIONS FOR PHYSICIANS WHEN PRESCRIBING EXERCISE TO OLDER ADULTS

■ Assess preferences: would they prefer to do something on their own or join a group?

■ Address fear of falling: encourage patients to start slowly and build up strength, advise them to wear proper footwear, and assure them that being more active will help them be less at risk for falling. Recommend safe routes for walking.

■ Recommend aerobic, strength-training, flexibility, and balance exercises: walking is the easiest aerobic activity for older adults to do and has strength benefits for the lower extremities. Carrying shopping bags and going up stairs can add to the strength component.

■ Suggest using a pedometer for self-monitoring and goal setting.

■ Refer interested individuals to local programs such as walking groups or exercise classes. Review a list of local programs and possibly provide maps to local exercise resources.

■ Encourage older adults to use walking aids to increase their confidence and facilitate walking in community environments.

■ Encourage older adults to walk instead of riding a scooter and to reduce time spent sitting and watching television.

References

Adler PA, Roberts BL: The use of Tai Chi to improve health in older adults. Orthop Nurs 25:122–126, 2006

American Geriatrics Society Panel on Exercise and Osteoarthritis: Exercise prescription for older adults with osteoarthritis pain: consensus practice recommendations. J Am Geriatr Soc 49:808–823, 2001

Ashworth NL, Chad KE, Harrison EL, et al: Home versus center based physical activity programs in older adults. Cochrane Database Syst Rev (1):CD004017, 2005

Ayabe M, Brubaker PH, Dobrosielski D, et al: Target step count for the secondary prevention of cardiovascular disease. Circ J 72:299–303, 2008

Baker MK, Atlantis E, Fiatarone Singh MA: Multi-modal exercise programs for older adults. Age Ageing 36:375–381, 2007

Batik O, Phelan EA, Walwick JA, et al: Translating a community-based motivational support program to increase physical activity among older adults with diabetes at community clinics: a pilot study of Physical Activity for a Lifetime of Success (PALS). Prev Chronic Dis 5:A18, 2008. Available at: http://www.cdc.gov/pcd/issues/2008/jan/07_0142.htm. Accessed June 26, 2009.

Belza B, Walwick J, Shiu-Thornton S, et al: Older adult perspectives on physical activity and exercise: voices from multiple cultures. Prev Chronic Dis 1:A09, 2004. Available at: http://www.cdc.gov/pcd/issues/2004/oct/04_0028.htm. Accessed June 26, 2009.

Belza B, Shumway-Cook A, Phelan EA, et al: The effects of a community-based exercise program on function and health in older adults: the Enhance Fitness Program. J Appl Gerontol 25:291–306, 2006

Bertera EM, Bertera RL: Fear of falling and activity avoidance in a national sample of older adults in the United States. Health Soc Work 33:54–62, 2008

Bravata DM, Smith-Spangler C, Sundaram V, et al: Using pedometers to increase physical activity and improve health: a systematic review. JAMA 298:2296–2304, 2007

Brawley LR, Rejeski WJ, King AC: Promoting physical activity for older adults: the challenges for changing behavior. Am J Prev Med 25:172–183, 2003

Centers for Disease Control and Prevention (CDC): Prevalence of no leisure-time physical activity—35 states and the District of Columbia, 1988–2002. MMWR Morb Mortal Wkly Rep 53:82–86, 2004

Chad KE, Reeder BA, Harrison EL, et al: Profile of physical activity levels in community-dwelling older adults. Med Sci Sports Exerc 37:1774–1784, 2005

Colcombe S, Kramer AF: Fitness effects on the cognitive function of older adults: a meta-analytic study. Psychol Sci 14:125–130, 2003

Cotman CW, Berchtold NC, Christie L: Exercise builds brain health: key roles of growth factor cascades and inflammation. Trends Neurosci 30:464–472, 2007

Cress ME, Buchner DM, Prohaska T, et al: Best practices for physical activity programs and behavior counseling in older adult populations. J Aging Phys Act 13:61–74, 2005

Crews D: Artificial environments and an aging population: designing for age-related functional losses. J Physiol Anthropol Appl Human Sci 24:103–109, 2005

Croteau KA, Richeson NE, Vines SW, et al: Effects of a pedometer-based physical activity program on older adults' mobility-related self-efficacy and physical performance. Activities, Adaptation, and Aging 28:19–33, 2004

Croteau KA, Richeson NE, Farmer BC, et al: Effect of a pedometer-based intervention on daily step counts of community-dwelling older adults. Res Q Exerc Sport 78:401–406, 2007

Cunningham GO, Michael YL: Conepts guidng the study of the impact of the built environment on physical activity for older adults: a review of the literature. Am J Health Promo 18:435–443, 2004

Dinan S, Lenihan P, Tenn T, et al: Is the promotion of physical activity in vulnerable older people feasible and effective in general practice? Br J Gen Pract 56:791–793, 2006

Dunn MZ: Psychosocial mediators of a walking intervention among African American women. J Transcult Nurs 19:40–46, 2008

Eakin EG, Mummery K, Reeves MM, et al: Correlates of pedometer use: results from a community-based physical activity intervention trial (10,000 Steps Rockhampton). International Journal of Behavioral Nutrition and Physical Activity 4:31, 2007; doi: 10.1186/1479-5868-4-31. Available at: http://www.ijbnpa.org/content/4/1/31. Accessed June 26, 2009.

Engel L, Lindner H: Impact of using a pedometer on time spent walking in older adults with type 2 diabetes. Diabetes Educ 32:98–107, 2006

Fisher KJ, Li F: A community-based walking trial to improve neighborhood quality of life in older adults: a multilevel analysis. Ann Behav Med 28:186–194, 2004

Fontana JA, Colella C, Wilson BR, et al: The energy costs of a modified form of T'ai Chi exercise. Nurs Res 49:91–96, 2000

Gooberman-Hill R, Ebrahim S: Making decisions about simple interventions: older people's use of walking aids. Age Ageing 36:569–573, 2007

Hendrie HC, Albert MS, Butters MA, et al: The NIH Cognitive and Emotional Health Project: report of the Critical Evaluation Study Committee. Alzheimers Dement 2:12–32, 2006

Hirvensalo M, Heikkinen E, Lintunen T, et al: The effect of advice by health care professionals on increasing physical activity of older people. Scand J Med Sci Sports 13:231–236, 2003

Hughes SL, Seymour RB, Campbell RT, et al: Long-term impact of Fit and Strong! on older adults with osteoarthritis. Gerontologist 46:801–814, 2006

Joseph A, Zimring C: Where active older adults walk: understanding the factors related to path choice for walking among active retirement community residents. Environ Behav 39:75–105, 2007

Joseph A, Zimring C, Harris-Kotejin L, et al: Presence and visibility of outdoor and indoor physical activity features and participation in physical activity among older adults in retirement communities. Journal of Housing for the Elderly 19:141–165, 2005

Kahn EB, Ramsey LT, Brownson RC, et al: The effectiveness of interventions to increase physical activity: a systematic review. Am J Prev Med 22 (suppl 4):73–107, 2002

Kealey M, Kruger J, Hunter R, et al: Engaging older adults to be more active where they live: audit tool development. Prev Chronic Dis 2:1–2, 2005. Available at: http://www.cdc.gov/pcd/issues/2005/apr/04_0142q.htm. Accessed June 26, 2009.

Kerr J, Eves F, Carroll D: Six-month observational study of prompted stair climbing. Prev Med 33:422–427, 2001

Kerse N, Elley CR, Robinson E, et al: Is physical activity counseling effective for older people? A cluster randomized, controlled trial in primary care. J Am Geriatr Soc 53:1951–1956, 2005

King AC, Rejeski WJ, Buchner DM: Physical activity interventions targeting older adults: a critical review and recommendations. Am J Prev Med 15:316–333, 1998

King WC, Brach JS, Belle S, et al: The relationship between convenience of destinations and walking levels in older women. Am J Health Promot 18:74–82, 2003

King WC, Belle SH, Brach JS, et al: Objective measures of neighborhood environment and physical activity in older women. Am J Prev Med 28:461–469, 2005

Kolt GS, Schofield GM, Kerse N, et al: Effect of telephone counseling on physical activity for low-active older people in primary care: a randomized, controlled trial. J Am Geriatr Soc 55:986–992, 2007

Lee Y, Park KH: Health practices that predict recovery from functional limitations in older adults. Am J Prev Med 31:25–31, 2006

Lees E, Taylor WC, Hepworth JT, et al: Environmental changes to increase physical activity: perceptions of older urban ethnic-minority women. J Aging Phys Act 15:425–438, 2007

Li F, Fisher KJ, Bauman A, et al: Neighborhood influences on physical activity in middle-aged and older adults: a multilevel perspective. J Aging Phys Act 13:87–114, 2005

Lockett D, Willis A, Edwards N: Through seniors' eyes: an exploratory qualitative study to identify environmental barriers to and facilitators of walking. Can J Nurs Res 37:48–65, 2005

McDermott AY, Mernitz H: Exercise and older patients: prescribing guidelines. Am Fam Physician 74:437–444, 2006

Michael YL, Green MK, Farquhar SA: Neighborhood design and active aging. Health Place 12:34–40, 2006

Mowen A, Orsega-Smith E, Payne L, et al: The role of park proximity and social support in shaping park visitation, physical activity, and perceived health among older adults. J Phys Act Health 4:167–179, 2007

Nelson ME, Rejeski WJ, Blair SN, et al: Physical activity and public health in older adults: recommendation from the American College of Sports Medicine and the American Heart Association. Med Sci Sports Exerc 39:1435–1445, 2007

National Institute for Health and Clinical Excellence, Public Health Collaborating Centre Physical Activity and the Environment: Reviews, 2006

Ogilvie D, Foster CE, Rothnie H, et al; Scottish Physical Activity Research Collaboration: Interventions to promote walking: systematic review. BMJ 334(7605):1204, 2007; DOI: 10.1136/bmj.39198.722720.BE. Available at: http://www.bmj.com/cgi/content/full/334/7605/1204. Accessed June 26, 2009.

Paterson DH, Jones GR, Rice CL: Ageing and physical activity: evidence to develop exercise recommendations for older adults. Can J Public Health 98:S69–S108, 2007

Patterson PK, Chapman NJ: Urban form and older residents' service use, walking, driving, quality of life, and neighborhood satisfaction. Am J Health Promot 19:45–52, 2004

Prohaska T, Belansky E, Belza B, et al: Physical activity, public health, and aging: critical issues and research priorities. J Gerontol B Psychol Sci Soc Sci 61:S267–S273, 2006

Ravaglia G, Forti P, Lucicesare A, et al: Physical activity and dementia risk in the elderly: findings from a prospective Italian study. Neurology 70:1786–1794, 2008

Reed J, Malvern L, Muthukrishnan S, et al: An ecological approach with primary-care counseling to promote physical activity. J Phys Act Health 5:169–183, 2008

Richardson CR, Newton TL, Abraham JJ, et al: A meta-analysis of pedometer-based walking interventions and weight loss. Ann Fam Med 6:69–77, 2008

Rosenberg D, Kerr J, Sallis JF, et al: Pedometer step counts and health status among older adults in retirement communities (abstract). Ann Behav Med 35(suppl):S64, 2008

Rosenberg D, Kerr J, Sallis JF, et al: Feasibility and outcomes of a multilevel place-based walking intervention for seniors: a pilot study. Health Place 15:173–179, 2009

Sallis JF, Kerr J: Physical activity and the built environment. President's Council on Physical Fitness and Sports 7:1–8, 2006

Sallis JF, King AC, Sirard JR, et al: Perceived environmental predictors of physical activity over 6 months in adults: activity counseling trial. Health Psychol 26:701–709, 2007

Sarkisian C, Prohaska TR, Davis C, et al: Pilot test of an attribution retraining intervention to raise walking levels in sedentary older adults. J Am Geriatr Soc 55:1842–1846, 2007

Schoenborn CA, Vickerie JL, Powell-Griner E: Health characteristics of adults 55 years and over: United States, 2000–2003. Adv Data April 11(370):1–31, 2006. Available at: http://www.cdc.gov/nchs/data/ad/ad370.pdf. Accessed June 26, 2009.

Schutzer KA, Graves BS: Barriers and motivations to exercise in older adults. Prev Med 39:1056–1061, 2004

Sjösten N, Kivelä SL: The effects of physical exercise on depressive symptoms among the aged: a systematic review. Int J Geriatr Psychiatry 21:410–418, 2006

Slingerland AS, van Lenthe FJ, Jukema JW, et al: Aging, retirement, and changes in physical activity: prospective cohort findings from the GLOBE study. Am J Epidemiol 165:1356–1363, 2007

Spirduso WW, Cronin DL: Exercise dose-response effects on quality of life and independent living in older adults. Med Sci Sports Exerc 33 (suppl 6):S598–S608, 2001

Stewart AL, Verboncoeur CJ, McLellan BY, et al: Physical activity outcomes of CHAMPS II: a physical activity promotion program for older adults. J Gerontol A Biol Sci Med Sci 56:M465–M470, 2001

Takeshima N, Rogers NL, Rogers ME, et al: Functional fitness gain varies in older adults depending on exercise mode. Med Sci Sports Exerc 39:2036–2043, 2007

Talbot LA, Gaines JM, Huynh TN, et al: A home-based pedometer-driven walking program to increase physical activity in older adults with osteoarthritis of the knee: a preliminary study. J Am Geriatr Soc 51:387–392, 2003

Tannenbaum C, Shatenstein B: Exercise and nutrition in older Canadian women: opportunities for community intervention. Can J Public Health 98:187–193, 2007

Taylor L, Whittington F, Hollingsworth C, et al: Assessing the effectiveness of a walking program on physical function of residents in an assisted living facility. J Community Health Nurs 20:15–26, 2003

Tudor-Locke C, Bassett DR: How many steps/day are enough? Preliminary pedometer indices for public health. Sports Med 34:1–8, 2004

Tudor-Locke C, Myers AM: Methodological considerations for researchers and practitioners using pedometers to measure physical (ambulatory) activity. Res Q Exerc Sport 72:1–12, 2001

Tully MA, Cupples ME, Hart ND, et al: Randomised controlled trial of home-based walking programmes at and below current recommended levels of exercise in sedentary adults. J Epidemiol Community Health 61:778–783, 2007

Vandelanotte C, Spathonis KM, Eakin EG, et al: Website-delivered physical activity interventions: a review of the literature. Am J Prev Med 33:54–64, 2007

Verhagen AP, Immink M, van der Meulen A, et al: The efficacy of Tai Chi Chuan in older adults: a systematic review. Fam Pract 21:107–113, 2004

Wang C, Collet JP, Lau J: The effect of Tai Chi on health outcomes in patients with chronic conditions: a systematic review. Arch Intern Med 164:493–501, 2004

Wilcox S, Dowda M, Griffin SF, et al: Results of the first year of Active for Life: translation of 2 evidence-based physical activity programs for older adults into community settings. Am J Public Health 96:1201–1209, 2006

Wilcox S, Dowda M, Leviton LC, et al: Active For Life: final results from the translation of two physical activity programs. Am J Prev Med 35:340–351, 2008

Wu G: Evaluation of the effectiveness of Tai Chi for improving balance and preventing falls in the older population—a review. J Am Geriatr Soc 50:746–754, 2002

Wyman JF, Croghan CG, Nachreiner NM, et al: Effectiveness of education and individualized counseling in reducing environmental hazards in the homes of community-dwelling older women. J Am Geriatr Soc 55:1548–1556, 2007

Recommended Web Sites

AARP, "Get Fit on Route 66": www.aarp.getfitonroute66.com

AARP, links to various tips for "Getting Motivated" to exercise:
www.aarp.org/health/fitness/get_motivated

National Blueprint: Increasing Physical Activity Among Adults Aged 50 and Over:
www.agingblueprint.org/apaLinks.cfm

National Council on Aging, Center for Healthy Aging: Model Health Programs for Communities, "Physical Activity" resources:
www.healthyagingprograms.com/content.asp?sectionid=73

International Society for Aging and Physical Activity: www.isapa.org/

Medline Plus, "Exercise for Seniors," links to various information pages:
www.nlm.nih.gov/medlineplus/exerciseforseniors.html

Silver Sneakers Fitness Program: www.silversneakers.com

AARP, "Step Up to Better Health" (walking program): www.stepuptobetterhealth.com

15 Diet, Nutritional Factors, and the Aging Brain

Cheryl L. Rock, Ph.D., R.D.

Nutrition is the process by which the human body utilizes food for the maintenance of health, for growth, and for the normal functioning of every organ and tissue. Decades of research have established the important role of diet and nutritional factors in the development and management of human disease, in addition to assembling an impressive amount of knowledge about meeting nutrient needs for normal function. In the older adult, nutritional requirements and considerations are typically influenced both by the physiological and metabolic changes normally associated with aging and by the presence of or risk for disease.

Although the biochemical and biological aspects of diet and nutrition constitute the base of knowledge in nutritional science, it is important to recognize that food has meaning, and that people eat food, not nutrients. Eating behaviors and food choices (including dietary supplement use) occur in the context of belief systems and individual preferences that arise from personal experience, anecdotal evidence, family interactions, and cultural influences. Nutrition is not a religion, despite belief systems that are often involved and as might be suggested by various advocates and zealots. However, the behavioral and psychosocial aspects of diet and nutrition can be as crucial as knowledge based on biomedical science, when this aspect of care is applied to promote health and reduce disease risk in the aging individual. In this chapter, I discuss the influence that nutrition has on the aging brain and provide dietary recommendations based on the empirical evidence.

Nutritional Requirements

The brain, similar to other organs and tissues, requires essential nutrients and dietary constituents for optimal function. Essential nutrients include water, substrates that are a source of energy (e.g., carbohydrates, fat), essential fatty acids, and indispensable amino acids, plus sources of nonspecific nitrogen, vitamins, minerals, ultratrace elements, and electrolytes (sodium, potassium, and chloride). Some characteristics of the brain differ from characteristics of other organs and tissues and influence response to dietary and nutritional factors. For example, brain function is dependent on a constant supply of glucose. Also, the availability, and thus the impact, of nutrients and other dietary constituents is regulated by the blood-brain barrier, as well as by the biochemical and cellular mechanisms that regulate tissue uptake and deposition of nutrients and other dietary constituents.

Water

Although not always considered in a discussion of nutritional requirements, water is an important nutrient, the adequate intake of which can be a problem for older individuals. Under normal circumstances, physiological adaptations and thirst enable free-living humans to maintain normal fluid balance despite an estimated turnover of 5%–10% each day (Sawka et al. 2005). An adequate intake has been established to be 3.7 L/day for adult men and 2.7 L/day for adult women (Food and Nutrition Board 2004). Fluid sources include drinking water and water from beverages and food; national survey data indicate that 80% of fluids typically come from beverages and 20% from food in the United States. These data suggest that under normal circumstances, 740 and 540 mL of fluids (including but not exclusively from drinking water) will meet water requirements for adult men and women, respectively. Physiological changes associated with aging (including a decline in the sensation of thirst and reduced appetite), problems with access to fluids, and cognitive disorders are among the factors that can sometimes make the maintenance of adequate hydration challenging for older individuals (Ferry 2005).

Energy Requirements

Energy requirements generally decline with aging, as a result of a lower level of physical activity and reduced lean body mass (the latter being the major determinant of resting energy expenditure). For example, data from doubly labeled water studies suggest that mean total daily energy expenditures are 2,404, 2,066, and 1,564 kcal/day for normal-weight women ages 31–50, 51–70, and 71 or older, respectively (Food and Nutrition Board 2002). For normal-weight men, these figures are 3,021, 2,469, and 2,238 kcal/day for the 31–50, 51–70, and 71 and older age groups, respectively. Micronutrient requirements do not similarly decline, so a more nutrient-dense diet is necessary to maintain good nutritional status when total food intake is reduced in association with aging.

Carbohydrates

A major source of energy provided by the diet, carbohydrates are generally classified as starches and sugars (mono- and disaccharides). The current recommended dietary allowance (RDA) for carbohydrates is set at 130 g/day based on the average minimum amount of glucose utilized by the brain (Food and Nutrition Board 2002). Added sugars are usually found in foods with lower nutrient density compared with foods that contain naturally occurring sugars (e.g., lactose in milk, fructose in fruits) and starches, so a maximal intake of no more than one-quarter of energy from added sugars is advised for all persons.

Fat

Fat is another major source of energy in the diet, and 20%–35% of energy intake from total fat, predominantly mono- and polyunsaturated fatty acids, is the current recommendation (Food and Nutrition Board 2002). Linoleic acid, an omega-6 polyunsaturated fatty acid, is an established essential fatty acid. Current evidence indicates that the long-chain omega-3 fatty acid docosahexaenoic acid (DHA) is also essential, for its role as a structural membrane lipid, particularly in nerve tissue and the retina. Other biological activities of DHA that are relevant to brain function include the inhibition of oxidative stress–induced expression of proinflammatory genes and apoptosis in the brain and retina (Innis 2007). DHA is obtained from the diet either as DHA itself or through intake of the precursor fatty acid, α-linolenic acid (ALA), and the intermediate compound, eicosapentaenoic acid. Rich sources of ALA include several types of nuts, especially walnuts (Feldman 2002), and soybean and canola oils; fatty fish is the richest dietary source of DHA (Innis 2007). Dietary restriction of these omega-3 fatty acids and the resulting reduction in brain DHA levels in animal models are associated with impaired cognitive and behavioral performance.

Protein

The RDA for protein for adult men and women is 0.8 g of good-quality protein per kilogram of body weight per day, and evidence does not suggest that protein requirements change with aging in adults (Food and Nutrition Board 2002). Higher-quality protein is that with better essential amino acid composition (e.g., protein from animals and their products) and high digestibility.

Vitamins

Vitamins are a heterogeneous group of small organic molecules with a wide range of biochemical activities that are required in small amounts for normal metabolism and cellular function. An important concept that has emerged over the past few years is that these micronutrients, because they are so biologically active, are likely to cause adverse effects at doses beyond the amounts that can be obtained from food sources and managed by physiological and biochemical regulatory mechanisms. The Institute of Medicine panels that review the literature and provide dietary reference intakes now evaluate data to identify tolerable upper intake levels (ULs)—the highest levels of daily nutrient intake that are likely to pose no risk of adverse health effects to almost all individuals in the general population—in addition to RDAs or adequate intake levels. Sufficient evidence has enabled a UL to be established for most of the essential vitamins and minerals (Food and Nutrition Board 1997, 2000, 2001). These levels and supporting data are especially useful when evaluating dietary supplement formulations and their safety (Hathcock et al. 2007).

For older adults, achieving and maintaining good vitamin D and vitamin B_{12} status can be difficult without consuming fortified foods or dietary supplements. The 2005 Dietary Guidelines for Americans from the U.S. Department of Agriculture and Department of Health and Human Services now recommend that older adults consume vitamin D–fortified foods and supplements to achieve a daily intake of 25 µg (1,000 IU), in contrast to the adequate intake level established in 1997, which was 15 µg/day (600 IU) for men and women over 70 years old (Johnson and Kimlin 2006). Vitamin D has numerous biological functions and activities beyond those that affect the skeletal system (facilitating calcium absorption and bone health). Vitamin D receptors and vitamin D–metabolizing enzymes have been found in many regions of the brain, including the hippocampus, and evidence from laboratory studies has established that vitamin D can affect brain function (Garcion et al. 2002). The relationship between vitamin D status and cognition has been investigated in a few observational studies, with inconsistent results. For example, low serum 25-hydroxyvitamin D concentrations (an acceptable indicator of overall status) was associated with low mood and worse cognitive performance in 80 older adults (age range=60–92), 40 of whom had been diagnosed with mild Alzheimer disease and 40 of whom did not have dementia (Wilkins et al. 2006). In contrast, no association between these serum levels and performance on psychometric tests was found in a large sample of individuals participating in a national survey, which included a subset of 4,809 individuals ages 60–90 years (McGrath et al. 2007). The concern with vitamin B_{12} is based on the increased prevalence of atrophic gastritis with hypochlorhydria in association with aging, which limits the bioavailability of the protein- and peptide-bound vitamin B_{12} as it occurs in food (Selhub et al. 2000). Individuals over age 50 years are advised to meet the RDA for vitamin B_{12} (2.4 µg/day) mainly by choosing foods fortified with the vitamin or a dietary supplement, which solves the potential problem with bioavailability. Ensuring good vitamin B_{12} status in older adults, particularly when maintaining good cognitive function is the goal, is of particular importance because deficiency in this vitamin is associated with impaired neuropsychiatric functions and dementia (Selhub et al. 2000). The prevalence of low serum vitamin B_{12} concentrations tends to decrease with age (Pfeiffer et al. 2005). None of the six randomized clinical trials of the effect of vitamin B_{12} supplementation (administered orally or intramuscularly) on cognitive function reported to date have found beneficial effects (reviewed in Balk et al. 2007). These studies, however, have been criticized for being underpowered or too short.

Minerals

Requirements for two minerals, calcium and iron, also differ in older adults. To maintain calcium balance, both men and women age 50 years and older require 1,200 mg/day, compared with 1,000 mg/day for younger adults (Food and Nutrition Board 1997). Dairy products, including low-fat and nonfat products, are excellent sources of calcium, and numerous food products (e.g., juice, bread, cereals) are now fortified with calcium. Iron requirements, in contrast, are considerably lower for women age 50 and older (8 mg/day) versus women younger than age 50 (18 mg/day), due to menopause-associated cessation of menstruation (Food and Nutrition Board 2001). Potential prooxidant effects of excess iron, which may increase the risk for cardiovascular disease and cancer, are a good rationale to avoid higher intake of iron than is necessary to maintain balance.

Bioactive Food Components

The complexity of foods and the number of biologically active compounds provided by the diet, in addition to essential nutrients, have become an area of intense interest that particularly relates to the relationship between diet and disease risk. Bioactive food components under study include phy-

TABLE 15-1. Mechanisms by which bioactive food components may play a role in disease prevention

Antioxidant activity

Effects on cell proliferation, differentiation, and apoptosis

Enzyme induction or inhibition and detoxification

Effects on immune function

Effects on angiogenesis and cell adhesion and invasion

Regulation of hormone metabolism

Antibacterial and antiviral effects

---

tochemicals such as carotenoids, flavonoids, organosulfur compounds, isothiocyanates, indoles, monoterpenes, and phenolic acids, as well as probiotics. The interest is fueled by observational studies that have linked food choices and the overall dietary pattern with risk and progression of cancer and cardiovascular disease (Kris-Etherton et al. 2002). The epidemiological evidence is strongly supported by cell culture and laboratory animal studies, in which various bioactive food components have demonstrated diverse biological activities that have been shown to be involved in disease progression at the molecular and cellular level. Table 15–1 lists various mechanisms by which bioactive food components may play a role in disease prevention. A basic premise of current nutritional recommendations is that nutrient needs should be met primarily through food consumption, because this strategy enables the potential beneficial effects of the nonnutrient, bioactive components in foods to reduce the risk and progression of disease.

Moreover, the activities and effects of these dietary constituents, especially phytochemicals, may explain why dietary supplement formulations containing isolated micronutrients have generally not been demonstrated to reduce the risk for cancer or preinvasive lesions (Davies et al. 2006), despite fairly consistent associations between lower risk and higher intake of foods that contain those micronutrients. These nonnutrient constituents may influence different molecular and biochemical pathways, so although they may have a small effect independently, together (as present in food) they can produce an effect that is substantial enough to be clinically significant. Potential synergy of micronutrients and phytochemicals also has been suggested (R.H. Liu 2004). One would expect a similar situation in the evaluation of the relationship between diet and neurocognitive disease as seen in observational studies and the negative results from studies of dietary supplements. Another relevant issue is that interactions between bioactive food components and genetic factors are highly likely and should be examined when evaluating the response to dietary factors (Milner 2004). The molecular targets of various biological activities often involve metabolic pathways and metabolizing enzymes for which polymorphisms, as well as epigenetic effects, determine the contribution of a dietary or nutritional factor to disease risk.

Although this is currently an area of intense research efforts, much remains to be learned about the bioavailability and metabolism of the phytochemicals of interest and other nonnutrient bioactive food components in the human biological system. An example that is relevant to brain function is the phytochemical curcumin (a component of the spice turmeric, an ingredient of curry powder), which has been shown to have several biological effects such as anti-inflammatory, antioxidant, and hypolipidemic activity (Tayyem et al. 2006). Curcumin administration has been found to attenuate cognitive deficits, neuroinflammation, and plaque pathology in animal models of Alzheimer disease (Frautschy et al. 2001). However, the bioavailability, specific tissue targets, and biologically effective doses of curcumin in humans have yet to be identified (Lao et al. 2006).

Dietary Supplements

The Dietary Supplement Health and Education Act (DSHEA) of 1994 provides the following definition of a dietary supplement: a product, other than tobacco, intended to supplement the diet that contains at least one or more of the following ingredients: a vitamin, a mineral, an herb or other botanical, an amino acid, or a dietary substance for use to supplement the diet by increasing the total dietary intake; or a concentrate, metabolite, constituent, or extract, or combination of any of the previously mentioned ingredients. With regard to regulation, dietary supplements are classified as food products although they are labeled as dietary supplements.

As established by the DSHEA, dietary supplements have minimal requirements for premarketing notification of and review by the U.S. Food and Drug Administration (FDA) and are not required to have formal, premarketing FDA evaluation and approval, in contrast to the regulations for food additives and new drugs. Risk-benefit analysis is neither mandatory nor routinely conducted for these products, and postmarketing surveillance is not required. The burden of proof for demonstrating safety or lack thereof lies solely with the FDA, rather than with the manufacturer. Risks associated with dietary supplements include vitamin and mineral excess and toxicity, other adverse biological events (e.g., biochemical and pathophysiological changes), interactions with drugs, and interference with diagnostic tests, as well as economic burden.

There are a few clearly established indications for dietary supplementation. For example, one indication would be to meet nutrient needs when intake or absorption from food sources is known to be problematic, as discussed above for vitamin D and vitamin B_{12} in the elderly (see "Vitamins"). Most standard multivitamin and mineral formulations provide recommended (and not excessive) levels to meet nutrient requirements without risk of toxicity. Notably, encouraging older patients to eat fortified foods is an alternative strategy that avoids the extra expense and compliance issues involved with taking pills.

Some dietary supplements have been shown to be beneficial for a few conditions in randomized clinical trials (NIH State-of-the-Science Panel 2007). Examples are fish oil supplements to prevent new cardiovascular events, and calcium supplementation to reduce the risk for recurrence of adenomatous polyps. Current evidence from randomized clinical trials does not support the usefulness of multivitamins in promoting improved immune system function, or the usefulness of antioxidant supplements in reducing the risk for cardiovascular disease or in preventing or treating cancer. In some trials, supplementation actually was found to increase risk for poorer disease outcome and mortality (Huang et al. 2007). Thus, to reduce the risk for adverse events due to excess intake, the dosage used should not exceed the UL (the tolerable upper intake level set by the Institute of Medicine).

Diet and Alzheimer Disease

Alzheimer disease is the primary cause of dementia in the elderly, and current knowledge of the pathophysiology of Alzheimer disease suggests several mechanisms by which numerous dietary and nutritional factors could affect both the risk and progression of the disease. The primary mechanisms and pathways by which nutritional factors could affect the process of neurodegeneration are via altering oxidative stress, improving vascular function, and reducing inflammation. To date, a fair amount of evidence from observational studies, cell culture and laboratory animal studies, and a few clinical trials has been collected. In the evaluation of clinical and epidemiological studies, it should be recognized that the apolipoprotein E gene (*APOE*) ε4 allele, a genetic risk factor for Alzheimer disease, may modify the effects of dietary factors on risk (see Chapter 11, "Influence of Dietary Factors on Brain Aging and the Pathogenesis of Alzheimer Disease," this volume). Several comprehensive reviews have concluded that although some of the evidence is supportive of the potential for dietary factors to be protective, available data do not support specific conclusions about or dietary recommendations for the primary prevention of Alzheimer disease or slowing its progression (reviewed and summarized in Luchsinger and Mayeux 2004; Luchsinger et al. 2007; Nourhashemi et al. 2000; Staehelin 2005; Steele et al. 2007).

Oxidative stress results from an imbalance between the generation of reactive oxygen species and the ability of the organism to dispose of them. Micronutrients and dietary constituents that exhibit antioxidant activities include tocopherols (vitamin E), carotenoids, vitamin C, and flavonoids and lignans (in vegetables, fruits, and legumes). β-Amyloid protein, which is accumulated in the brains of Alzheimer disease patients, has been observed to be toxic in neuronal cell cultures via increased oxidative stress, and in laboratory experiments vitamin E has been shown to prevent the oxidative damage caused by β-amyloid protein (Christen 2000; Grundman 2000). Furthermore, supplementation with vitamin E, the most potent antioxidant in the human biological system, has been shown to increase concentrations of this vitamin in the brain (Vatassery et al. 1988). As noted earlier (see section "Nutritional Requirements"), this is a crucial factor because availability to the target tissue can be a limiting factor for demonstrating a clinically significant effect of various dietary constituents. Results from observational studies examining dietary intake of antioxidants or antioxidant supplement use and the risk for Alzheimer disease are inconsistent (Luchsinger and Mayeux 2004).

The effect of vitamin E supplementation on the progression of Alzheimer disease has been tested in two placebo-controlled, double-blind randomized clinical trials. In one trial, placebo or vitamin E (2,000 IU/day) and/or selegiline was administered to patients with moderate Alzheimer disease ($N=$ 341), and although the vitamin E supplementation was found to increase time to institutionalization, cognitive outcomes were not affected over a 2-year follow-up period (Sano et al. 1997). In a more recent trial, individuals with amnestic, mild cognitive impairment ($N=769$), who have a substantially increased risk for Alzheimer disease compared with elderly individuals without this impairment, were randomly assigned to receive 2,000 IU of vitamin E per day, donepezil (a cholinesterase inhibitor), or placebo (Petersen et al. 2005). Vitamin E supplementation did not affect the primary outcome at 2-year follow-up, which was the probability of developing Alzheimer disease, or measures of cognition and function used in the study.

Vegetables and fruits in the diet provide numerous antioxidants, such as vitamin C, carotenoids, and other phytochemicals. Markers of oxidative stress have been observed to decline in association with increased vegetable and fruit intake in feeding studies (Broekmans et al. 2000; Thompson et al. 2005). A notable characteristic of the Mediterranean diet, which has been associated with lower risk for Alzheimer disease (Scarmeas et al. 2006), is that it is rich in vegetables and fruits.

High plasma homocysteine concentration has been found to be associated with increased risk for dementia and Alzheimer disease in observational studies (Seshadri et al. 2002), and good nutritional status for three vitamins (vitamin B_6, vitamin B_{12}, and folate) is crucial to promote normal one-carbon metabolism that reduces homocysteine levels. The requirement for vitamin B_6 is fairly easy to meet with the typical U.S. diet, so inadequate intake of this vitamin is rare. However, suboptimal folate (and, in the elderly, vitamin B_{12}) status has been more commonly observed, although the situation for folate has been improving since the FDA mandated folate fortification of all cereal-grain products several years ago. Observational data from epidemiological studies of folate or vitamin B_{12} status and the risk for Alzheimer disease are mixed (reviewed in Luchsinger et al. 2007). In a placebo-controlled randomized clinical trial testing the effects of vitamin B_{12}, vitamin B_6, and folate supplementation in participants age 65 years and older with elevated homocysteine concentrations ($N=276$, cognitive function did not change even though the regimen effectively reduced homocysteine levels at 2-year follow-up (McMahon et al. 2006).

Inflammatory reactions have been proposed to contribute to neuronal loss in Alzheimer disease, and this is another mechanism by which diet might affect the risk for and progression of Alzheimer disease (Lau et al. 2007). Diets poor in omega-3 fatty acids, vegetables, and fruits have been observed to promote inflammatory markers (reviewed in Giugliano et al. 2006). In fact, patients with Alzheimer disease have been found to have lower levels of DHA in plasma and brain tissue compared with age-matched controls (Florent-Bechard et al. 2007), although the observational data have not consistently shown an association between intake of fish or omega-3 fatty acids and risk for Alzheimer disease (reviewed in Luchsinger et al. 2007). Notably, the effect of increased consumption of both fish and omega-3 fatty acids in reducing the risk for and mortality associated with cardiovascular disease is well established, based on data from both observational studies and clinical trials (Lichtenstein et al. 2006). Improvement in vascular function would be expected to be similarly beneficial for brain function, although a specific effect on risk for Alzheimer disease has not been demonstrated. In overweight or obese individuals, weight loss also has been observed to reduce inflammatory markers (Devaraj et al. 2006).

Alcohol is a neurotoxin when administered at intoxicating doses; however, epidemiological studies have shown moderate consumption to be associated with a lower risk of Alzheimer disease and overall dementia (for review, see Orgogozo et al. 1997; moderate consumption in this French study was defined as three to four glasses of wine per day). The American Heart Association's current recommendations for reducing the risk of heart disease advise that a moderate level of consumption (≤ 2 drinks per day) may be beneficial for those who consume alcohol (Lichtenstein et al. 2006), due to beneficial effects on vascular function and associations with a reduced risk for cardiovascular disease.

Caloric Restriction

In several animal models, including primates, caloric restriction prolongs longevity, apparently through a reduction in both oxidative stress and inflammation (Holloszy and Fontana 2007). A delay in the appearance of degenerative brain disease has also been observed in these animal studies (Nourhashemi et al. 2000), which suggests that a long-term regimen of caloric restriction may specifically be beneficial in reducing the risk for cognitive changes associated with Alzheimer disease and other forms of dementia. As recently reviewed by Speakman and Hambly (2007), results from animal studies suggest that the benefits of caloric restriction are related to the extent and timing of the strategy. For example, these investigators calculated (based on laboratory animal study data) that a caloric restriction of 30% (consuming 30% fewer calories than are estimated to be expended) in a 48-year-old man with a normal life expectancy of 78 years could increase his life expectancy by 2.8 years. Also, caloric restriction does not promote diminished hunger, even in the long term, which suggests that discomfort would be expected to accompany this practice. In primates, a caloric restriction of 30% has been shown to promote reduced lean muscle mass in addition to reduced fat mass (Blanc et al. 2003).

More positive arguments about the potential usefulness of caloric restriction are that a restriction of even 20% has been shown to promote favorable changes in various risk factors (e.g., elevated levels of blood lipids, blood glucose, and inflammatory markers) in short-term clinical studies (Everitt and Le Couteur 2007). Even intermittent caloric restriction in middle-aged rats has been shown to promote favorable changes in oxidative stress and other biomarkers (Sharma and Kaur 2007). Thus, this remains an intriguing area of research. Although this strategy may be potentially useful in extending the life span and postponing the onset of age-related degenerative diseases, sustained purposeful undereating (while still maintaining good nutritional status) is a difficult lifestyle for most individuals. An emphasis on nutrient-dense food choices becomes even more important under conditions of caloric restriction than it is under normal circumstances of aging.

Nutritional Management Issues in Dementia

Specific nutritional problems often arise in association with the onset and progression of impaired neurocognitive functions and dementia. Individuals with dementia are at high risk for malnutrition due to pathophysiological changes that affect eating behavior and food intake and due to reliance on assistance from family members or caregivers to ensure adequate intake. Aging is normally associated with a decline in odor detection; changes in the processing of olfactory information that occur in Alzheimer disease can further compound the problem of loss of the sense of smell (Nordin et al. 1995).

Weight loss in association with dementia is common, and recent evidence based on data obtained using state-of-the-art technologies to measure energy expenditure and body composition provides some insight into the etiology and management of such weight loss. Body weight is determined by the amount of energy consumed versus the amount of energy expended, so the focus of research has been to identify the primary etiological factors that could influence both sides of this equation. Current findings suggest that increased energy expenditure (perhaps due to pacing or wandering) or a hypermetabolic state does not explain weight loss in Alzheimer disease patients. In fact, a higher level of physical activity has been found to be associated with the prevention of skeletal muscle loss, and skeletal muscle loss, which is frequently observed in patients with Alzheimer disease patients, is a major factor in the increased risk of decubitus ulcers, infection, and mortality (Poehlman and Dvorak 2000).

Evidence now indicates that the weight loss commonly observed in patients with dementia is attributable mainly to insufficient energy intake relative to expenditure. A longitudinal study in a cohort of patients with probable Alzheimer disease examined the relationships between nutritional factors, including weight loss, and several patient, caregiver, and disease-related behavioral and psychosocial factors (Gillette-Guyonnet et al. 2000). In that study, greater severity of dementia and caregiver burden and stress were identified as predictive of weight loss. This finding suggests that a potential intervention is to identify and assist caregivers who feel overburdened or are not able or willing to devote the time and effort necessary to ensure that the patient consumes an adequate amount of food.

Dietary Guidelines and Recommendations

Table 15–2 lists current dietary recommendations of the U.S. Department of Agriculture (U.S. Department of Health and Human Services 2005), which are quite appropriate and applicable for promoting successful aging, including optimizing brain function. The first priority is to meet nutrient needs, because the brain, like all organs, needs fuel and essential nutrients in ade-

TABLE 15–2. Current dietary guidelines

1. Consume adequate nutrients within energy (calorie) requirements
2. Achieve and maintain a healthy weight
3. Be physically active each day
4. Consume vegetables, fruits, and whole grains and fat-free or low-fat milk or equivalent dairy products
5. Choose a diet that is low in saturated fat (and cholesterol) and moderate in total fat
6. Include nutrient- and fiber-rich carbohydrate sources
7. Consume <2,300 mg of sodium (approximately 1 tsp salt) per day
8. Drink alcoholic beverages sensibly and in moderation

Source. Adapted from U.S. Department of Health and Human Services 2005.

quate amounts in order to function. Nutrient-dense foods (those providing protein, vitamins, minerals, and other beneficial food components such as fiber and phytochemicals) that are low in saturated fat and added sugars should constitute the majority of the food choices. Vitamin D– and vitamin B_{12}–fortified foods or vitamin D and B_{12} supplements are recommended for older adults (U.S. Department of Health and Human Services 2005).

Achieving and maintaining a healthy weight are accomplished by balancing caloric intake with caloric expenditure. Current research suggests that a low-energy-density, high-fiber diet is the dietary pattern most consistently associated with optimal weight management throughout adulthood (Bell and Rolls 2001; Ledikwe et al. 2007; S. Liu et al. 2003). Healthy weight management is also facilitated by daily physical activity (see Chapter 14, "Creating Environments to Encourage Physical Activity"), and current recommendations are for at least 30 minutes of moderate-intensity physical activity, above the usual lifestyle activity, on most days of the week (U.S. Department of Health and Human Services 2005). A higher level of physical activity (60–90 minutes daily) is recommended to promote weight loss and to prevent regaining weight, based on current evidence (U.S. Department of Health and Human Services 2005). Stretching for flexibility and resistance or strength training, in addition to cardiovascular or aerobic exercise, are also encouraged.

The recommended dietary pattern is high in vegetables, fruits, and whole grains, with low-fat or nonfat dairy products. At least 2–3 cups of vegetables and 1½–2 cups of fruit are the levels recommended, with vegetables and fruits consumed at every meal and for snacks. Vegetables and fruits contain numerous dietary constituents that may play a role in promoting normal cognitive function, such as essential vitamins and minerals and bioactive food components that may reduce oxidative stress and inflammatory phyto-chemicals. Additionally, these are low-energy-density foods that promote satiety and thus form the basis of a diet that is low in energy density.

Colorful vegetables and fruits, such as dark green and orange vegetables and orange or red fruits, are typically those with the highest amounts of phyto-chemicals. Fresh, frozen, or canned—raw, cooked, or dried—vegetables and fruits are all good sources; they do not need to be raw to be good choices. Cooking vegetables and fruits, especially with methods such as microwaving or steaming, enables some of the constituents to be more bioavailable and thus better absorbed. Practical strategies include adding vegetables to other foods, such as pasta and rice dishes, pizza, sandwiches, soups, salads, quick breads, and muffins. Fruits can be added to cereal, mixed dishes, salads, quick breads, and muffins. Keeping prewashed and ready-to-eat (or frozen) vegetables and fruits handy for snacks and to add to foods facilitates increased consumption. Whole fruits (instead of juices) add more fiber and fewer calories to the diet. When fruit juice is chosen, the best choice is 100% fruit juice, especially nutrient-rich juices such as orange juice, rather than fruit drinks.

Whole-grain products are also encouraged, and three or more ounce-equivalents daily is the current recommendation. Whole grains are rich in a variety of compounds (in addition to fiber) that exhibit various biological activities, including hormonal and antioxidant effects. For example, whole-grain products contain antioxidants, such as phenolic acids, flavonoids, and tocopherols, in addition to lignans, phytosterols, and unsaturated fatty acids (Slavin 2003). Choosing whole grains and whole-grain food products as a source of fiber, rather than relying on fiber supplements, adds nutritional value to the diet.

Refined grains have been milled, which removes the bran and germ. Examples of refined grain products include white flour, degermed cornmeal, white bread, and white rice. In the United States, most refined grain products have been enriched, which means that several vitamins (thiamin, riboflavin, niacin, and folic acid) and iron are added back to the product after processing. Thus, these products are not completely without nutritional value, but many of the potentially helpful constituents (e.g., fiber, phytochemicals) are not added back. The best choices are made by reading food labels, especially ingredient lists, to assess whole-grain content: whole grain or whole wheat should be listed as a major ingredient. Approximately one-half of the white flour in many baked goods can be replaced with whole-grain wheat or oat flour. Eating whole-grain foods (e.g., ready-to-eat cereal, crackers, popcorn) for a snack, instead of refined grain products, is another useful strategy.

The benefits of a diet low in saturated fat (and cholesterol) for vascular function are well established (Lichtenstein et al. 2006). Meat and meat products are the major sources of saturated fat in the diet, and reducing saturated fat intake to less than 10% of total calories is recommended. Choose the leanest meat or pork, trim all visible fat before cooking, and broil, grill, roast, poach, or boil meat, pork, or poultry. Boneless, skinless chicken and turkey cutlets are the leanest poultry choices. Fish, beans, nuts, eggs, and low-fat dairy foods are all good sources of protein that can replace meat in the diet. Beans, such as dried beans, pinto beans, lentils, and soybeans, are high in fiber and numerous phytochemicals. Nuts are a good meat replacement because the type of fat contained in nuts is primarily unsaturated fat.

Conclusion

Current evidence suggests that diet and nutritional factors can have an important impact on the aging brain. A healthy dietary pattern can be achieved— one that considers a given individual's food preferences and capabilities— across the many food choices and products that currently constitute the U.S. food supply. Referral to a registered dietitian, who is credentialed and trained in nutritional science, food science, and behavioral counseling, is recommended for those who need individualized assistance in the practical aspects of establishing a healthy diet, such as reading food labels and planning menus.

KEY POINTS

▪ The brain requires essential nutrients and dietary constituents, as other organs and tissues do, for optimal function.

▪ Most standard multivitamin and mineral formulations provide recommended (and not excessive) levels to meet nutrient requirements without risk of toxicity.

▪ The primary mechanisms and pathways by which nutritional factors could affect the process of neurodegeneration are via altering oxidative stress, improving vascular function, and reducing inflammation.

▪ In several animal models, including primates, caloric restriction prolongs longevity, apparently through a reduction in both oxidative stress and inflammation.

▪ Referral to a registered dietitian, who is credentialed and trained in nutritional science, food science, and behavioral counseling, is recommended for those who need individualized assistance in the practical aspects of establishing a healthy diet.

References

Balk EM, Raman G, Tatsioni A, et al: Vitamin B6, B12, and folic acid supplementation and cognitive function. Arch Intern Med 167:21–30, 2007

Bell EA, Rolls BJ: Energy density of foods affects energy intake across multiple levels of fat content in lean and obese women. Am J Clin Nutr 73:1010–1018, 2001

Blanc S, Schoeller D, Kemnitz J, et al: Energy expenditure of rhesus monkeys subjected to 11 years of dietary restriction. J Clin Endocrinol Metab 88:16–23, 2003

Broekmans WM, Klöpping-Ketelaars IA, Schuurman CR, et al: Fruits and vegetables increase plasma carotenoids and vitamins and decrease homocysteine in humans. J Nutr 130:1578–1583, 2000

Christen Y: Oxidative stress and Alzheimer disease. Am J Clin Nutr 71:621S–629S, 2000

Davies AA, Smith GD, Harbord R, et al: Nutritional interventions and outcome in patients with cancer or preinvasive lesions: systematic review. J Natl Cancer Inst 98:961–973, 2006

Devaraj S, Kasim-Karakas S, Jialal I: The effect of weight loss and dietary fatty acids on inflammation. Curr Atheroscler Rep 8:477–486, 2006

Everitt AV, Le Couteur DG: Life extension by caloric restriction in humans. Ann NY Acad Sci 1114:428–433, 2007

Feldman EB: The scientific evidence for a beneficial health relationship between walnuts and coronary heart disease. J Nutr 132:1062S–1101S, 2002

Ferry M: Strategies for ensuring good hydration in the elderly. Nutr Rev 63:S22–S29, 2005

Florent-Bechard S, Malaplate-Armand C, Koziel V, et al: Towards a nutritional approach for prevention of Alzheimer's disease. J Neurol Sci 262:27–36, 2007

Food and Nutrition Board, Institute of Medicine: Dietary Reference Intakes for Calcium, Phosphorus, Magnesium, Vitamin D, and Fluoride. Washington, DC, National Academy Press, 1997

Food and Nutrition Board, Institute of Medicine: Dietary Reference Intakes for Vitamin C, Vitamin E, Selenium, and Carotenoids. Washington, DC, National Academy Press, 2000

Food and Nutrition Board, Institute of Medicine: Dietary Reference Intakes for Vitamin A, Vitamin K, Arsenic, Boron, Chromium, Copper, Iodine, Iron, Manganese, Molybdenum, Nickel, Silicon, Vanadium, and Zinc. Washington, DC, National Academy Press, 2001

Food and Nutrition Board, Institute of Medicine: Dietary Reference Intakes for Energy, Carbohydrate, Fiber, Fat, Fatty Acids, Cholesterol, Protein, and Amino Acids. Washington, DC, National Academy Press, 2002

Food and Nutrition Board, Institute of Medicine: Dietary Reference Intakes for Water, Potassium, Sodium, Chloride, and Sulfate. Washington, DC, National Academy Press, 2004

Frautschy SA, Hu W, Kim P, et al: Phenolic anti-inflammatory antioxidant reversal of Abeta-induced cognitive deficits and neuropathology. Neurobiol Aging 22:993–1005, 2001

Garcion E, Wion-Barbot N, Montero-Menei CN, et al: New clues about vitamin D functions in the nervous system. Trends Endocrinol Metab 3:100–105, 2002

Gillette-Guyonnet S, Nourhashemi F, Andrieu S, et al: Weight loss in Alzheimer disease. Am J Clin Nutr 71:637S–642S, 2000

Giugliano D, Ceriello A, Esposito K: The effects of diet on inflammation. J Am Coll Cardiol 48:677–685, 2006

Grundman M: Vitamin E and Alzheimer disease: the basis for additional clinical trials. Am J Clin Nutr 71:630S–636S, 2000

Hathcock JN, Shao A, Vieth R, et al: Risk assessment for vitamin D. Am J Clin Nutr 85:6–18, 2007

Holloszy JO, Fontana L: Caloric restriction in humans. Exp Gerontol 42:709–712, 2007

Huang HY, Caballero B, Chang S, et al: Multivitamin/mineral supplements and prevention of chronic disease: executive summary. Am J Clin Nutr 85:265S–268S, 2007

Innis SM: Dietary (n-3) fatty acids and brain development. J Nutr 137:855–859, 2007

Johnson MA, Kimlin MG: Vitamin D, aging, and the 2005 Dietary Guidelines for Americans. Nutr Rev 64:410–421, 2006

Kris-Etherton PM, Hecker KD, Bonanome A, et al: Bioactive compounds in foods: their role in the prevention of cardiovascular disease and cancer. Am J Med 113:71S–88S, 2002

Lao CD, Ruffin MT 4th, Normolle D, et al: Dose escalation of a curcuminoid formulation. BMC Complement Altern Med 6:10, 2006

Lau FC, Shukitt-Hale B, Joseph JA: Nutritional intervention in brain aging: reducing the effects of inflammation and oxidative stress. Subcell Biochem 42:299–318, 2007

Ledikwe JH, Rolls BJ, Smiciklas-Wright H, et al: Reductions in dietary energy density are associated with weight loss in overweight and obese participants in the PREMIER trial. Am J Clin Nutr 85:1212–1221, 2007

Lichtenstein AH, Appell LJ, Brands M, et al: Diet and lifestyle recommendations revision 2006: a scientific statement from the American Heart Association Nutrition Committee. Circulation 114:82–96, 2006

Liu RH: Potential synergy of phytochemicals in cancer prevention: mechanism of action. J Nutr 134:3479–3485, 2004

Liu S, Willett WC, Manson JE, et al: Relation between changes in intakes of dietary fiber and grain products and changes in weight and development of obesity among middle-aged women. Am J Clin Nutr 78:920–927, 2003

Luchsinger JA, Mayeux R: Dietary factors and Alzheimer's disease. Lancet Neurol 3:579–587, 2004

Luchsinger JA, Noble JM, Scarmeas N: Diet and Alzheimer's disease. Curr Neurol Neurosci Rep 7:366–372, 2007

McGrath J, Scragg R, Chant D, et al: No association between serum 25-hydroxyvitamin D3 level and performance on psychometric tests in NHANES III. Neuroepidemiology 29:49–54, 2007

McMahon JA, Green TJ, Skeaff CM, et al: A controlled trial of homocysteine lowering and cognitive performance. N Engl J Med 354:2764–2772, 2006

Milner JA: Molecular targets for bioactive food components. J Nutr 134:2492S–2498S, 2004

NIH State-of-the-Science Panel: National Institutes of Health State-of-the-Science Conference Statement: multivitamin/mineral supplements and chronic disease prevention. Am J Clin Nutr 85:257S–264S, 2007

Nordin S, Monsch AU, Murphy C: Unawareness of smell loss in normal aging and Alzheimer's disease: discrepancy between self-reported and diagnosed smell sensitivity. J Gerontol B Psychol Sci Soc Sci 50:P187–P192, 1995

Nourhashemi F, Gillette-Guyonnet S, Andrieu S, et al: Alzheimer disease: protective factors. Am J Clin Nutr 71:643S–649S, 2000

Orgogozo JM, Dartigues JF, Lafont S, et al: Wine consumption and dementia in the elderly: a prospective community study in the Bordeaux area. Rev Neurol (Paris) 153:185–192, 1997

Petersen RC, Thomas RG, Grundman M, et al: Vitamin E and donepezil for the treatment of mild cognitive impairment. N Engl J Med 352:2379–2388, 2005

Pfeiffer CM, Caudill SP, Gunter EW, et al: Biochemical indicators of B vitamin status in the US population after folic acid fortification: results from the National Health and Nutrition Examination Survey 1999–2000. Am J Clin Nutr 82:442–450, 2005

Poehlman ET, Dvorak RV: Energy expenditure, energy intake, and weight loss in Alzheimer disease. Am J Clin Nutr 71:650S–655S, 2000

Sano M, Ernesto C, Thomas RG, et al: A controlled trial of selegiline, alpha-tocopherol, or both as treatment for Alzheimer's disease. N Engl J Med 336:1216–1222, 1997

Sawka MN, Cheuvront SN, Carter R 3rd: Human water needs. Nutr Rev 63:S30–S39, 2005

Scarmeas N, Stern Y, Tang MX, et al: Mediterranean diet and risk for Alzheimer's disease. Ann Neurol 59:912–921, 2006

Selhub J, Bagley LC, Miller J, et al: B vitamins, homocysteine, and neurocognitive function in the elderly. Am J Clin Nutr 71:614S–620S, 2000

Seshadri S, Beiser A, Selhub J, et al: Plasma homocysteine as a risk factor for dementia and Alzheimer's disease. N Engl J Med 346:476–483, 2002

Sharma S, Kaur G: Intermittent dietary restriction as a practical intervention in aging. Ann NY Acad Sci 1114:419–427, 2007

Slavin J: Why whole grains are protective: biological mechanisms. Proc Nutr Soc 62:129–134, 2003

Speakman JR, Hambly C: Starving for life: what animal studies can and cannot tell us about the use of caloric restriction to prolong human lifespan. J Nutr 137:1078–1086, 2007

Staehelin HB: Micronutrients and Alzheimer's disease. Proc Nutr Soc 64:565–570, 2005

Steele M, Stuchbury G, Munch G: The molecular basis of the prevention of Alzheimer's disease through healthy nutrition. Exp Gerontol 42:28–36, 2007

Tayyem RF, Heath DD, Al-Delaimy WK, et al: Curcumin content of turmeric and curry powders. Nutr Cancer 55:126–131, 2006

Thompson HJ, Heimendinger J, Sedlacek S, et al: 8-Isoprostane F2alpha excretion is reduced in women by increased vegetable and fruit intake. Am J Clin Nutr 82:768–776, 2005

U.S. Department of Health and Human Services and U.S. Department of Agriculture: Dietary Guidelines for Americans 2005 (HHS Publ No HHS-ODPHP-2005-01-DGA-A). Washington, DC, U.S. Department of Health and Human Services, 2005. Available at: http://www.health.gov/dietaryguidelines/dga2005/document/pdf/DGA2005.pdf. Accessed February 1, 2008.

Vatassery GT, Brin MF, Fahn S, et al: Effect of high doses of dietary vitamin E on the concentrations of vitamin E in several brain regions, plasma, liver, and adipose tissue of rats. J Neurochem 51:621–623, 1988

Wilkins CH, Sheline YI, Roe CM, et al: Vitamin D deficiency is associated with low mood and worse cognitive performance in older adults. Am J Geriatr Psychiatry 14:1032–1040, 2006

Recommended Readings and Web Sites

Ferry M: Strategies for ensuring good hydration in the elderly. Nutr Rev 63:S22–S29, 2005

Huang HY, Caballero B, Chang S, et al: Multivitamin/mineral supplements and prevention of chronic disease: executive summary. Am J Clin Nutr 85:265S–268S, 2007

NIH State-of-the-Science Panel: National Institutes of Health State-of-the-Science Conference Statement: multivitamin/mineral supplements and chronic disease prevention. Am J Clin Nutr 85:257S–264S, 2007

Scarmeas N, Stern Y, Tang MX, et al: Mediterranean diet and risk for Alzheimer's disease. Ann Neurol 59:912–921, 2006

U.S. Department of Agriculture: MyPyramid.gov. Available at: http://www.mypyramid.gov. Accessed April 6, 2009.

16 Pharmacological Approaches to Successful Cognitive and Emotional Aging

Thomas Meeks, M.D.

One need only recall Ponce de León's search for the Fountain of Youth to recognize that the desire for some substance that would reverse the effects of aging has long existed. Although this yearning has largely been fanciful or even reflective of the ageist attitudes in Western societies, modern medicine has indeed turned to pharmaceuticals as remedies for a wide spectrum of age-related illnesses or symptoms. Despite ancient sayings regarding the value of prevention, Western medicine has been slower in looking toward pharmacological and other means of maintaining wellness and preventing illness. This is a wise and needed shift in the Western medical frame of reference. In this chapter I review existing evidence regarding curative (which are rare), palliative, and preventive means to promote healthy aging of the brain and mind. My aim is not to deny that age-related changes in brain function inevitably occur or to undervalue some positive aspects of the aging brain (e.g., more effective emotional regulation). Yet some facts remain unchanged no matter how much one respects and values the place of older adults in society: 1) the brain loses neurons and overall volume with increasing age, impacting cognitive and emotional functioning; 2) cognitive disorders such as dementia increase in incidence in a nearly exponential pattern after age 60; and 3) psychosocial stressors specific to older adults (e.g., forced moves, multiple bereavements, loss of functional independence, increasing medical burden, loss of social support systems) may challenge even the most resilient of persons. This chapter outlines what is known about pharmacological means, both traditional Western and alternative medications, of promoting successful cognitive and emotional aging.

Successful Cognitive Aging: Preventive Agents

Complementary and Alternative Medications

Many products considered as dietary supplements or herbs, which are not under the regulation of the U.S. Food and Drug Administration (FDA), have been touted to have various antiaging effects. It is not hard to find hundreds of products in an Internet search that tout their ability to reverse or prevent the ravages of aging on memory and other cognitive functions. Many such products contain a wide variety of chemical compounds, at times with little rationale for their selection or specific combination.

The primary messages of this chapter regarding such products are as follows:

1. No individual nonprescription herbal or biological supplement has been shown to have definitive benefits in delaying the onset of cognitive problems (with memory often receiving the most attention).
2. No combination of these various agents has been shown to be effective (or safe; e.g., free of drug–drug interactions) for delaying the onset of cognitive problems.
3. Being outside of the purview of the FDA, manufacturers of such products can make nonspecific claims (e.g., "to promote improved thinking") without supportive empirical, peer-reviewed evidence, and the products are not subject to the same regulations that prescription medications are regarding the standardization of the products that are listed as active ingredients. In other words, what you see on the label may not be what you get when you ingest any given product.

Nonetheless, there are some interesting and promising lines of research regarding various alternative medicines (including several dietary ingredients) and their role in promoting cognitive health and perhaps decreasing the chance of developing a cognitive disorder in late life. Some examples of such preliminary research are summarized in Table 16–1.

TABLE 16–1.   Alternative biological or dietary agents proposed to promote healthy cognitive aging as forms of prevention

Biological/dietary agent	Evidence for/against[a]
B vitamins (e.g., folate and vitamin B12)	Overall, epidemiological data linking B vitamin intake with cognitive outcomes are weak, unless there is an obvious deficiency in a certain vitamin; clinical trials have generally not been very sound methodologically and do not currently indicate any role for B vitamins in preserving cognition among healthy older adults.
Curcumin (a chemical in turmeric, an ingredient in curry)	Epidemiological evidence suggests lower than expected rates of AD in India, where curry is prevalent in the diet, and curcumin in animals has shown antioxidant, anti-inflammatory, and antiamyloid properties. Prospective research is lacking to establish a true cause-and-effect relationship between curcumin and healthier cognitive aging.
Ginkgo biloba	A large prevention trial is under way in Europe, but one randomized, controlled trial has already failed to show benefits.
Mediterranean diet	• High intake of vegetables, legumes, fruits, and cereals • High intake of unsaturated fatty acids (mostly in the form of olive oil), but low intake of saturated fatty acids • Moderately high intake of fish • Low to moderate intake of dairy products (mostly cheese or yogurt) • Low intake of meat and poultry • Regular but moderate amount of ethanol, primarily in the form of wine and generally during meals Some reports of association with lower risk of developing AD and lower rates of death among persons who already have AD. Multiple components make it difficult to know which dietary choices are most crucial.

TABLE 16–1. Alternative biological or dietary agents proposed to promote healthy cognitive aging as forms of prevention *(continued)*

Biological/dietary agent	Evidence for/against[a]
Omega-3 fatty acids (e.g., fish oil)	Shown to have anti-inflammatory properties. Several epidemiological studies have shown an association between increased fish consumption (especially so-called fatty fish such as salmon) and reduced AD risk. Low serum levels of omega-3 fatty acids have also been linked cross-sectionally with AD. No prospective trials exist to validate the notion that omega-3 fatty acids promote healthy cognitive aging in cognitively intact older adults.
Resveratrol (in red wine, grapes, cranberries, and peanuts)	A potent antioxidant, and anti-inflammatory agent. Epidemiological studies suggest an association between moderate red wine consumption and lowered risk of AD. No prospective studies to prove a cause-and-effect relationship between resveratrol and healthier cognitive aging.
Vitamin E (α-tocopherol)	Vitamin E is among a host of antioxidant nutrients (including vitamins A and C). A study in persons with MCI showed no benefit of vitamin E in preventing dementia. No solid evidence suggests vitamin E is helpful in promoting healthy cognitive aging in normal older adults.

Note. AD=Alzheimer disease; MCI=mild cognitive impairment.
[a]See Meeks and Jeste 2009 for review of studies on which evidence is based.

Traditional Western Medications

Like herbs and dietary supplements, no prescription medication has un-equivocally shown benefit in preserving cognitive function among healthy older adults. Case-control studies (which look backward in time and are thus less convincing in establishing cause and effect) have suggested that use of nonsteroidal anti-inflammatory agents such as ibuprofen (Motrin, Advil) is associated with a lower risk of developing dementia (Szekely et al. 2004). Prospective studies of the use of these agents in cognitive disorders have been less impressive (ADAPT Research Group et al. 2008). Even if these agents might confer some decreased risk of developing Alzheimer disease (which does appear to involve inflammation as part of the pathology that causes nerve cell death), they have significant side effects among older adults, including possible increased cardiovascular disease, kidney damage, and gastrointestinal (GI) bleeding. In fact, a prospective trial using rofecoxib (Vioxx), an anti-inflammatory drug that was pulled from the American market because of apparent cardiovascular side effects, found that it actually tended to increase rates of dementia among susceptible persons with baseline mild cognitive impairment (Thal et al. 2005).

Case-control evidence also exists for statin medications (the most commonly used drugs to treat abnormal cholesterol levels), suggesting that they possibly decrease the risk of developing Alzheimer disease (Rockwood et al. 2002). These medications have been shown to affect the formation of amyloid-β plaques, one of the cellular hallmarks of Alzheimer disease (Höglund et al. 2007). However, the use of statins simply to decrease dementia risk in persons without abnormal lipid levels cannot currently be justified. Nevertheless, this line of inquiry brings up what is probably the most important way in which currently available pharmacological agents may be helpful in preventing dementia—via decreasing risk factors for cerebrovascular disease (CVD) and stroke. CVD and Alzheimer disease have a complex relationship with each other. CVD may cause a purely vascular dementia but it also appears to increase the risk of Alzheimer disease. Thus, proactive management of vascular risk factors, including hypertension, diabetes mellitus, smoking, and dyslipidemia, may very well help preserve cognitive function. For instance, a large European study showed that treatment of hypertension with a calcium channel blocker decreased the odds of developing dementia (Trompet et al. 2008). Other studies suggest that different classes of anti-hypertension drugs (e.g., angiotensin-converting enzyme inhibitors and diuretics), when used to control hypertension, may also decrease the risk of developing dementia (Guo et al. 1999; Rozzini et al. 2006).

Although modification of vascular risk factors other than hypertension has not been shown as definitively to alter dementia risk in prospective studies, the idea that adequately treating diabetes mellitus (also a risk factor for Alzheimer disease, independent of its effects on CVD), nicotine dependence, and dyslipidemia could alter the risk for dementia seems intuitive, and such treatment would also reap a variety of other health benefits for affected persons. The use of aspirin is commonplace in older adults to prevent vascular disease and could also theoretically alter the risk for dementia.

Another line of preventive research regarding cognition and cognitive decline in older adults has focused on a prodromal state of cognitive decline, most often termed *mild cognitive impairment* (MCI). MCI typically refers to demonstrable memory impairment older adults (relative to normative scores of peers matched for age and education) that does not cause functional disability. This definition, of course, assumes that there is not another clear explanation for the memory impairment (e.g., depression, delirium). Increasingly, the term *mild cognitive impairment* has also been applied to deficits in cognitive domains other than memory, so-called *nonamnestic MCI*. MCI is an interesting condition in which to try preventive interventions because persons who meet diagnostic criteria for amnestic MCI have an elevated risk of developing dementia—around 10%–15% per year (Petersen and Negash 2008)—and further tissue damage may be avoided.

Probably the most logical pharmacological interventions to test in MCI are those already approved to treat dementia, and in fact most therapeutic trials in subjects with MCI have examined acetylcholinesterase inhibitors (see "Successful Cognitive Aging: Curative or Palliative Agents, Traditional Western Medications" below for a detailed explanation of these drugs), the first medications approved to treat Alzheimer disease. Unfortunately, the evidence of benefit for these drugs in treating MCI has been disappointing. Although one study of donepezil (Aricept) showed a delay of progression to dementia in the first year among persons with MCI, the outcomes at 3 years were no different between those treated with drug versus placebo (Petersen et al. 2005). Negative study results with other cholinesterase inhibitors have since been reported (Feldman et al. 2007; Winblad et al. 2008). The aforementioned donepezil study also included a treatment arm with high-dose vitamin E, but this treatment likewise failed to show benefits for older adults with MCI. Similarly, a study comparing a walking intervention with vitamin B supplements for persons with MCI failed to show any delay in progression to dementia with the vitamin supplements (van Uffelen et al. 2008). Several smaller, pilot-level studies of other pharmacological agents have reported some positive cognitive effects in subjects with MCI, but all of these studies are very preliminary and the agents need more extensive study to verify any possible benefits. These experimental agents include triflusal (an anti-inflammatory drug), nilvadipine (a calcium channel blocker), fluoxetine (a selective serotonin reuptake inhibitor), raloxifene (a selective estrogen receptor modulator), and intranasal insulin.

Successful Cognitive Aging: Curative or Palliative Agents

Complementary and Alternative Medications

Ginkgo biloba extract at dosages of 120–240 mg/day is the most studied and most widely used biological supplement for the prevention of dementia. As with most botanical products, the ginkgo plant has many potentially bioactive compounds. The most common standardized extract of ginkgo is called *EGb 761* and can be given orally or intravenously. Several mechanisms of action for ginkgo in dementia have been proposed. It has antioxidant properties, may enhance cerebral blood flow via antagonism of platelet-activating factor and alterations in vascular tone, and appears to enhance glucose metabolism. Many of the early studies with ginkgo enrolled participants with a somewhat vague diagnosis of "cerebral insufficiency," limiting interpretations that can be made from these trials.

A recent systematic review of *Ginkgo biloba* extract for treating "cognitive impairment" and dementia (Birks and Grimley Evans 2007) examined 35 randomized, double-blind trials and concluded that Clinical Global Impression Scale scores showed improvement at 24 weeks in high-dosage (>200 mg/day) studies; all dosages were associated with improved cognitive scores at week 12 but not at week 24. Surprisingly, lower-dosage studies showed improvement on activities of daily living measures but high-dosage studies did not; overall, the level of evidence was still deemed "inconsistent and unconvincing." The review also revealed no difference in overall adverse effects between ginkgo and placebo, but there were possible side effects, including GI upset, skin reactions, headache, and bleeding complications.

Moreover, ginkgo may have important interactions with prescription anticoagulant medications. The potential for herb–drug interactions has become increasingly recognized as a potentially problematic consequence of using herbs, and this issue is one that physicians may forget to ask about, and patients may forget or decide not to reveal their use of herbal supplements. Ginkgo may often be used, without a physician's knowledge, along with prescription dementia medications, but the efficacy and safety of this combination are unknown. Overall, the body of evidence thus far for *Ginkgo biloba* extract as a cognitive treatment for dementia indicates that even though it has some possible benefits on cognition in Alzheimer disease and vascular dementia, the effects are less convincing than those of prescription dementia medications (which themselves have relatively modest effects).

Huperzine A is a plant-based chemical derived from a club moss (*Huperzia serrata*) that has been used for centuries in China as a folk medicine for a variety of ailments. Huperzine A has shown inhibition of acetylcholinesterase, the same enzyme targeted by prescription drugs for dementia, in the laboratory. Other research indicates that huperzine A reduces generation of amyloid-β, the protein fragment that accumulates and possibly initiates the cascade of cell death in Alzheimer disease; that it has antioxidant properties; and that it inhibits cell death (Ma et al. 2007). A randomized, controlled trial in China with more than 200 participants tested 0.2–0.4 mg of huperzine A versus placebo among persons with possible or probable Alzheimer disease (Zhang et al. 2002). The results were promising, with improvement seen in cognition, measures of activities of daily living, and neuropsychiatric symptoms (e.g., depression, delusions, repetitive activities). Huperzine A is currently in clinical trials that should provide more definitive answers regarding its benefits and risks in Alzheimer disease. Adverse effects likely resemble those of prescription acetylcholinesterase inhibitors (e.g., GI upset, insomnia).

Along with vitamins A and C, vitamin E is well known for its antioxidant properties and has thus been studied for its potential therapeutic benefits for a wide variety of illnesses, including cardiovascular disease, cancer, and Alzheimer disease. Vitamin E became commonly used in the mainstream treatment of Alzheimer disease because of a landmark study showing that high-dose vitamin E (α-tocopherol 1,000 IU twice daily) delayed time to institutionalization and helped preserve activities of daily living over a 2-year period in a study of persons with moderate Alzheimer disease (Sano et al. 1997). Enthusiasm for its use has waned, however, since evidence from a meta-analysis (mostly among persons without dementia) showed a slightly increased risk of mortality with high-dose (>400 IU/day) vitamin E versus placebo (relative risk of death = 1.04) (Miller et al. 2005). The reason for this increase in mortality was not clear, but otherwise the most problematic side effects of vitamin E are GI upset and bleeding/bruising.

Traditional Western Medications

The tremendous impact of dementias includes impaired patient and caregiver quality of life, increased need for institutional care, a rising rate of dementia as the cause of death among older adults, and a growing financial health care burden. These issues have sparked considerable interest in research to discover better treatments and ultimately a cure for these devastating illnesses. Because Alzheimer disease accounts for two-thirds or more of dementias and because relatively more is understood about the pathways leading to its development, the preponderance of the research has focused on this form of dementia. For decades, it has been known that the neurotransmitter acetylcholine (ACh) is important in normal memory function and is affected early in the course of Alzheimer disease. This led to the development of dozens of investigational compounds for Alzheimer disease that aimed to restore normal functioning in the ACh neuronal pathways. Several initial trials proved disappointing but eventually, in 1993, the first FDA-approved drug to treat the symptoms of Alzheimer disease—tacrine (Cognex)—came onto the U.S. market. Tacrine works by inhibiting acetylcholinesterase, an enzyme responsible for degrading the majority of ACh released into the synapse between certain nerve cells. Because tacrine blocks the degradation of ACh, levels of ACh are effectively increased in the synapse, which translates into some clinical improvements in cognition. Because of its short half-life (creating a need for multiple daily dosing) and associated liver toxicity, tacrine soon fell out of favor, replaced by three newer drugs with similar mechanisms of action that now dominate the American prescription drug market for Alzheimer disease: donepezil (Aricept), galantamine (Razadyne, formerly Reminyl), and rivastigmine (Exelon).

There are some potential differences in side effects (e.g., nausea, muscle cramps) from one acetylcholinesterase inhibitor to another, as well as other differences in how they are metabolized by the body, but largely all three drugs are thought, on average, to be equally (but modestly) effective. Any given individual may fare better with one drug over another for currently unknown reasons. What these drugs have been demonstrated to do is, over the course of several months (with relatively few studies extending beyond 1 year), to slightly improve the average scores for patients with Alzheimer disease on tests of memory and other types of cognition in comparison with placebo treatment (Raina et al. 2008). In some investigations, these drugs have also shown a temporary slowing of the progression of disease severity (generally on the order of months), improvements in daily functioning, and possibly the ability to delay placement of patients in institutional settings. What is less clear is to what extent these medications help with behavioral and psychological symptoms of dementia and what their average maximal duration of benefit is. Even though Alzheimer disease is such a devastating and prevalent illness with relatively few other treatment options, the enthusiasm for use of acetylcholinesterase inhibitors is nonetheless lukewarm at best, as they seem to offer a temporary Band-Aid that ultimately does not affect the course of the illness.

Recently, the FDA approved rivastigmine for the treatment of dementia related to Parkinson disease also, the first FDA indication for a drug to treat dementia not related to Alzheimer disease. Some research indicates that rivastigmine may also be helpful in treating dementia with Lewy bodies (a syndrome with overlapping features of Parkinson disease and Alzheimer disease) and perhaps even vascular dementia (which may be related to the fact that many patients with clinically diagnosed vascular dementia also show Alzheimer-type changes in the brain) (Vincent and Lane 2003; Wesnes et al. 2002). No drug has been proven effective in the treatment of the rarer form of dementia known as *frontotemporal dementia.* Of course, there are other rare causes of dementia that are usually screened for by competent clinicians evaluating a person with cognitive symptoms and that would respond to very specific drug therapies (e.g., vitamin B_{12} for pernicious anemia, levothyroxine for hypothyroidism).

The slow progress in treating Alzheimer disease after decades of focusing on the manipulation of cholinergic functioning led researchers to turn to other avenues of investigation. The only FDA-approved drug for Alzheimer disease that is not an acetylcholinesterase inhibitor is memantine (Namenda), which despite its being approved in the United States (in 2003) is not as novel as it may seem, having been on the market in Europe for many years previously. Memantine is a weak inhibitor of a receptor for another neurotransmitter, glutamate. In excess, glutamate can cause massive influx of calcium into neurons, which results in cell death; this is called *excitotoxicity* because glutamate is the primary excitatory neurotransmitter in the brain. Memantine may thus block glutamate when it is in a state of excess and thereby prevent pathological nerve cell death. Despite some excitement for a dementia drug with a novel mechanism of action, memantine is only FDA approved for moderate to severe Alzheimer disease and, like its predecessors, appears to have only modest effects on cognitive functioning and activities of daily living, although some evidence indicates it may work synergistically with cholinesterase inhibitors to produce somewhat larger improvements than either agent alone (Tariot et al. 2004). All three cholinesterase inhibitors are FDA-approved for treating mild-to-moderate Alzheimer disease, and donepezil is also now FDA-approved for treating moderate-to-severe Alzheimer disease.

It is probably obvious after reviewing the existing medications used in the treatment of dementia that all currently effective agents fall more in line with palliative than curative care. A cure for dementia remains a daunting challenge for the scientific community, but there are some promising pharmacological approaches under development, primarily for Alzheimer disease for reasons discussed above. The potential new treatments are exciting in part because many are targeting cellular changes that are fundamentally closer to the actual direct causes of Alzheimer disease. The most common examples of these are drugs that target the development of amyloid plaques, long known to be a hallmark of Alzheimer disease when brain tissue is examined postmortem. When the protein amyloid-β is degraded by certain pathways, it creates relatively insoluble protein fragments. It is thought that a cardinal cellular event that initiates the pathological changes of Alzheimer disease is the accumulation of these insoluble protein fragments, with subsequent inflammation and ultimately nerve cell death. Figure 16–1 illustrates some of the cellular events related to the development of Alzheimer disease and where in this chain of events certain drugs under development are being targeted for action (van Marum 2008).

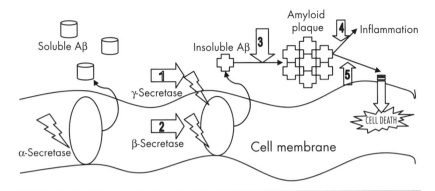

FIGURE 16–1. Proposed cellular pathways involved in Alzheimer disease and potential new drug targets.

1: Inhibition of formation of insoluble amyloid-β (Aβ) via inhibiting the enzyme γ-secretase

2: Inhibition of formation of insoluble Aβ via inhibiting the enzyme β-secretase

3: Inhibition of aggregation of insoluble Aβ into plaques by

Immunotherapy (e.g., antibodies that attach to and rid insoluble Aβ)

Promoting enzymes that degrade insoluble Aβ (e.g., insulin-degrading enzyme)

Chelating agents that specifically block insoluble Aβ aggregation

4: Anti-inflammatories to prevent inflammatory cascade and cell death

5: Antioxidants to prevent free radical damage and cell death

Source.   Adapted from Bourgeois et al. 2008.

Successful Emotional Aging

The notion of using pharmacological compounds to promote healthy *emotional* aging is somewhat different than using such agents for healthy cognitive aging. There are some well-established changes in cognition that occur with normal aging, and the prevalence of cognitive disorders increases dramatically with age. However, research to date indicates that many emotional disorders (e.g., major depression, anxiety disorders) are actually less prevalent in older adults than in younger and middle-aged populations (Blazer 1985). Thus, widespread use of pharmacological agents as a preventive measure to maintain emotional health in aging persons does not appear to be appropriate, especially because minimizing the number of medications an older person takes is often a goal of geriatricians and geriatric psychiatrists. Nonetheless, a significant number of older adults are afflicted with emotional disorders such as major depression (or, more commonly, subsyndromal depression; see discussion under "Traditional Western Medications" below), anxiety disorders, and insomnia. Some of the commonly used alternative and conventional medications for such disorders are briefly reviewed below.

Complementary and Alternative Medications

St. John's wort is probably the best known example of an herb (*Hypericum perforatum*) proposed to treat depression. This plant's extract has at least seven different chemical groups that may exert biological effects. Several possible antidepressant mechanisms of action have been proposed for St. John's wort (Bennett et al. 1998), most involving modulation of neurotransmitter (e.g., serotonin, norepinephrine) functioning similar to the mechanism of prescription antidepressants. A recent systematic review (Linde et al. 2005) analyzed 37 trials and found a marginally significant benefit for St. John's wort over placebo in the largest trials restricted to evaluating treatment for major depression, whereas its superiority over placebo was greater in smaller trials and in trials with less standardized definitions of the depressive disorder. The largest and most publicized trial of St. John's wort in depression (Hypericum Depression Trial Study Group 2002) was conducted by the National Institute of Mental Health (NIMH), which compared the herb to placebo and sertraline (Zoloft). Although St. John's wort had no better efficacy than placebo, the trial was difficult to interpret in that the FDA-approved antidepressant sertraline was also no more effective than placebo.

Only one randomized, controlled trial of St. John's wort among older adults could be found, a German study comparing 800 mg/day of an extract of St. John's wort versus 20 mg/day of fluoxetine (Prozac) among persons experiencing a mild or moderate depressive episode (Harrer et al. 1999). The two treatments were equally effective, but the study had several design weaknesses. The ability of St. John's wort to cause serious herb–drug interactions (e.g., with medications for human immunodeficiency virus or organ transplantation) has been increasingly recognized (Zhou and Lai 2008). Reported side effects of St. John's wort include GI upset and photosensitivity, though little is known about possible side effects unique to older adults.

S-adenosyl-L-methionine (SAMe) is involved in important chemical reactions in the central nervous system, including some related to the synthesis of neurotransmitters important for mood regulation (e.g., serotonin and norepinephrine) (Almeida et al. 2005); it is also a compound in the chemical cycle involving homocysteine, folate (vitamin B_9), and vitamin B_{12}, which have been implicated in mood and cognitive disorders; for example, elevated homocysteine levels and decreased folate levels have been reported in studies of late-life depression (Almeida et al. 2008). Folate itself appeared to have modest benefit as an augmentation to antidepressant treatment in two randomized, controlled trials (not specifically for older adults) (Taylor et al. 2004). SAMe demonstrated superior efficacy compared with placebo for depression in a recent meta-analysis, although many studies included in this analysis had significantly limited methodology (Bressa 1994). Early trials of

SAMe used intravenous formulations because only recently has a stable oral formulation been available. Effective dosages have ranged from 200 to 1,600 mg/day in general adult populations (with the higher range usually needed for oral doses), and 1,600 mg/day of oral SAMe costs hundreds of dollars per month with currently available over-the-counter preparations in the United States—a serious practical barrier to its widespread use. Reported side effects include insomnia, anorexia/GI upset, anxiety, and mania. Ongoing NIMH studies are testing SAMe in head-to-head trials with prescription antidepressants and as an augmentation to prescription antidepressants, but no trials are known that focus exclusively on older adults.

Fish oil has become a popular supplement (as have other supplements with omega-3 fatty acids) because of its reported benefits for blood lipid levels and vascular disease (Juturu 2008). Omega-3 fatty acids have also been tested for possible effects on mood and cognition because they have anti-inflammatory properties and may significantly alter the makeup of neuronal cell membranes. The evidence regarding their potential benefits in individuals with a variety of neuropsychiatric conditions, including depression, bipolar disorder, dementia, and schizophrenia, remains insufficient to justify their widespread use for prevention or treatment of neuropsychiatric conditions (Freeman et al. 2006).

Traditional Western Medications

A discussion of the myriad prescription medications used for depression, anxiety, and insomnia in older adults is beyond the scope of this chapter. The most widely used prescription medications for both depression and anxiety disorders are probably familiar to most readers—selective serotonin reuptake inhibitors (e.g., fluoxetine [Prozac], paroxetine [Paxil], sertraline [Zoloft], citalopram [Celexa], and escitalopram [Lexapro]). There is no evidence that these medications have any role as preventive treatments to promote successful emotional aging in the general population, although certain medical and psychosocial stressors common among older adults have received increasing attention as possible indications for using these medications prophylactically. Examples include their use in individuals post–myocardial infarction or poststroke, both conditions that are often accompanied by significant depressive symptoms and in which depression has been linked to worse outcomes, including higher mortality rates (Carney and Freedland 2009; Starkstein et al. 2008). Furthermore, the majority of the cases of clinically significant depressive disorders among older adults actually do not meet criteria for major depression and are often lumped together under the name *subsyndromal depression*. Although persons with subsyndromal depression are at increased risk for developing major depression, the role of antidepressants in treating these symptoms or preventing the conversion to major depression remains unclear. Psychosocial stressors among older adults that warrant close attention for the need for depression treatment (be it psychotherapy or antidepressants or both) include bereavement, acting as a caregiver for an ill family member, and moving into an institutional setting; however, prophylactic use of antidepressant medications in these situations has not been explored to any significant extent.

One other instance in which pharmacotherapy may be helpful in promoting both successful cognitive and emotional aging involves sleep disturbance (Ancoli-Israel and Ayalon 2006). Insomnia may be a symptom of both depression and anxiety, but when insomnia occurs alone it is still a significant risk factor for the later development of major depression. Sleep disturbance may also contribute to cognitive impairments. The best initial line of treatment for primary insomnia in older adults involves education regarding sleep hygiene, and/or psychotherapy such as cognitive-behavioral therapy. However, in some circumstances (lack of available psychosocial treatments or presence of refractory symptoms), short-term use of prescription sleep aids (e.g., zolpidem [Ambien]) may be helpful and could potentially help avert the development of more severe emotional and cognitive consequences. Prescription sleep aids, however, are not without side effects in older adults and a careful risk-benefit analysis should precede their prescription. Ironically, over-the-counter sleep aids can be more harmful than prescription sleep aids for older adults, as the active ingredient is often diphenhydramine (the active ingredient in Benadryl), which blocks ACh—the neurotransmitter vital in memory functioning discussed above (see "Successful Cognitive Aging: Curative or Palliative Agents, Traditional Western Medications")— and often has a long half-life that causes sleepiness to linger throughout the next day.

Conclusion

As the mind-set of Western medicine moves to a focus on prevention, so, we hope, will the funding and time devoted to research on successful cognitive and emotional aging. Currently, evidence for using any prescription drug or over-the-counter dietary supplement to promote healthier aging of the brain is lacking. There are several promising areas of research in this regard, but until prospective clinical trials using the gold standard of randomized, double-blinded, placebo-controlled methods are conducted and replicated, the use of any of the biological agents discussed here for successful cognitive or emotional aging in healthy older adults remains experimental. Persons who have already developed certain disorders (e.g., Alzheimer disease, major depression, primary insomnia) may benefit from certain prescription medications, but there is still room to improve upon the success rates of existing therapies. Based on current evidence, no "alternative" herbal or supplemental treatment can be reasonably recommended in lieu of prescription drugs for diagnosable cognitive and/or emotional disorders among older adults. Although high hopes remain for future medications that are more effective and/or act earlier in the course of illness to help ward off severe symptoms, the limitations of current pharmacological therapies for successful cognitive and emotional aging point to the importance of remembering that psychosocial and other nonpharmacological therapies have benefits in this arena (see, e.g., Chapter 17, "Cognitive Interventions").

KEY POINTS

▮ No drug/biological compound can be said irrefutably to enhance successful cognitive or emotional aging.

▮ No complementary or alternative medication (e.g., herbs) has sufficient proof of improving any aging-related syndrome affecting the brain to be widely recommended.

▮ Promising research on both naturally occurring and pharmacologically derived compounds may soon provide some options for proactively promoting successful cognitive and/or emotional aging, especially in vulnerable or at-risk populations.

▮ Treatments under development that are targeting very specific molecular changes associated with Alzheimer disease may be among the first compounds to prevent cognitive decline among select older adults.

▮ Research on preventive effects of medications is more difficult, costly, and time-consuming than research on treatments of established conditions but may ultimately prove to have large public health significance for the growing population of older adults interested in preserving brain health.

References

ADAPT Research Group, Martin BK, Szekely C, et al: Cognitive function over time in the Alzheimer's Disease Anti-inflammatory Prevention Trial (ADAPT): results of a randomized, controlled trial of naproxen and celecoxib. Arch Neurol 65:896–905, 2008

Almeida OP, Flicker L, Lautenschlager NT, et al: Contribution of the MTHFR gene to the causal pathway for depression, anxiety and cognitive impairment in later life. Neurobiol Aging 26:251–257, 2005

Almeida OP, McCaul K, Hankey GJ, et al: Homocysteine and depression in later life. Arch Gen Psychiatry 65:1286–1294, 2008

Ancoli-Israel S, Ayalon L: Diagnosis and treatment of sleep disorders in older adults. Am J Geriatr Psychiatry 14:95–103, 2006

Bennett DA Jr, Phun L, Polk JF, et al: Neuropharmacology of St John's wort (Hypericum). Ann Pharmacother 32:1201–1208, 1998

Birks J, Grimley Evans J: Ginkgo biloba for cognitive impairment and dementia. Cochrane Database Syst Rev Apr 18 (2):CD003120, 2007

Birks J, Grimley Evans J: Ginkgo biloba for cognitive impairment and dementia. Cochrane Database Syst Rev (1):CD003120, 2009

Blazer D: The epidemiology of psychiatric disorders in the elderly. J Am Geriatr Soc 33:226–227, 1985

Bourgeois JA, Seaman JS, Servis ME: Delirium, dementia, and amnestic and other cognitive disorders, in The American Psychiatric Publishing Textbook of Psychiatry, 5th Edition. Edited by Hales RE, Yudofsky SC, Gabbard GO. Washington, DC, American Psychiatric Publishing, 2008, pp 303–363

Bressa GM: S-adenosyl-L-methionine (SAMe) as antidepressant: meta-analysis of clinical studies. Acta Neurol Scand Suppl 154:7–14, 1994

Carney RM, Freedland KE: Treatment-resistant depression and mortality after acute coronary syndrome. Am J Psychiatry 166:410–417, 2009

Feldman HH, Ferris S, Winblad B, et al: Effect of rivastigmine on delay to diagnosis of Alzheimer's disease from mild cognitive impairment: the InDDEx Study. Lancet Neurol 6:501–512, 2007

Freeman MP, Hibbeln JR, Wisner KL, et al: Omega-3 fatty acids: evidence basis for treatment and future research in psychiatry. J Clin Psychiatry 67:1954–1967, 2006

Guo Z, Fratiglioni L, Zhu L, et al: Occurrence and progression of dementia in a community population aged 75 years and older: relationship of antihypertensive medication use. Arch Neurol 56:991–996, 1999

Harrer G, Schmidt U, Kuhn U, et al: Comparison of equivalence between the St John's wort extract LoHyp-57 and fluoxetine. Arzneimittelforschung 49:289–296, 1999

Höglund K, Blennow K: Effect of HMG-CoA reductase inhibitors on beta-amyloid peptide levels: implications for Alzheimer's disease. CNS Drugs 21:449–462, 2007

Hypericum Depression Trial Study Group: Effect of Hypericum perforatum (St John's wort) in major depressive disorder: a randomized controlled trial. JAMA 287:1807–1814, 2002

Juturu V: Omega-3 fatty acids and the cardiometabolic syndrome. J Cardiometab Syndr 3:244–253, 2008

Linde K, Mulrow CD, Berner M, et al: St John's wort for depression. Cochrane Database Syst Rev Apr 18 (2):CD000448, 2005

Ma X, Tan C, Zhu D, Gang DR, Xiao P. Huperzine A from Huperzia species—an ethno-pharmacolgical review. J Ethnopharmacol. 2007 Aug 15;113(1):15-34.

Meeks TW, Jeste DV: Complementary and alternative medicine in geriatric psychiatry, in Kaplan & Sadock's Comprehensive Textbook of Psychiatry, 9th Edition. Edited by Sadock BJ, Sadock VA, Ruiz P. Baltimore, MD, Lippincott Williams & Wilkins, 2009

Miller ER 3rd, Pastor-Barriuso R, Dalal D, et al: Meta-analysis: high-dosage vitamin E supplementation may increase all-cause mortality. Ann Intern Med 142:37–46, 2005

Petersen RC, Negash S: Mild cognitive impairment: an overview. CNS Spectr 13:45–53, 2008

Petersen RC, Thomas RG, Grundman M, et al; Alzheimer's Disease Cooperative Study Group: Vitamin E and donepezil for the treatment of mild cognitive impairment. N Engl J Med 352:2379–2388, 2005

Raina P, Santaguida P, Ismaila A, et al: Effectiveness of cholinesterase inhibitors and memantine for treating dementia: evidence review for a clinical practice guideline. Ann Intern Med 148:379–397, 2008

Rockwood K, Kirkland S, Hogan DB, et al: Use of lipid-lowering agents, indication bias, and the risk of dementia in community-dwelling elderly people. Arch Neurol 59:223–227, 2002

Rozzini L, Chilovi BV, Bertoletti E, et al: Angiotensin converting enzyme (ACE) inhibitors modulate the rate of progression of amnestic mild cognitive impairment. Int J Geriatr Psychiatry 21:550–555, 2006

Sano M, Ernesto C, Thomas RG, et al: A controlled trial of selegiline, alpha-tocopherol, or both as treatment for Alzheimer's disease. The Alzheimer's Disease Cooperative Study. N Engl J Med 336:1216–1222, 1997

Starkstein SE, Mizrahi R, Power BD: Antidepressant therapy in post-stroke depression. Expert Opin Pharmacother 9:1291–1298, 2008

Szekely CA, Thorne JE, Zandi PP, et al: Nonsteroidal anti-inflammatory drugs for the prevention of Alzheimer's disease: a systematic review. Neuroepidemiology 23(4):159–169, 2004

Tariot PN, Farlow MR, Grossberg GT, et al; Memantine Study Group: Memantine treatment in patients with moderate to severe Alzheimer disease already receiving donepezil: a randomized controlled trial. JAMA 291:317–324, 2004

Taylor MJ, Carney SM, Goodwin GM, et al: Folate for depressive disorders: systematic review and meta-analysis of randomized controlled trials. J Psychopharmacol 18:251–256, 2004

Thal LJ, Ferris SH, Kirby L, et al; Rofecoxib Protocol 078 Study Group: A randomized, double-blind, study of rofecoxib in patients with mild cognitive impairment. Neuropsychopharmacology 30:1204–1215, 2005

Trompet S, Westendorp RG, Kamper AM, et al: Use of calcium antagonists and cognitive decline in old age. The Leiden 85-Plusstudy. Neurobiol Aging 29:306–308, 2008

van Marum RJ: Current and future therapy in Alzheimer's disease. Fundam Clin Pharmacol 22:265–274, 2008 van Uffelen JG, Chinapaw MJ, van Mechelen W, et al: Walking or vitamin B for cognition in older adults with mild cognitive impairment? A randomised controlled trial. Br J Sports Med 42:344–351, 2008

Vincent S, Lane R: Rivastigmine in vascular dementia. Int Psychogeriatr 15 (suppl 1): 201–205, 2003

Wesnes KA, McKeith IG, Ferrara R, et al: Effects of rivastigmine on cognitive function in dementia with Lewy bodies: a randomised placebo-controlled international study using the cognitive drug research computerised assessment system. Dement Geriatr Cogn Disord 13:183–192, 2002

Winblad B, Gauthier S, Scinto L, et al; GAL-INT-11/18 Study Group: Safety and efficacy of galantamine in subjects with mild cognitive impairment. Neurology 70:2024–2035, 2008

Zhang Z, Wang X, Chen Q, et al: Clinical efficacy and safety of huperzine alpha in treatment of mild to moderate Alzheimer disease, a placebo-controlled, double-blind, randomized trial. Zhonghua Yi Xue Za Zhi 82:941–944, 2002

Zhou SF, Lai X: An update on clinical drug interactions with the herbal antidepressant St John's wort. Curr Drug Metab 9:394–409, 2008

Recommended Readings

Depp CA, Glatt SJ, Jeste DV: Recent advances in research on successful or healthy aging. Curr Psychiatry Rep 9:7–13, 2007

Meeks TW, Jeste DV: Complementary and alternative medicine in geriatric psychiatry, in Kaplan & Sadock's Comprehensive Textbook of Psychiatry, 9th Edition. Edited by Sadock BJ, Sadock VA, Ruiz P. Baltimore, MD, Lippincott Williams & Wilkins, 2009

Patterson C, Feightner JW, Garcia A, et al: Diagnosis and treatment of dementia, 1: risk assessment and primary prevention of Alzheimer's disease. CMAJ 178:548–556, 2008

Smits F, Smits N, Schoevers R, et al: An epidemiological approach to depression prevention in old age. Am J Geriatr Psychiatry 16:444–453, 2008

Thachil AF, Mohan R, Bhugra D: The evidence base of complementary and alternative therapies in depression. J Affect Disord 97:23–35, 2007

17

Cognitive Interventions
Traditional and Novel Approaches

Ipsit V. Vahia, M.D.
Ashley Cain, B.S.
Colin A. Depp, Ph.D.

A s described in many other chapters in this book, a large body of literature indicates that cognitive abilities account for a substantial amount of variability in longevity and the capacity of older individuals to function independently. Estimating what is typical (or successful) in regard to cognitive aging is incredibly complex, with interacting influences of neuronal loss, compensation, cognitive and brain reserve, and genetic risks. Amid this complexity, there appears to be growing evidence from observational studies that environmental, and thus potentially modifiable, factors influence the course of cognitive aging. There are also hopeful signs from animal experiments that show the cognitive-enhancing effect of enriched environments, and human neuroimaging studies that seem to demonstrate a surprising degree of neuroplasticity retained into older age (Studenski et al. 2006).

These findings translate to optimism that cognitive training can boost memory and other cognitive functions in older age, optimism that can be seen in the recent boom in age-targeted brain-training games. Some of this hopefulness needs to be tempered by the data on how well these interventions work, how long the effects last, and whether they improve real-world functioning in addition to performance in laboratory testing. Nevertheless, cognitive training is an emerging area of interest in promoting healthy aging, spurred by the massive National Institutes of Health (NIH)–funded Advanced Cognitive Training for Independent and Vital Elderly (ACTIVE) study (Jobe et al. 2001). There is also a fascinating expansion in what falls under the umbrella of cognitive training, with social activities, physical exercise, and even acting classes or intergenerational programs as potential means for enhancing cognitive abilities in older people. In this chapter, we briefly review the data on the impact of lifetime cognitive engagement on outcomes in observational studies, discuss the various forms of traditional cognitive training interventions that have been evaluated in older adults and review the available evidence for their effectiveness, and then describe novel, nontraditional approaches to enhancing cognitive functioning.

Observational Studies of Lifetime Cognitive Engagement

Of little doubt in aging research is that variability in phenotypes increases with age, and cognitive functions are no exception. Whether engagement in intellectual activities over the life course accounts for some of this variability has long been of research interest. In 44 B.C.E., Cicero hypothesized, in an essay titled *De Senectute,* that behavioral and environmental factors influence mental capacities in older age: "memory is impaired, that is, if you do not exercise it." In popular media, this "use it or lose it" paradigm is commonly seen in recommendations to do crossword puzzles or engage in cognitively challenging activities. As described eloquently by Brickman and colleagues in Chapter 9 ("Cognitive and Brain Reserve"), the twin concepts of cognitive reserve and brain reserve are predicated, to some extent, on the degree to which environmental influences impact the trajectories of cognitive aging.

Longitudinal, observational studies have indicated that greater educational attainment, working in more cognitively challenging professions, and engaging in more active leisure time pursuits relate to decreased risk of cognitive impairment and dementia. In a review of 34 studies on the impact of education on cognitive changes, Anstey and Christensen (2000) found a protective effect for education on broad measures of cognitive functioning, with inconsistent relationships between educational attainment and more fine-grained neuropsychological domains. In the 10-year Canadian Study of Health and Aging (Kröger et al. 2008), which followed more than 4,000 older adults, jobs worked in earlier life were assigned a degree of cognitive complexity, and those older adults who had held more cognitively complex positions (such as working with people or things) were less likely to have dementia at year 10. In a study or more than 700 older individuals who underwent annual clinical evaluations for up to 5 years (Wilson et al. 2007), at 5-year follow-up individuals who were initially judged to be cognitively inactive were 2.6 times more likely to have developed Alzheimer disease. Interestingly, a neuropathological study in available postmortem cases found no association between cognitive activity scores and presence of amyloid plaques and neurofibrillary tangles (Wilson et al. 2007). Participation in leisure time activities has been examined as a potential moderator of cognitive decline as well. Verghese et al. (2003) followed 469 older adults over age 75 with no dementia at baseline and assessed the amount of participation in leisure activities, both cognitive and physical in nature. At 5-year follow-up, playing board games, playing a musical instrument, and reading were associated with a reduced risk of dementia. In a similar study, television watching had a negative effect and was associated with greater decline in cognitive functioning (Wang et al. 2006). Importantly, recent longitudinal studies have controlled for baseline cognitive functioning and cognitive activity participation, reducing the problem of reverse causality (i.e., poor cognition leading to lower cognitive activity participation).

Some intriguing neuroimaging and animal studies have shown the impact of specific intellectual activities on the brain. Using structural magnetic resonance imaging (MRI), the hippocampal volumes of taxicab drivers in London were estimated (Maguire et al. 2000). Because of the complexity of London's streets, it was hypothesized that if mental maps of the city were needed to perform the task of cab driving, brain structure would be impacted by length of time in the position. Indeed, hippocampal volume was positively correlated with the number of years spent as a cabdriver. In animal studies, a surprisingly consistent finding is that neurogenesis continues to occur in the hippocampus in adult animals, and that environmental exposure can modulate this neurogenesis. Experiments with adult mice randomized to live in habitats with a running wheel showed neuropathological evidence for greater long-term potentiation in the dentate gyrus than in mice that did not have access to a running wheel (Kuhn et al. 1996). The fact that neurogenesis can be observed in older animals, and impacted by environmental changes, shows the remarkable and continuing capacity of the brain for plasticity.

Criticisms about the evidence for the impact of intellectual engagement on human cognitive aging do exist, however. As Salthouse (2006) explained, convincing evidence of the effect of cognitive stimulation would entail demonstrating 1) a negative relationship between cognitive stimulation and age, 2) a positive relationship between cognitive stimulation and cognitive functioning, and 3) an interaction between the first two such that cognitive stimulation changes the rate of cognitive aging. In their 2002 study, Salthouse et al. found little evidence that cognitive stimulation affects the rate of cognitive aging. In observational studies, there is a considerable problem of self-selection, in that it is quite plausible that more cognitively adept people choose to (or are able to) work in more challenging jobs and engage in cognitively enriching activities. Another issue is the quantification of cognitive stimulation retrospectively—there is imprecision in assigning levels of cognitive stimulation to specific jobs or to crossword puzzles, for example. Another source of imprecision is the variation in actual exposure to cognitive stimulation in seemingly well-defined variables such as education. Manly (2005) provided compelling data about the relatively poor quality of education that older African Americans received as children prior to the civil rights movement, even for those whose years of education attained were equivalent to those of their white counterparts. As Salthouse (2006) pointed out, the ideal test of the use-it-or-lose-it hypothesis in regard to intellectual activities would be to randomly assign individuals to either a lifetime of carefully codified mental engagement or one that was less enriched. No such study can be realistically conducted.

In sum, the evidence from observational studies suggests that cognitive engagement throughout the life course has bearing on cognitive aging, as suggested by Cicero thousands of years ago. Specific lifestyle factors include educational attainment and occupational challenges, but also more discretionary activities such as leisure time pursuits. Cognitive health thus appears to depend on, to an extent, what one does with one's brain during the life span. Due to self-selection and imprecision in estimating the amount of cognitive stimulation engaged in, it is unclear just how much influence cognitive engagement has on late-life cognitive functioning. It is also unclear whether the same degree of plasticity is retained throughout the life span—that is, whether cognitive stimulation initiated in older age can produce the same beneficial effects as stimulation at a younger age. This brings us to the next question covered in this chapter—whether interventions can be effective in changing the rate of cognitive aging, via cognitive training.

Cognitive Interventions: Traditional Approaches

Cognitive training programs typically focus on specific domains of functioning such as memory, attention, and problem solving but can also examine cognitively mediated domains of functioning such as basic and instrumental activities of daily living. Much of the literature on cognitive rehabilitation and training focuses on the enhancement of cognitive functioning after neurological injury (e.g., stroke or traumatic brain injury). For the populations with impaired cognitive functioning, training can be divided into three subdomains:

- Restorative approaches/cognitive training
- Compensatory approaches/rehabilitation
- Cognitive stimulation interventions

Restorative strategies seek to improve cognitive functioning, with the ultimate goal of returning functioning to its premorbid level (Sitzer et al. 2006). Teaching memory enhancement techniques such as training in mnemonics would fall under this category. Compensatory strategies are used to improve cognitive functioning by teaching new ways to perform cognitive tasks to compensate for any cognitive deficits. An example would be the use of a pillbox with a set of medication reminders for an individual recovering from a stroke. Finally, cognitive stimulation encompasses a broader and less standardized set of interventions, which may include activity therapy, reminiscence, and reality orientation therapies that have long been used in institutional settings.

For the purposes of this chapter, we focus on research on interventions enhancing cognitive functioning with restorative and compensatory approaches. We also focus on two studies that have been influential in determining whether cognitive training can alter the course of "normal" cognitive aging, which has been the subject of more recent interest (Espeland and Henderson 2006). We first review the nature and results of the two clinical trials, the ACTIVE study (Jobe et al. 2001) and a study of brain plasticity training (Mahncke et al. 2006), and then describe the specific interventions that were used.

Cognitive Training: The ACTIVE Study

The most ambitious, and likely the most informative, examination of the effect of cognitive training on cognitively intact older people has been the multisite, randomized, controlled NIH-funded trial, the ACTIVE study (Jobe et al. 2001). The aims of this trial were to determine whether three cognitive training interventions, shown to improve performance on basic measures of cognition in laboratory and small field conditions, would translate to improvement on measures of cognitively demanding daily activities in a large sample of older adults without dementia ($N=2,832$). Participants were randomly assigned to one of four groups:

- Memory training
- Reasoning training
- Speed of processing training
- Control subjects

The goal of the memory training intervention was to transfer mnemonic training to everyday cognitive tasks. The goal of the reasoning training was to improve the ability to solve problems that require linear thinking and follow a serial pattern or sequence. The speed of processing intervention's goal was to improve performance on one or more attentional tasks and improve the speed of visual searching in each group. The initial training phase consisted of ten 60- to 75-minute sessions over a 6-week period in small group settings, led by a certified trainer. A subset of participants also received booster training 11 months after completing the initial training phase (Jobe et al. 2001).

At 2-year follow-up, cognitive interventions had improved participants' performance on measures specific to the cognitive ability for which they were trained (e.g., memory training on memory measures); however, these results did not generalize to performance on everyday activities at 2 years. Willis et al. (2006) conducted a 5-year follow-up study and found that compared with the control subjects, subjects who had received cognitive training reported less difficulty in performing the instrumental activities of daily living. However, only for those in the reasoning group was there a significant effect. In terms of performance-based measures, those in the speed of processing group who had received the booster training showed a significant effect. Similar to the 2-year follow-up results, the 5-year results showed that compared with the control subjects, individuals who received any form of cognitive training retained their improved performance on measures specific to the cognitive ability for which they were trained. Wolinsky et al. (2006) examined the ability of the ACTIVE cognitive training trial to protect against decline in health-related quality of life. They found at the 2-year follow-up that the speed of processing intervention had a protective effect against declines in this area, but no effect was found for the memory or reasoning interventions. However, in the 5-year follow-up all three interventions showed a protective effect against declines in health-related quality of life.

Edwards et al. (2005) further examined speed of processing training on a more targeted sample than in the ACTIVE study. They selected only individuals who showed speed of processing difficulty but otherwise had intact mental status. Their findings were similar to those in the studies previously mentioned. They found that compared to those in the control group (*n*=63), subjects who received the speed of processing training (*n*=63) improved their performance on a measure of that cognitive ability (the Useful Field of View Test), and this transferred to improved performance on the timed Instrumental Activities of Daily Living Test.

Brain Plasticity Training

Mahncke et al. (2006) reported a new cognitive training program based on brain plasticity for memory enhancement in healthy older adults. Older adults, over the age of 60 (N=182), were randomly assigned to one of three groups:

1. The experimental training group, in which subjects used a computer-based Posit Science program consisting of six exercises that progressively increased in difficulty as the user's ability improved (n=62)
2. The active control group (n=61), in which subjects used a computer-based educational program where they were given information and then quizzed on what is recommended for cognitive health
3. The no-contact control group (n=59) of subjects who received no study activities

The experimental training consisted of 60-minute sessions, five times per week, for 8–10 weeks. Participants in the experimental training group had significant improvement in task-specific performance in speed of processing, spatial syllable match memory, forward word recognition span, and working and narrative memory tasks. The active control group and no-contact control group showed no significant improvements in memory function (Mahncke et al. 2006).

Summary of Major Trial Results

Taken together, the ACTIVE study (Jobe et al. 2001; Willis et al. 2006) and the brain plasticity training trial (Mahncke et al. 2006) support the following conclusions:

1. Cognitive interventions can be associated with improvements in cognition.
2. These improvements appear to be specific to the kind of intervention tested, and they appear to be somewhat durable as much as 5 years post-training.
3. Improvements in measures of functioning are less impressive than those detected with cognitive measures.

In the next section we describe the specific techniques used in these two studies.

Domain-Targeted Cognitive Training Techniques

Memory Training

Memory training in the ACTIVE trial consisted of multiple different mnemonic strategies, specifically focusing on verbal episodic memory. Mnemonic strategies were used for remembering and organizing things such as grocery shopping, recalling text material like that on medication labels, and recalling main ideas and details of stories. One such strategy taught participants how to organize material into categories and associate them with visual images to aid in the recall of the material (Ball et al. 2002). A variety of mnemonic memory strategies have also been used in other cognitive training studies (Rebok et al. 2007). In *method of loci* training or *loci mnemonics*, participants create a mental map and associate each landmark or object on the map with an item on a list of words to be memorized, creating a visual image association (Yesavage and Rose 1983). When asked to recall the list, they take a mental "walk" through the map, visit each location that was paired with the items on the list, and use the visual cues at each location to recall the associated words on the list.

Reasoning Training

Reasoning training is designed to teach participants strategies for finding patterns in letter, number, or word sequences and improve their ability to recognize the next item in the series (Willis and Schaie 1986). In the ACTIVE trial, Ball et al. (2002) also included reasoning problems that involve activities of daily living like travel schedules or prescription medication regimens. Reasoning training emphasizes three strategies to help identify patterns: visual scanning of the series, saying the series aloud, and underlining repeated letters. Participants then generate a hypothesis about the pattern type and keep track of all repetitions that follow this pattern in the series, which then enables them to determine the next item in the series that follows the pattern rule (Willis and Schaie 1986).

Speed of Processing Training

The aim of speed of processing training is to improve the fluid ability of mental processing speed so that one can process more and more information over shorter periods of time (Ball et al. 2007). Trainer-guided practice with computerized tasks is used. These tasks involve target detection, identification, discrimination, and localization. Participants are given feedback after each trial, and the tasks gradually increase in difficulty (complexity and speed) based on each individual's performance. Tasks include *central tasks* such as indicating the presence or absence of targets, identifying targets, or performing same/different discriminations of targets. The main goal of this training procedure is to improve cognitive processing speed by gradually increasing the difficulty of the task while decreasing the display speed (Ball et al. 2007).

Brain Plasticity Training

This training program, used in the Mahncke et al. (2006) trial, consists of six exercises that gradually increase in difficulty as the participant's performance improves. The six exercises are performed on a computer and require participants to do the following: 1) indicate the sequence of a frequency-modulated sweep and whether it is upward or downward; 2) identify a syllable from a similar pair (e.g., *ba* vs. *da*); 3) match similar consonant-vowel-consonant words on a spatial grid (e.g., *bad, dad*); 4) indicate the sequence of the same short consonant-vowel-consonant words; 5) follow spoken instructions by clicking and dragging icons on a computer screen; and 6) listen to a short narrative and answer questions about it.

Other Cognitive Training Approaches

Face/Name Association

In face/name association training, participants are shown an unfamiliar face paired with a name. They are instructed to come up with a visual association for the name (e.g., Smith = blacksmith = anvil). Participants then pick a prominent feature on the face to focus on. The visual name associate and the prominent feature are then paired, so that when the participant is confronted with the face again, the prominent feature will serve as a cue to the paired name (Brooks et al. 1999).

Strategic Training

Strategic training involves matching strategies to specific real-world tasks. For example, for tasks in which participants have to remember a list of words, they are taught how to associate the items. For tasks in which participants have to remember a face/name association, they are instructed on techniques used to generate the corresponding image. The idea behind this type of training is that participants will learn how to use the best strategy appropriate for the type of memory task they are presented with (Cavallini et al. 2003).

Implementation Intentions

Chasteen et al. (2001) examined the use of implementation intentions to improve prospective memory in older adults. This technique involves the mental rehearsal of a plan or desired behavior, so that when the person encounters certain situational cues in the future, the behavior is more automatic. Those participants who performed the implementation strategy, as opposed to those who were simply instructed on what to do, were more than twice as likely to perform the intended behavior (e.g., writing the day of the week at the top of each page). These strategies may be useful in improving prospective memory in older adults for instrumental activities of daily living such as taking medication.

Overall Effectiveness of Cognitive Training

Meta-analyses assessing the impact of cognitive training in older adults indicate that improvements in cognitive functioning are attainable. In 31 memory training studies sampling healthy older adults, effect size for pre-post gains in memory performance in experimental groups was 0.73, whereas it was approximately 0.37 in control groups (Verhaeghen et al. 1992). Greater gains were seen for group interventions that had shorter durations. In addition, those interventions that included pretraining about age-related cognitive decline, and interventions in individuals who were younger and more cognitively intact, appeared to be more effective. A more recent meta-analysis, which includes the results of the ACTIVE and brain plasticity trials, compared posttreatment effect sizes between control groups and experimental conditions in eight trials (Valenzuela 2008). The mean effect size was 0.6 in favor of the cognitive training conditions. In a meta-analysis of 17 trials that examined the efficacy of cognitive training for individuals with Alzheimer disease, the mean effect size was 0.47, with considerable variation across differing outcome measures (Sitzer et al. 2006). These estimates typically derive from immediate posttraining performance, so the effect sizes at longer-term follow-up are unclear. Nevertheless, there is accumulating evidence that improvement in cognitive test performance can be accomplished through cognitive training.

Consideration for Outcomes

The primary outcome in most cognitive training studies is performance on objective measures of cognitive performance, as described above. Although these measures provide standardized and reliable estimates of cognitive abilities, there are three problems that may affect the interpretation of clinical trials: 1) practice effects, 2) ceiling effects, and 3) transfer of training issues:

1. Improvements in neuropsychological test scores do occur as a result of repeated exposure to stimuli; practice effects may thus inflate the impact of cognitive training.
2. "Normal" cognitive aging encapsulates a highly heterogeneous group, with some older adults performing at extremely high levels with little room for improvement on standardized tests. Inclusion of these high performers in clinical trials may attenuate the effect of cognitive training.
3. The relevance of neuropsychological tests to everyday functioning and well-being can be questioned (the so-called transfer of training issue). If improvements observed on cognitive measures do not translate to im-

provement in performance of everyday tasks, then the rationale for cognitive training is diminished.

A key contribution of the ACTIVE trial was the inclusion of performance-based and self-rated functional measures, which assess the transfer of skills to improvements in everyday life. The effect sizes of the ACTIVE interventions on "distal" outcomes related to functioning were smaller than those seen on neuropsychological measures. Future cognitive interventions will need to improve the transfer of training to functioning. Conversely, some trials assessing cognitive training interventions have included measures of depression and subjective memory complaints, and improvements have been seen (Rebok et al. 2007). It is important to measure whether older people seem to derive an emotional benefit from engaging in cognitive training, perhaps through experiencing "normalization" of age-associated cognitive changes or greater perceived control over the circumstances.

Innovations in the Format of Training

The most common format for cognitive training in the past has been in group settings with the intervention delivered by a trained professional—participants are taught strategies, practice them, and are provided corrective feedback by the instructor. Alternatives to this format have been evaluated. Baltes et al. (1989) developed a cognitive training program to improve fluid intelligence (e.g., processing speed) in older adults and examined whether older adults were able to improve their cognitive skills and problem-solving strategies on their own, not just through guided practice techniques. Participants were divided into three groups: a control group, subjects who received tutor-guided training, and those who implemented self-guided training. In both experimental conditions, the materials and training length were the same and focused on training in figural relations. However, with self-guided training, participants were given minimal instruction and told to work on practice problems on their own. Results indicated that those in the self-guided training group were able to produce training gains comparable to those achieved with tutor-guided training. The investigators found no evidence that tutor-guided training was superior, and therefore concluded that older adults are able to achieve training gains on their own.

Recent training approaches, such as those used in the brain plasticity training trial described earlier (Mahncke et al. 2006; see also sections "Cognitive Interventions: Traditional Approaches, Brain Plasticity Training" and

"Nontraditional Approaches to Cognitive Training), have employed computerized methods of delivering interventions. As reviewed by Rebok et al. (2007), other approaches may use collaborative training, CD-ROMs, or videotape/audiotape approaches. These approaches have the potential benefit of increasing the practicality of the interventions. For instance, in collaborative training, both members of a married couple attend cognitive training and they support each other in the maintenance of skills. In the brain plasticity training study (Mahncke et al. 2006), a key innovation was the use of an adaptive computerized approach, in which training is modified based on the individual's performance and is made progressively more difficult.

All of the modifications described above on the traditional group-format delivery of cognitive training are geared to fitting training to individual preferences and capabilities, as well as moving training out of the laboratory.

Cognitive Training for Memory-Impaired Individuals

Administering cognitive training programs to individuals with already existing cognitive impairment (e.g., mild cognitive impairment [MCI] or Alzheimer disease) has theoretical appeal. Particularly among individuals with MCI, training would ideally delay the onset of conversion to frank dementia and potentially help individuals retain their independence. A handful of studies have administered cognitive training interventions to individuals with MCI, in both computerized and traditional formats, and improvements in subjective memory and some objective measures have been seen (Belleville et al. 2006). As with normal aging, given that MCI is by definition not associated with marked deficits in functioning, the functional impact of these interventions is less impressive. These studies were small and often not adequately powered to determine whether a preventive effect on the onset of dementia could be attained with cognitive training. Recent studies have examined the potential synergistic effect of cognitive training and cholinesterase inhibitors for people with Alzheimer disease (Yesavage et al. 2007). Similar to hypotheses about the potential ability of antidepressants to increase capacity to adopt new coping mechanisms, it is hypothesized that cholinesterase inhibitors may increase the ability of persons with MCI to retain cognitive skills. However, the evidence for the preventive impact of either intervention alone remains somewhat slim, so it is currently unclear whether combining treatments would be efficacious (see Chapter 16, "Pharmacological Approaches to Successful Cognitive and Emotional Aging," this volume).

Nontraditional Approaches to Cognitive Training

In contrast to traditional approaches to cognitive training, which focus on tasks that enhance specific cognitive domains, an alternative approach involves structured global activities that require engagement of multiple cognitive domains. The term *nontraditional approach* has been used to describe cognitive training methods designed on this basis. Using the nontraditional approach, interventions requiring active engagement with multimodal activities have been developed (Park et al. 2007).

Interventions Based on Performing Arts, Fine Arts, and Literary Skills

Noice and colleagues (2004) have reported the results of theater training for a sample of 124 community-dwelling older adults. The authors chose acting because it requires engagement of cognitive, emotional, and physiological faculties. In this study, 44 participants were enrolled in a theater training course, 44 were enrolled in a visual arts course, and 36 served as no-intervention control subjects. The theater and visual arts courses consisted of nine sessions of training in a month. The visual arts course involved a discussion of art and the meaning of paintings and so forth. The theater course consisted of various acting exercises that were designed to engross the participants in the drama of the scene, creating alterations in their cognitive/psychological demeanor. The participants in this group did not engage in creating works of art. At the conclusion of the study, the theater group demonstrated significant improvement over the no-treatment group in the cognitive domains of recall and problem solving and in psychological well-being. Additionally, the theater group scored significantly higher than the visual arts group in problem solving and psychological well-being. At 4-month follow-up, the problem-solving and memory effects showed no decline, and the recall scores actually improved over time. A similar study conducted by the same authors in a sample drawn from retirement homes showed a similar positive effect on cognition with the acting intervention, and the individuals in this study were older, were less well educated, and lived in subsidized, primarily low-income, retirement homes (Noice and Noice 2009).

A study currently under way at the University of Illinois is evaluating the effects of learning to quilt or learning digital photography on cognition in older adults (Park et al. 2007). The study sample consists of older adults who live alone, and treatment is being compared with a wait-list control condition. While the results of this study are awaited, it demonstrates the feasibility of testing broad-based interventions that require engagement of multiple cognitive domains.

In a pilot study, de Medeiros and colleagues (2007) examined whether participation in a structured autobiographical writing workshop would affect cognitive performance. The authors assessed 18 high-functioning older adults with an MMSE score greater than 25. (The study involved physicians or physicians' spouses.) The participants were enrolled in a workshop that taught participants various writing techniques in eight weekly 90-minute sessions. This pilot study showed that the intervention was associated with increases in verbal learning, processing speed, and attention. The authors also noted a decrease in idea density and grammatical complexity, suggesting that participants learned to simplify their writing style. Although this was a noncontrolled study, it demonstrated the positive effects of lifelong learning.

In summary, existing studies using interventions based on multidimensional creative tasks have demonstrated improvement in cognitive function. Importantly, these studies attest to the feasibility of learning new skills in late life. Broader studies are needed to determine the interactive and independent effects of cognitive, emotional, and physiological elements of such tasks.

Community-Oriented Social Programs

Based on the literature suggesting the protective effects of cognitive stimulation, two senior-focused social programs have been assessed for its impact on cognitive functioning. *Senior Odyssey* is an adaptation of a program that was initially developed for grade-school children, focusing on presenting novel problems and encouraging group collaboration in forming creative solutions. Examples might be working as a team to create a play to describe a historical event, or building a bridge with balsa wood. Steps in the process tap into executive functions and planning, working memory, and prospective memory, with novelty of the task a key feature (Stine-Morrow et al. 2007). Initial findings from a sample of 95 older adults participating in the program suggest that greater maintenance of processing speed is achieved in comparison with a control group.

Another innovative program that could enhance cognition through stimulation is the *Experience Corps*, an intergenerational program in Baltimore, Maryland. Older adults are trained to enter public schools and provide instruction in literacy and math skills to students, in collaboration with teachers. In addition to providing a meaningful contribution to the community, this program can improve older adults' cognitive functioning: participants showed improvements in executive functioning and memory. Additionally, participants spent less time watching TV and more time engaged in cognitively demanding activities as a result of the program (Studenski et al. 2006).

Although both the Experience Corps and Senior Odyssey programs are less well researched than traditional cognitive training, they have the advantage of directly reducing cognitive inactivity as well as providing meaningful social interaction to older adults. In addition, intergenerational approaches affect the participants' well-being, as discussed in Chapter 20 ("Gaining Wisdom Through Multiage Learning: The Story of The Intergenerational School").

Combining Physical Activity With Cognitive Training

Oswald et al. (2006) conducted a study to examine the effects of cognitive, psychoeducational, physical, and combination (psychoeducational and physical; cognitive and physical) training on cognitive and physical functioning, physical health, independent living, and well-being. They examined the training's effects after 5 years and found significant effects for those participants exposed to the cognitive and physical training.

- Cognitive training consisted of training in three areas: memory, attention, and fluid abilities. In memory training, participants were taught techniques for short-term storage and retrieval of visual, numerical, or verbal targets as well as long-term storage via verbal categorization, elaboration, or visual imaging to remember more complex information. They used visual search tasks (locating a specific number or letter as quickly as possible in a row or diagram of letters or numbers) to train for attention and fluid abilities.
- Psychoeducational training was designed to improve one's ability to deal with everyday life demands (e.g., getting adequate nutrition in old age, taking prescription medications, compensating for decreased physical strength, and coping with loss of social contacts) through lectures, group discussions, exercises, handouts, etc.
- Physical training involved training to improve balance and perceptual and motor coordination using a variety of gymnastic exercises and games such as table tennis.

Subjects participated in training sessions every week, for 30 sessions, in a small group format. Physical training sessions lasted 45 minutes each, and cognitive and psychoeducational training sessions lasted 90 minutes. Participants in the combination cognitive and physical training group showed greater sustained improvement than the control group 5 years later in both domains. Investigators also found that the combined physical and cognitive training intervention was associated with improvements in everyday functioning (e.g., functional tasks like using the telephone) and health status.

Computer Games and Cognitive Function

Some studies have examined computer games as a modality for assessment of cognitive function in the elderly (Basak et al. 2008). Jimison and colleagues (2007) have described a set of standardized adaptive computer games designed to assess cognitive performance in a home environment. The authors stress the importance of monitoring cognition in a home setting and state that with appropriate software and network support, using games may be an effective way of monitoring changes in cognitive function remotely. There has been commentary on the potential use of computer games as a therapeutic intervention for psychiatric disorders as well (Wilkinson et al. 2008). No data exist at this time to determine the efficacy of such modalities, however.

In the commercial realm, the "brain training" industry has grown by leaps and bounds in the past several years. The market for such games is expected to reach billions of dollars in the next several decades. The Posit Science Corporation has introduced a game named *HiFi* (Miller 2005). This game involves several scenarios based on senior-friendly themes, which involve the utilization of specific neural mechanisms. For example, one of the tasks aims to associate images with auditory signals, requiring exercise of auditory, visual, and association pathways. A game titled *Brain Age* (and its follow-up, *Brain Age 2*), by Nintendo Co., Ltd., aims to improve prefrontal function through a series of tasks that require prefrontal activation. Given the evidence for the beneficial effect of physical activity on cognitive functioning (see Chapter 14, "Creating Environments to Encourage Physical Activity"), there is increasing interest in interventions that may combine cognitive and physical aspects. One of the more interesting developments in this arena is the emergence of so-called *exergames*, such as one available on the Nintendo Wii. These games provide a degree of cognitive stimulation as well as physical activity that may be adapted to suit older people with physical disabilities. A significant amount of media attention has been placed on the increasing use of these games in assisted living facilities and the increasing sales of these devices to the older segment of the population. At the time of this writing, however, efficacy of these tasks had not been tested in any large, well-designed clinical trial. Nevertheless, the surge in popularity of these games suggests that a considerable number of older adults are actively interested in improving their cognitive capacities and/or delaying the onset of dementia.

Meditation

The term *meditation* describes a broad group of complex training regimens that aim at optimizing emotional and cognitive regulation through attentional tasks (Lutz et al. 2008). Meditation is an ancient technique (Jeste and Vahia 2008) and has been used to achieve various goals, including promotion of well-being. Research on the impact of meditation on health and medicine has been criticized for lack of a common theoretical perspective (Ospina et al. 2007). Nevertheless, functional MRI studies have demonstrated neurocircuitry and neurochemical changes in response to meditation, suggesting that pathways and chemicals that affect the brain aging process may be modified using meditation (Doraiswamy and Xiong 2007). Meditation has also been shown to reduce central nervous system cortisol levels, suggesting that it may cause a resultant increase in brain-derived neurotrophic factor levels that results in a neuroprotective effect (Doraiswamy and Xiong 2007). Mindfulness meditation, a related form, has been described as effective for controlling stress (Jain et al. 2007), improving emotional regulation (Miller et al. 1995), and providing psychosomatic effects such as relief of pain (Gardner-Nix et al. 2008). In a study comparing transcendental meditation, mindfulness meditation, relaxation training, and no treatment for elderly persons (Alexander et al. 1989), the transcendental meditation group improved most on measures of cognitive flexibility, learning tasks, behavioral flexibility, and systolic blood pressure. The mindfulness meditation group did better on measures of perceived control and word fluency. Both groups did better than the relaxation and no-treatment groups. Although the literature on meditation's effects is limited, scattered, and impaired by a lack of consistency and rigorous methodology, available evidence suggests that meditation has potential usefulness in improving both cognitive and emotional functioning of older persons.

Conclusion

Observational studies and animal models have produced a great deal of optimism that cognitive health can be enhanced through cognitive stimulation. That brain plasticity is retained in older animals suggests that older people may benefit from initiating cognitively challenging activities and interventions. Although there are caveats to the data, cognitive stimulation does appear to interact with dementia risk. Furthermore, formal cognitive training methods do appear to enhance cognitive functioning and, to a lesser extent, the ability to perform daily activities. New directions in cognitive training may enable greater transfer of training to enhance functioning, and there is an increasingly broad array of activities, such as social programs, training in the arts, meditation, and computer games, that are being evaluated for their cognition-enhancing effects (see Table 17–1). It is certain there will be many ways of training your brain in the future.

TABLE 17–1. Empirically studied training techniques

Training technique	Reference	Description
Speed of processing training	Ball et al. 2007	Tasks involve target detection, identification, discrimination, and localization; the aim is to increase speed of responding to stimuli
Reasoning training	Willis and Schaie 1986	Teaches participants strategies for finding patterns in letter, number, or word sequences and improving their ability to recognize the next item in the series
Memory training	Jobe et al. 2001	ACTIVE study approach: different mnemonic strategies, specifically focusing on verbal episodic memory, used for remembering and organizing lists, recalling text, and recalling main ideas and details of stories
Face/name association		Participants assign a semantic associate to the name and pair it with a prominent feature on the face, to later serve as a cue when asked to recall the name when confronted with the face
Method of loci training	Yesavage and Rose 1983	Participants create a mental map and associate each landmark or object on the map with an item on a list of words to be memorized
Brain plasticity training	Mahncke et al. 2006	Six computerized exercises that gradually increase in difficulty as participants' abilities improve
Strategic training	Cavallini et al. 2003	Involves using several different strategies for different tasks so that participants learn how to use the best strategy appropriate for the type of memory task they are presented with

TABLE 17–1. Empirically studied training techniques *(continued)*

Training technique	Reference	Description
Implementation intentions	Chasteen et al. 2001	Mental rehearsal of a plan or desired behavior, so that when the person encounters certain situational cues in the future, the behavior is more automatic
Meditation and yoga	Alexander et al. 1989	Aim to optimize emotional and cognitive regulation through specialized attentional tasks
Senior Odyssey	Stine-Morrow et al. 2007	Team-based approach involving solving novel problems
Experience Corps	Studenski et al. 2006	Intergenerational program matching seniors with youth; tutoring in classroom skills
Autobiographical writing	de Medeiros et al. 2007	Teaching and practice of narrative forms to tell one's life story

Note.   ACTIVE=Advanced Cognitive Training for Independent and Vital Elderly.

KEY POINTS

- Cognitive stimulation over the life span, through education, work complexity, and cognitively engaging leisure activities, appears to reduce the risk of developing dementia risk.

- The magnitude of the benefit of cognitive stimulation is unclear due to confounding factors and imprecision in assessing cognitive engagement.

- Cognitive training appears to enhance cognitive performance, and, to a lesser extent, everyday functioning, in healthy seniors.

- Nontraditional methods of cognitive enhancement include meditation, computer games, intergenerational programs, and autobiographical writing.

References

Alexander CN, Langer EJ, Newman RI, et al: Transcendental meditation, mindfulness, and longevity: an experimental study with the elderly. J Pers Soc Psychol 57:950–964, 1989

Anstey K, Christensen H: Education, activity, health, blood pressure and apolipoprotein E as predictors of cognitive change in old age: a review. Gerontology 46(3):163–167, 2000

Ball K, Berch DB, Helmers KF, et al; Advanced Cognitive Training for Independent and Vital Elderly Study Group: Effects of cognitive training interventions with older adults: a randomized controlled trial. JAMA 288:2271–2281, 2002

Ball K, Edwards JD, Ross LA: The impact of speed of processing training on cognitive and everyday functions. J Gerontol B Psychol Sci Soc Sci 62:19–31, 2007

Baltes PB, Sowarka D, Kliegl R: Cognitive training research on fluid intelligence in old age: what can older adults achieve by themselves? Psychol Aging 4:217–221, 1989

Basak C, Boot WR, Voss MW, et al: Can training in a real-time strategy video game attenuate cognitive decline in older adults. Psychol Aging 23:765–777, 2008

Belleville S, Gilbert B, Fontaine F, et al: Improvement of episodic memory in persons with mild cognitive impairment and healthy older adults: evidence from a cognitive intervention program. Dementia Geriatr Cogn Disord 22:486–499, 2006

Brooks JO 3rd, Friedman L, Pearman AM, et al: Mnemonic training in older adults: effects of age, length of training, and type of cognitive pretraining. Int Psychogeriatr 11:75–84, 1999

Brooks JO 3rd,

Cavallini E, Pagnin A, Vecchi T: Aging and everyday memory: the beneficial effect of memory training. Arch Gerontol Geriatr 37:241–257, 2003

Chasteen AL, Park DC, Schwarz N: Implementation intentions and facilitation of prospective memory. Psychol Sci 12:457–461, 2001

de Medeiros K, Kennedy Q, Cole T, et al: The impact of autobiographic writing on memory performance in older adults: a preliminary investigation. Am J Geriatr Psychiatry 15:257–261, 2007

Doraiswamy PM, Xiong GL: Does meditation enhance cognition and brain longevity? Ann NY Acad Sci September 28, 2007 (Epub ahead of print)

Edwards JD, Wadley VG, Vance DE, et al: The impact of speed of processing training on cognitive and everyday performance. Aging Ment Health 9:262–271, 2005

Espeland MA, Henderson VW: Preventing cognitive decline in usual aging. Arch Intern Med 166:2433–2434, 2006

Gardner-Nix J, Backman S, Barbati J, et al: Evaluating distance education of a mindfulness-based meditation programme for chronic pain management. J Telemed Telecare 14:88–92, 2008

Jain S, Shapiro SL, Swanick S, et al: A randomized controlled trial of mindfulness meditation versus relaxation training: effects on distress, positive states of mind, rumination, and distraction. Ann Behav Med 33:11–21, 2007

Jeste DV, Vahia IV: Comparison of the conceptualization of wisdom in ancient Indian literature with modern views: focus on the Bhagavad Gita. Psychiatry 71:197–209, 2008

Jimison HB, Pavel M, Bissell P, et al: A framework for cognitive monitoring using computer game interactions. Stud Health Technol Inform 129:1073–1077, 2007

Jobe JB, Smith DM, Ball K, et al: ACTIVE: a cognitive intervention trial to promote independence in older adults. Control Clin Trials 22:453–479, 2001

Kröger E, Andel R, Lindsay J, et al: Is complexity of work associated with risk of dementia? The Canadian Study of Health and Aging. Am J Epidemiol 167:820–830, 2008

Kuhn HG, Dickinson-Anson H, Gage FH: Neurogenesis in the dentate gyrus of the adult rat: age-related decrease of neuronal progenitor proliferation. J Neurosci 16:2027–2033, 1996

Lutz A, Slagter HA, Dunne JD, et al: Attention regulation and monitoring in meditation. Trends Cogn Sci 12:163–169, 2008

Maguire EA, Gadian DG, Johnsrude IS, et al: Navigation-related structural change in the hippocampi of taxi drivers. Proc Natl Acad Sci USA 97:4398–4403, 2000

Mahncke HW, Connor BB, Appelman J, et al: Memory enhancement in healthy older adults using a brain plasticity–based training program: a randomized, controlled study. Proc Natl Acad Sci USA 103:12523–12528, 2006

Manly JJ: Advantages and disadvantages of separate norms for African Americans. Clin Neuropsychol 19:270–275, 2005

Miller G: Society for Neuroscience meeting: computer game sharpens aging minds. Science 310:1261, 2005

Miller JJ, Fletcher K, Kabat-Zinn J: Three-year follow-up and clinical implications of a mindfulness meditation–based stress reduction intervention in the treatment of anxiety disorders. Gen Hosp Psychiatry 17:192–200, 1995

Noice H, Noice T: An arts intervention for older adults living in subsidized retirement homes. Neuropsychol Dev Cogn B Aging Neuropsychol Cogn 16:56–79, 2009

Noice H, Noice T, Staines G: A short-term intervention to enhance cognitive and affective functioning in older adults. J Aging Health 16:562–585, 2004

Ospina MB, Bond K, Karkhaneh M, et al: Meditation practices for health: state of the research. Evid Rep Technol Assess (Full Rep) (155):1–263, 2007

Oswald W, Gunzelmann T, Rupprecht R, et al: Differential effects of single versus combined cognitive and physical training with older adults: the SimA study in a 5-year perspective. Eur J Ageing 3:179–192, 2006

Park DC, Gutchess AH, Meade ML, et al: Improving cognitive function in older adults: nontraditional approaches. J Gerontol B Psychol Sci Soc Sci 62:45–52, 2007

Rebok GW, Carlson MC, Langbaum JBS: Training and maintaining memory abilities in healthy older adults: traditional and novel approaches. J Gerontol B Psychol Sci Soc Sci 62 (spec no 1):53–61, 2007

Salthouse TA: Mental exercise and mental aging. Perspect Psychol Sci 1:68–87, 2006

Salthouse TA, Berish DE, Miles JD: The role of cognitive stimulation on the relations between age and cognitive functioning. Psychol Aging 17:548–557, 2002

Sitzer DI, Twamley EW, Jeste DV: Cognitive training in Alzheimer's disease: a meta-analysis of the literature. Acta Psychiatr Scand 114:75–90, 2006

Stine-Morrow EA, Parisi JM, Morrow DG, et al: An engagement model of cognitive optimization through adulthood. J Gerontol B Psychol Sci Soc Sci 62:62–69, 2007

Studenski S, Carlson MC, Fillit H, et al: From bedside to bench: does mental and physical activity promote cognitive vitality in late life? Sci Aging Knowledge Environ 2006:pe21, 2006

Valenzuela MJ: Brain reserve and the prevention of dementia. Curr Opin Psychiatry 21:296–302, 2008

Verghese J, Lipton RB, Katz MJ, et al: Leisure activities and the risk of dementia in the elderly. N Engl J Med 348:2508–2516, 2003

Verhaeghen P, Marcoen A, Goossens L: Improving memory performance in the aged through mnemonic training: a meta-analytic study. Psychol Aging 7:242–251, 1992

Wang JYJ, Zhou DHD, Li J, et al: Leisure activity and risk of cognitive impairment: the Chongqing aging study. Neurology 66:911–913, 2006

Wilkinson N, Ang RP, Goh DH: Online video game therapy for mental health concerns: a review. Int J Soc Psychiatry 54:370–382, 2008

Willis SL, Schaie KW: Training the elderly on the ability factors of spatial orientation and inductive reasoning. Psychol Aging 1:239–247, 1986

Willis SL, Tennstedt SL, Marsiske M, et al: Long-term effects of cognitive training on everyday functional outcomes in older adults. JAMA 296:2805–2814, 2006

Wilson RS, Scherr PA, Schneider JA, et al: Relation of cognitive activity to risk of developing Alzheimer disease. Neurology 69:1911–1920, 2007

Wolinsky FD, Unverzagt FW, Smith DM, et al: The effects of the ACTIVE cognitive training trial on clinically relevant declines in health-related quality of life. J Gerontol B Psychol Sci Soc Sci 61:S281–S287, 2006

Yesavage JA, Rose TL: Concentration and mnemonic training in elderly subjects with memory complaints: a study of combined therapy and order effects. Psychiatry Res 9:157–167, 1983

Yesavage J, Hoblyn J, Friedman L, et al: Should one use medications in combination with cognitive training? If so, which ones? J Gerontol B Psychol Sci Soc Sci 62:11–18, 2007

Recommended Readings

Ball K, Berch DB, Helmers KF, et al; Advanced Cognitive Training for Independent and Vital Elderly Study Group: effects of cognitive training interventions with older adults: a randomized controlled trial. JAMA 288:2271–2281, 2002

Mahncke HW, Connor BB, Appelman J, et al: Memory enhancement in healthy older adults using a brain plasticity–based training program: a randomized, controlled study. Proc Natl Acad Sci USA 103:12523–12528, 2006

Park DC, Gutchess AH, Meade ML, et al: Improving cognitive function in older adults: nontraditional approaches. J Gerontol B Psychol Sci Soc Sci 62:45–52, 2007

Salthouse TA: Mental exercise and mental aging. Perspect Psychol Sci 1:68–87, 2006

18

Aging, Cognition, and Technology

Sara J. Czaja, Ph.D.
Raymond L. Ownby, M.D., Ph.D., M.B.A.

Although researchers in many disciplines are interested in changes that occur in mental abilities as people age, *cognitive aging* researchers have studied in detail how various cognitive abilities change over time during the life span. The abilities studied have included obvious targets such as short- and long-term memories in both verbal and spatial domains, but have also included other abilities such as everyday problem solving, perception of social situations, and expertise in specific fields of endeavor such as playing chess (Roring and Charness 2007). In addition, much attention has been given to issues surrounding the measurement of cognition and, more recently, to the identification of strategies to prevent or remediate age-related cognitive decline (e.g., Green and Bavelier 2008; Valenzuela and Sachdev 2009). In short, the literature on this topic is vast and evolving.

Cognitive aging research has substantial implications for understanding how to help older adults maintain their functional status over time. To the extent that changes in abilities are related to declines in functional performance on such key activities as instrumental activities of daily living, understanding how abilities change over time may be an essential first step in maintaining older adults in the community. Greater understanding of how older adults' cognitive abilities interact with their functioning in everyday tasks may inform interventions to allow them to perform better on a daily basis. Numerous studies have suggested that with appropriate design and support for cognitive limitations, older adults may function at levels similar to those of younger individuals.

If, for example, the memory demands of interacting with technologies such as the Internet are kept to a minimum, older adults may be better able to successfully use these technologies to perform everyday activities. Similarly, reducing the cognitive demands associated with medication adherence may help alleviate problems with nonadherence among older people, who on average tend to take more medications than younger adults. Knowledge of these issues may also help in the development of strategies to foster communication between family members or health care professionals and older people. With advancements in computing technologies, there are also a myriad of technologies available that can help older adults adapt to the environment, such as technologies that enhance the ability to sense and integrate information and select appropriate actions (Czaja and Moon 2003). Electronic memory aids have been successfully used as a compensatory approach to provide reminders to individuals with prospective memory problems (Inglis et al. 2003). However, taking advantage of these advances will require understanding of the effects of aging on cognition, because such effects are often dependent on the context and the cognitive demands inherent in that context. It will also require a user-centered design approach, in which the needs and preferences of older people are considered in the design process.

Our intent in this chapter is to demonstrate the importance of age-related changes in cognition to the performance of everyday tasks, and how understanding these relationships can help foster independence and quality of life among older adults. We emphasize information technologies because technology is ubiquitous in most settings and is involved in the performance of most routine activities. Furthermore, technology aids may help support cognitive functions among older people.

Brief Overview of Aging and Cognition

Existing research on aging and cognition (e.g., Park 1992, 1999) has shown that many cognitive abilities such as processing speed, working memory, and spatial cognition decline with age. Declines are especially apparent when tasks are complex or use unfamiliar stimuli (see, e.g., Park 1992, 1999). Generally, performance for activities that involve new learning or problem solving peaks when individuals are in their twenties or thirties, then gradually declines with increasing age (Park 1999; Schaie 1996). Knowledge, or what is referred to as *crystallized intelligence,* however, either remains relatively stable or increases throughout the life span at least until age 70 (Schaie 1996). Many studies have found age differences on measures of component cognitive abilities that reflect processing, or the *fluid* aspects of intelligence, and on the performance of laboratory-based tasks that draw on these abilities (e.g., Fisk and Rogers 1991; Schaie 1996). There are also numerous studies reporting age-related differences in skill acquisition. These studies have generally indicated that older adults learn new skills more slowly than younger adults and do not reach the same levels of performance (e.g., Charness and Campbell 1988; Jenkins and Hoyer 2000; Salthouse 1994).

However, it is also well established that there is wide interindividual and intraindividual variability in cognitive aging. *Interindividual variability* refers to differences among individuals and reflects the fact that although, on average, older people perform less well than younger people on cognitive tasks, there are wide individual differences among older people in the extent to which they experience cognitive decline. *Intraindividual variability* refers to differences within an individual as shown on multiple tasks at a single measurement occasion (e.g., a spatial task vs. a reasoning task), or on a single task over multiple measurement occasions (i.e., differences in performance that arise from practice) (Hultsch et al. 2008). Overall, this variability indicates that age-related cognitive decline is not inevitable and is perhaps due to lifestyle and environmental factors.

Laboratory Testing Versus Everyday Functioning

One important issue to consider is the relevance of findings from laboratory studies of cognitive aging to everyday tasks within real-world contexts. To the extent that competence in everyday activities is a manifestation of underlying basic abilities, one would expect that older people would perform at lower levels than younger people if a task relies on abilities for which there are age-related declines (e.g., Marsiske and Willis 1998; Schaie and Willis 1993).

In fact, research has generally shown that age-related differences in performance on everyday tasks are explained to some degree by differences in age-related cognitive abilities such as working memory, processing speed, and reasoning. For example, studies have shown that variance in cognitive abilities is an important predictor of performance of instrumental activities of daily living (Marsiske and Willis 1998), medication adherence (Park 1999), use of computer application programs such as text editing (e.g., Charness et al. 2001), performance of technology-based work tasks (e.g., Czaja and Sharit 1993; Czaja et al. 2001; Ownby et al. 2008), use of interactive telephone menu systems (e.g., Sharit et al. 2003), performance of Internet search tasks (Sharit et al. 2008), and health knowledge (e.g., Beier and Ackerman 2003).

However, it has also been shown that domain-specific knowledge is important to the performance of everyday activities. *Domain knowledge* refers to knowledge specific to a content or task area. Investigators have usually found that domain knowledge is also an important contributor to performance on tasks. For example, investigators have shown that domain knowledge contributes to success in the performance of chess (Chase and Simon 1973), bridge (Engle and Bukstel 1978), and other cognitively demanding tasks. Hambrick and Engle (2002) found that prior knowledge about baseball had a strong facilitative effect on memory performance for a baseball-related recall task, independent of working memory and age. In fact, in this study, domain knowledge had a much stronger effect on memory performance than working memory. They also found that those with greater working memory benefited the most from higher domain knowledge and that overall the younger adults had the best performance. Beier and Ackerman (2005) found that prior knowledge was an important predictor of learning new information about cardiovascular disease and xerography. In a series of studies, we (e.g., Czaja and Sharit 1998; Czaja et al. 2001; Nair et al. 2007; Sharit et al. 2008) also found that prior experience with computers in addition to cognitive abilities was an important predictor of performance on subsequent computer-based tasks. These findings are cause for optimism, suggesting that to the extent that older people are familiar with a problem domain and are able to draw on domain-specific knowledge, age differences in performance should be reduced. Thus, training and task practice are important potential strategies for remediating age-related declines in cognitive abilities.

A cogent example of these hypothesized relationships can also be drawn from research on aging and work performance. Work behaviors require a broad range of motor and cognitive skills, and a number of studies have shown that cognitive abilities are related to job performance (e.g., Schmidt and Hunter 1992). Thus, on average, one would expect to find age-related declines in work performance; however, in general there is little evidence that older workers are less productive than younger workers (e.g., Avolio et al. 1990). One explanation is that ability measures are not tapping the abilities needed for particular jobs. In fact, little is currently known about the mapping of specific abilities to specific everyday tasks such as work tasks. Another explanation is that the measures fail to capture the complexity of work situations.

For many types of work tasks, older people may be able to draw on their expertise and contextual support to compensate for age-related declines in abilities. In this regard, Schmidt and Hunter (1998) conducted a meta-analysis and found that job knowledge was a better predictor of job performance than cognitive abilities. It may also be that tasks that are well learned do not require people to work at their maximum capacity, and thus age differences will only be observed when the tasks are unfamiliar and require new learning.

Potential Implications of Cognitive Aging on Technology Use

Overall, the current findings regarding cognitive aging have vast implications for the increasing numbers of older people in our society, especially the "older old" (age 85 and older), for whom we anticipate the greatest degree of cognitive decline and onset of cognition-related disorders. This is especially true given the increased reliance on information and computing technologies in most settings. Technology is also increasingly being used in the home (e.g., home security systems, microwave ovens, medical devices) and in service environments (e.g., automated teller machines [ATMs], ticket kiosks at airports). Technology is also pervading the health care arena and is increasingly being used for service delivery, in-home monitoring, interactive communication (e.g., between patient and physician), transfer of health information, and peer support. Developments in technology also offer great potential in terms of augmenting the cognitive functioning and independence of older adults.

Although the use of technology among older adults is increasing there is still a "digital divide." More than 32 million older people (55+ years) in the United States have a computer at home, compared with 62 million people ages 35–54 years. Similarly, although use of the Internet among older adults is increasing, it is still far lower than that by adults in younger age groups. In 2005, about 26% of individuals age 65 and older were Internet users as compared with 67% of individuals ages 50–64 and 80% of those ages 30–49. Furthermore, adults age 65 and older are much less likely than younger individuals to have a high-speed Internet connection (Pew Internet and American Life Project 2005). They are also less likely to use other forms of technology such as videocassette recorders (VCRs) or digital video disc (DVD) players and ATMs than are younger adults (Czaja et al. 2006).

Not being able to use technology puts older adults at a disadvantage in terms of their ability to live and function independently and to successfully negotiate the built environment. For example, as the Internet and other forms of information technologies are increasingly being used as a vehicle for providing health care information and services, people who cannot adapt to these technologies are likely to experience disparities in access to health care. Furthermore, they will not be able to realize the full benefits of technology. To maximize the use of technology by older adults and its benefits for them, we need to understand factors that influence their ability to successfully use the new technologies, so that programs can be developed to ensure that persons of all ages can use technology safely and effectively. Older adults commonly report that they would be more receptive to using new technologies if they were given adequate training and support (Rogers and Fisk 2000).

Generally, the use of technologies requires new learning and draws on cognitive abilities. Also, given that technology is not static, people continually confront the need to learn new systems or activities at multiple points during their lives. Human–technology interaction is fundamentally an information-processing task. In most cases during an interaction with technology, the user is required to search for and identify displayed information, select responses based on this information, recall commands and operating procedures associated with those responses, and execute the response (Proctor and Vu 2003). As noted earlier (see section "Laboratory Testing and Everyday Functioning"), several studies (e.g., Charness et al. 2001; Czaja and Sharit 1998; Czaja et al. 2001; Ownby et al. 2008) have shown that cognitive abilities such as working memory, attention, and spatial abilities are important predictors of performance of technology-based tasks. Issues of aging and cognition are therefore especially relevant when considering the use of technology.

Aging and Support for Everyday Task Performance

A critical issue is the extent to which age-related differences in abilities are modifiable or can be attenuated through interventions such as training or cognitive support aids. As noted earlier (see section "Brief Overview of Cognitive Aging"), there are wide individual differences in cognitive abilities among older adults, suggesting that in fact cognitive functioning and declines in cognition are modifiable through cognitive support aids and training. The current literature examining these issues is overall fairly encouraging. For example, we found that a graphical aid providing a hierarchical depiction of the menu structure of a telephone voice menu system reduced age differences in performance (Sharit et al. 2003). It may be that the aid reduced demands on working memory and enabled the older adults to plan ahead prior to using the menu system. Other studies have shown that older adults benefit from simple support aids such as reminder messages, especially if these messages are structured so that they draw on familiar cognitive schemata (Morrow et al. 1998). These simple aids can be used to remind people of appointments or medication regimens. Other research in this area is examining more sophisticated forms of cognitive aids such as artificial intelligence systems incorporated in devices that help remind older adults when to perform certain tasks or plan and execute needed activities. However, most research in this area has targeted populations with cognitive decline from causes such as stroke or traumatic brain injury; there is only limited effort being directed specifically at older adults without such conditions.

In terms of training, current data suggest that older adults can, in fact, learn new skills that can be improved through training manipulations. For example, Bherer and colleagues (2005) recently demonstrated that dual-task performance could be moderated by training. Specifically, they found that both younger and older adults could learn to perform the task combination, a tone and letter discrimination task, faster and more accurately and that the improvements in performance generalized to new task combinations. Many other studies involving laboratory-based tasks indicate that older adults can learn new skills and that training manipulations such as self-pacing facilitate performance. An important question is whether and to what extent these findings generalize to tasks that are representative of current everyday activities such as learning to interact with new technologies.

Before discussing what we know about aging and learning to use new technologies, it is important to understand that skill acquisition is a wide behavioral domain that involves perceptual, cognitive, and motor processes and is learned behavior. The emphasis on these various processes varies according to the task in question. Furthermore, there has been only limited research on the degree to which older adults can acquire new skills outside of the laboratory environment and retain these skills over time (Rogerset al. 1996). The term *older adults* is also somewhat ambiguous and very broad, especially given the increased number of people living into their eighth and ninth decades.

Research on Training to Use Technology

With the above caveats in mind, what is generally known is that older people can learn to perform new tasks and use new equipment and technologies, but it may take them longer and they may require more practice. Also, our data show that older adults are receptive to using new technologies but they may have less initial comfort with respect to interacting with new technology systems and less confidence about their abilities to successfully do so (Czaja et al. 2006). Thus it is critically important that when introducing older adults to technology applications or adaptive technologies, they be provided with appropriate training and support.

A number of studies (e.g., Charness et al. 1992; Mead and Fisk 1998; Morrell et al. 1995) have examined the ability of older adults to learn to use other forms of technology such as ATMs, home medical devices, and computer applications such as text editing. These studies varied with respect to training strategies, such as conceptual versus procedural training; they also examined the influence of other variables, such as attitudes toward computers and computer anxiety, on learning success. Overall, the results of these studies indicate that older adults are, in fact, able to learn to use new technology such as computers. However, they are typically slower to acquire new skills than younger adults and generally require more help and hands-on practice. Also, older adults often achieve lower levels of performance than younger adults.

The literature also indicates that training interventions can be successful in terms of improving performance of learners of all ages and points to the importance of matching training strategies with the characteristics of the learner. For example, Mead and Fisk (1998) found that action training was superior to concept training for teaching older adults how to use an ATMs. They also found that action training resulted in better retention performance. Mykityshyn et al. (2002) compared the differential benefits of instructional materials, a user manual versus an instructional video, for younger and older adults learning to use a home medical device. These researchers followed established training principles for designing both the written and the video instructions. The results indicate that the type of instructional material was critical for older adults' performance, with the instructional video being superior for them. The authors stress the importance of age-related usability testing for training materials and stress that recommendations from the literature cannot simply be implemented to design a training program for a particular task or situation, but rather should serve as a starting point for the design of training materials.

We completed several studies (e.g., Czaja and Sharit 1998; Czaja et al. 2001; Sharit et al. 2008) that examined the ability of older individuals to perform computer-based tasks that are common in work settings. Overall, the data from these studies indicate that older adults are willing and able to learn to perform such tasks; however, the older adults achieved lower levels of performance than younger adults, especially on measures of speed. However, importantly, the data also show that even after training, performance continued to improve with practice, and that prior computer experience was an important predictor of performance. These findings indicate the importance of providing older adults with sufficient practice and training on the actual use of a technology as well as instruction on the procedural elements of a task. Finally, we also found that cognitive abilities are important predictors of performance. In fact, in a recent study (Sharit et al. 2008) we found that older adults who had higher levels of cognitive abilities, such as inferencing and working memory, performed at the same level as a group of younger adults on an Internet-based health information–seeking task. These findings underscore the important role of providing cognitive support as a potential means of enhancing the performance of older people.

Conclusion and Recommendations

Clearly, within the domain of aging, cognition, and technology, the topics of training, cognitive aiding, and functional competence warrant further study. A number of issues are unresolved. For example, it is not clear what type of training approach is optimal for older adults for a given task domain. A variety of training techniques, such as activity learning, modeling, conceptual training, and self-paced instruction, have been explored with varying degrees of success. The potential use of technology as a training aid also needs to be examined. For example, older people may benefit from using online, home-based training programs that enhance procedural skills for tasks or strategies for remembering important events (Fisk et al. 2009). However, careful attention needs to be given to the design of the training programs. More research is also needed to clarify whether in fact there are age group × training technique interactions, in order to help clarify the types of training strategies and formats that are most beneficial to older adults. It is also important to examine the extent to which skills are retained over time. The issue of transfer of training is also critical, given, for example, the wide varieties of technology that are available.

More research is needed to better understand whether and to what extent training to enhance cognitive abilities enhances performance on functional tasks. Some promising research results suggest that training to promote cognitive skills such as speed of processing and attention can result in improvements in these skills (Willis et al. 2006). However, more research is needed to determine how training in these skills results in improvements in functional task performance. Work in this area is only at the beginning stages.

Much more work is also needed in the design and evaluation of adaptive technologies. Although several technology-based cognitive aids have been proposed to help offset age-related declines in cognition, more attention needs to be given to the design and evaluation of these systems from the perspective of older adults. Many of these systems were designed to aid people with cognitive impairments resulting from causes such as stroke or traumatic brain injury. More careful attention needs to be given to the specific needs and preferences of older adults who are using the systems.

Finally, the influence of contextual variables on learning success—variables such as access to technology, peer support, and other individual characteristics such as self-efficacy and motivation—also needs to be explored.

KEY POINTS

■ The primary aim of cognitive training and adaptive technologies in aging research is to enhance functioning, and a major task is to understand how training transfers to real-world functioning.

■ The use of technologies requires cognitive resources, and training that is adapted to older adults to use new technologies may be needed to reduce the technology gulf between older and younger adults.

■ Adaptive technologies such as memory aids may be useful for enhancing functioning, but these technologies need to be adapted to the needs and preferences of older adults.

■ Older adults appear to retain reserve capacity in adopting new skills, and there will likely be a role for technology in teaching these skills.

References

Avolio BJ, Waldman DA, McDaniel MA: Age and work performance in nonmanagerial jobs: the effects of experience and occupational type. Acad Manage J 33:407–422, 1990

Beier ME, Ackerman PL: Determinants of health knowledge: an investigation of age, gender, abilities, personality and interests. J Pers Soc Psychol 16:615–628, 2003

Beier ME, Ackerman PL: Age, ability and the role of prior knowledge on the acquisition of new domain knowledge: promising results in a real-world learning environment. Psychol Aging 20:341–355, 2005

Bherer L, Kramer AF, Peterson MS, et al: Training effects on dual-task performance: are there age-related differences in plasticity of attention control? Psychol Aging 20:695–709, 2005

Charness N, Campbell JID: Acquiring skill at mental calculation in adulthood: a task decomposition. J Exp Psychol Gen 117:115–121, 1988

Charness N, Schumann CE, Boritz GM: Training older adults in word processing: effects of age, training technique and computer anxiety. Int J Technol Aging 5:79–106, 1992

Charness N, Kelley CL, Bosman EA, et al: Word processing training and retraining: effects of adult age, experience, and interface. Psychol Aging 16:110–127, 2001

Chase WG, Simon HA: The mind's eye in chess, Visual Information Processing. Edited by Chase WG. New York, Academic Press, 1973, pp 215–281

Czaja SJ, Moen P: Technology and employment, in Technology and Adaptive Aging. Edited by Pew R, Van Hamel S. Washington, DC, National Research Council, 2004, pp 150–178

Czaja SJ, Sharit J: Ability-performance relationships as a function of age and task experience for a data entry task. J Exp Psychol Appl 4:332–351, 1998

Czaja SJ, Sharit J: Practically relevant research: capturing real world tasks, environments and outcomes. The Gerontologist 43:9–18, 2003

Czaja SJ, Sharit J, Ownby R, et al: Examining age differences in performance of a complex information search and retrieval task. Psychol Aging 16:564–579, 2001

Czaja SJ, Charness N, Fisk AD, et al: Factors predicting the use of technology: findings from the Center on Research and Aging and Technology Enhancement (CREATE). Psychol Aging 21:333–352, 2006

Engle RW, Bukstel LH: Memory processes among bridge players of different expertise. Am J Psychol 10:673–689, 1978

Fisk AD, Rogers W: Toward an understanding of age-related memory and visual search effects. J Exp Psychol Gen 120:131–149, 1991

Fisk AD, Rogers W, Charness N, et al (eds): Designing for Older Adults: Principles and Creative Human Factors Approaches, 2nd Edition. London, CRC Press, 2009

Green CS, Bavelier D: Exercising your brain: a review of human brain plasticity and training induced learning. Psychol Aging 23:692–702, 2008

Hambrick DZ, Engle RW: Effects of domain knowledge, working memory capacity, and age on cognitive performance: an investigation of the knowledge-is-power hypothesis. Cogn Psychol 44:339–387, 2002

Hultsch DE, Strauss E, Hunter MA, et al: Intra-individual variability, cognition, and aging, in The Handbook of Cognitive Aging, 3rd Edition. Edited by Craik FIM, Salthouse TA. New York, Psychology Press, 2008, pp 491–557

Inglis EA, Szmkowiak A, Gregor P, et al: Issues surrounding the user-centered development of a new interactive memory aid. Universal Access in an Information Society 2:226–234, 2003

Jenkins L, Hoyer WJ: Instance-based automaticity and aging: acquisition, reacquisition, and long term retention. Psychol Aging 15:551–565, 2000

Marsiske M, Willis SL: Practical creativity in older adults' everyday problem solving: life-span perspectives, in Creativity and Successful Aging: Theoretical and Empirical Approaches. Edited by Adams-Price CE. New York, Springer, 1998, pp 73–113

Mead SE, Fisk AD: Measuring skill acquisition and retention with an ATM simulator: the need for age-specific training. Human Factors 40:516–523, 1998

Morrell RW, Park DC, Mayhorn CB, et al: Older adults and electronic communication networks: learning to use ELDERCOMM. Paper presented at the annual meeting of the American Psychological Association, New York, August 1995

Morrow D, Leirer VO, Carver L, et al: Older and younger adults memory for health appointment information: implications for automated telephone messaging design. Journal of Experimental Psychology: Applied 4:352–374. 1998

Mykityshyn AL, Fisk AD, Rogers W: Learning to use a home medical device: mediating age-related differences with training. Hum Factors 44:354–364, 2002

Nair S, Czaja SJ, Sharit J: A multilevel modeling approach to examining: individual differences in skill acquisition for a computer-based task. J Gerontol B Psychol Sci Soc Sci 62 (spec no 1):85–96, 2007

Ownby RL, Czaja SJ, Loewenstein D, et al: Cognitive abilities that predict success in a computer-based training program. Gerontologist 48:170–180, 2008

Park DC: Applied cognitive aging research, in The Handbook of Aging and Cognition. Edited by Craik FIM, Salthouse TA. Hillsdale, NJ, Erlbaum, 1992, pp 449–494

Park DC: Aging and the controlled and automatic processing of medical information and medical intentions, in Processing of Medical Information in Aging Patients: Cognitive and Human Factors Perspectives. Edited by Park DC, Morrell RW, Shifren K. Mahwah, NJ, Erlbaum, 1999, pp 3–22

Pew Internet and American Life Project: Digital Divisions, 2005. Available at: http://www.pewinternet.org/pdfs/PIP_Digital_Divisions_Oct_5_2005.pdf.

Proctor RW, Vu KL: Human information processing: an overview for human-computer interaction, in The Human Computer Interaction Handbook: Fundamentals, Evolving Technologies and Emerging Applications. Edited by Jacko JA, Sears A. Mahwah, NJ, Erlbaum, 2003, pp 35–51

Rogers WA, Fisk AD, Mead SE, et al: Training older adults to use automatic teller machines. Hum Factors 38:425-433, 1996

Rogers WA, Fisk AD: Human factors, applied cognition, and aging, in The Handbook of Aging and Cognition, 2nd Edition. Edited by Craik FIM, Salthouse TA. Mahwah, NJ, Erlbaum, 2000, pp 559–592

Roring RW, Charness N: A multilevel model analysis of expertise in chess across the life span. Psychol Aging 22:291–299, 2007

Salthouse TA: Aging associations: influence of speed on adult aging differences in associative learning. J Exp Psychol Learn Mem Cogn 20:1486–1503, 1994

Schaie KW: Intellectual Development in Adulthood: The Seattle Longitudinal Study. New York, Cambridge University Press, 1996

Schaie KW, Willis SL: Age difference patterns of psychometric intelligence in adulthood: generalizability within and across domains. Psychol Aging 8:44–55, 1993

Schmidt FK, Hunter JE: Development of a causal model of processes determining job performance. Curr Dir Psychol Sci 1:89–92, 1992

Schmidt FK, Hunter JE: The validity and utility of selection methods in personnel psychology: practical and theoretical implications of 85 years of research. Psychol Bull 124:262–274, 1998

Sharit J, Czaja SJ, Nair S, et al: The effects of age and environmental support in using telephone voice menu systems. Hum Factors 45:234-251, 2003

Sharit J, Czaja SJ, Hernandez M, et al: An evaluation of performance by older persons on a simulated telecommuting task. J Gerontol B Psychol Sci Soc Sci 59:P305–P316, 2004

Sharit J, Hernandez M, Czaja SJ, et al: Investigating the roles of knowledge and cognitive abilities in older adult information seeking on the Web. Transactions of Computer-Human Interaction 15, 3:1–3.25, 2008

Valenzuela M, Sachdev P: Can cognitive exercise prevent the onset of dementia? Systematic review of randomized clinical trials with longitudinal follow-up. Am J Geriatr Psychiatry 17:179–187, 2009

Willis SL, Tennstedt SL, Marsiske M, et al; ACTIVE Study Group. JAMA 296:2805–2814, 2006

Recommended Readings

Fisk AD, Rogers W, Charness N, et al (eds): Designing for Older Adults: Principles and Creative Human Factors Approaches, 2nd Edition. London, CRC Press, 2009

Ownby RL, Czaja SJ, Loewenstein D, et al: Cognitive abilities that predict success in a computer-based training program. Gerontologist 48:170–180, 2008

Roring RW, Charness N: A multilevel model analysis of expertise in chess across the life span. Psychol Aging 22:291–299, 2007

19 Recognizing and Promoting Resilience

John Martin-Joy, M.D.
George E. Vaillant, M.D.

> It's not what happens to you, it's what you do with it.
>
> *Ben Aguilar, Core City man at age 67*

Over the past three decades, mental health clinicians have increasingly learned to appreciate the value of seeing strength amid pathology (Seligman 2002). Whereas clinical training focuses on problems and risks, researchers and theorists have noted that healthy outcomes do occur despite risk, and have been curious about why. In child psychology and psychiatry, for example, researchers have identified protective factors that are associated with resilience in at-risk children (Hauser et al. 2006; Rutter 1987). Such advances have built on a generation of work by psychoanalytic theorists, who have productively reworked Freudian thought by paying attention to areas of mental life that are not exclusively derived from conflict. As Erik Erikson (1968, p. 595) put it, if we know what may go wrong at each stage of the life

Work supported by research grant K05-MH00364 and MH42248 from the National Institute of Mental Health.

span, we should also be able to specify "what should have gone and can go right."

In contrast to child psychiatry, however, the study of old age has traditionally had less to say about resilience and more to say about stasis and decline. There are several reasons for this:

1. It has been unclear to what extent growth and development continue in late life. William James famously thought that personality development stops at age 30, and indeed some tests of personality do show a remarkable degree of consistency over the life span.
2. By definition, clinicians who treat older adults tend to see pathology, and may be tempted to conflate admittedly widespread dementia and depression with the normal aging process. At times, we may all be tempted to see old age exclusively as a story of loss, endings, and decline— Shakespeare's "Last scene of all…second childishness and mere oblivion, / Sans teeth, sans eyes, sans taste, sans everything" (*As You Like It* II.vii.163–166).
3. Until recently, we have had no way to correct our view using prospectively gathered empirical data from childhood to old age. This has made it difficult to judge on the basis of empirical evidence whether *successful aging* is simply an oxymoron, and whether some coping styles promote success in meeting the challenges of later life.

For all these reasons, it has remained unclear how a focus on resilience might inform clinical work with older adults.

In order to address the challenge of resilience, we use prospectively gathered empirical data from the Study of Adult Development, an ongoing 70+-year study designed to illuminate the unfolding of human strengths over the life span. The Study of Adult Development includes three cohorts of subjects who have been followed over extended periods of time: the College Study, a group of college sophomores selected in 1938–1942 and followed to the present; the Core City Study, a group of inner-city men selected as teenagers in the mid-1940s and followed to the present; and the Study of Gifted Women, a subgroup of California women with high intelligence who were selected as schoolgirls in the 1920s and then interviewed in late life. (See Vaillant 1993 and section "The Empirical Study of Coping Style"below for a fuller description of each cohort.) The College Study men and the Core City men were interviewed in depth at approximately ages 47 and 75, and were followed using questionnaires every 2 years from age 19 to the present. Because of its lengthy follow-up period, the Study of Adult Development is unique in its ability to examine psychological growth and change over time, including the issue of resilience.

In this chapter we focus on one special facet of resilience: the challenge of coping posed by Ben Aguilar, the Core City man quoted in our epigraph. (Aguilar's name and identifying information have been disguised, as have those of all research subjects presented in this chapter. Unless a citation is given, biographical vignettes on our subjects come from the research files of the Study of Adult Development.) Abandoned by his father, placed in foster care when he was 3 months old, then repeatedly beaten and neglected, Aguilar had more reason than most to feel that life is unjust. At age 15, he could not remember his own mother; in midlife, predictably, he suffered from depression and severe anxiety. At age 45, according to the Study of Adult Development interviewer, Aguilar suffered from headaches, vomiting, and a spastic colon when stressed, and worried "incessantly" about straying too far from competent medical care. The interviewer thought he was covertly asking for help. Yet at age 67 Aguilar was regularly volunteering at church and working with the elderly: his philosophy was to have a purpose in life, to learn from experience, and to achieve acceptance. As he said then, "It's not what happens to you, it's what you do with it."

To demonstrate that adaptive coping styles are not simply a figment of a deprived child's imagination, we present evidence to suggest that the choice of adaptive coping style is a key aspect of successful aging. Specifically, we show that coping styles (also known as *defense mechanisms* or *ego mechanisms of defense*) may be reliably rated, are associated with adult mental health in midlife, and predict successful aging at ages 70–80. Finally, we suggest ways that clinicians can promote adaptive coping styles and resilience in their older patients.

The Empirical Study of Coping Style

The psychoanalytic study of coping and defense began with Sigmund Freud. Freud first conceptualized defenses as tools the unconscious mind uses to ward off awareness of intolerable conflicts. For example, Freud's early patient Dora seemed to fend off all awareness of her sexual interest, a process Freud called *repression* (S. Freud 1905/1953). Freud first saw repression as the major tool that humans use to guard the boundary between conscious and unconscious life. In 1923, however, when he introduced the structural theory, Freud proposed a more complicated structure for the mind, with the ego mediating between the needs of the id (drives), the demands of the superego (conscience), and the ever-changing reality of other people (S. Freud 1923/1961). According to this theory, when reality changes, or when unacceptable conflicts threaten to emerge into awareness, the ego uses its specialized tools (defenses or coping styles) to adapt. Freud's daughter Anna, who helped systematize and elaborate the new ego psychology, presented a differentiated list of defenses as they were encountered in clinical situations and showed persuasively how they helped preserve patients' mental equilibrium (A. Freud 1937; Vaillant 1993).

When Erik Erikson (1950/1963) identified in sequence the adult strengths of identity, intimacy, generativity, and ego integrity, the longitudinal study of normal adult development acquired a theoretical foundation. The empirical study of coping, however, still faced significant obstacles. Among these were the fact that analysts used a bewildering array of names for different defenses; the reluctance of many analysts to accept evidence from outside the consulting room; the view of observable data as intrinsically superficial; and the related difficulty of using numbers to measure elusive intrapsychic phenomena. Erikson (1968, p. 595) himself serenely admitted that "I see no scientific merit in insisting on measuring what by its nature cannot be measured." It was not until the mid-1970s that the Study of Adult Development was able to address these problems adequately, by using clear definitions, observable behavior, and prospective study (Vaillant 1976).

Before coping styles could be put to use in the empirical study of aging, researchers had to address at least two challenges:

1. Coping styles have to be measured *reliably*. That is, different raters must be able to agree on what coping style they are seeing. At the level of individual defenses, achieving consistent reliability has proven to be a major challenge. However, in our laboratory's study of College Study men at age 47, suppression, humor, and anticipation proved highly reliable when clinical rating methods were used (Vaillant 1976; ($P<0.001$). Similarly, in the Study of Gifted Women, use of the Q-sort methods showed that suppression, humor, sublimation, and altruism were all highly reliable (Roston et al. 1992; $P<0.01$). The good news is that when viewed at the level of overall mature defenses, interrater reliability is consistently strong (e.g., 0.72 with $P<0.001$ as shown in Vaillant 1976).

2. Researchers have to be able to show that choice of coping style has *validity* and *clinical relevance*. Our study of college men (Vaillant 1976) showed strong positive associations between maturity of defenses assessed at age 47 and the independently rated realms of adult adjustment, marital success, psychiatric visits, and subjective happiness in midlife. (All were significant at the $P<0.001$ level.) In terms of specific coping styles, the correlation of defenses and outcomes varied somewhat. But later work confirmed positive associations between overall mature defenses and key aspects of mental health, this time in Core City men (Vaillant and Drake 1985). Positive associations were found between maturity of defenses and global mental health, Eriksonian stage achieved, high in-

come, and high social competence. Negative associations were observed between mature defenses and sociopathy, low adult social class, never having been married, and the presence of a personality disorder.

Since 1976, researchers have expanded the scope of inquiry on coping, showing that coping styles naturalistically group into clusters, map onto overall mental health, and predict clinical outcome (reviewed in Vaillant 1992b). In addition, our work has shown that severe childhood deprivation does not consistently correlate with mature defenses but that adult social class does—suggesting that mature coping style may even "make a causal contribution to upward social mobility" (Vaillant and Drake 1985, p. 599). In recognition of these and other advances, the *Diagnostic and Statistical Manual of Mental Disorders,* 4th Edition (DSM-IV), included an optional axis for defense assessment (American Psychiatric Association 1994, p. 752).

To study coping, the Study of Adult Development took advantage of 70 years of data gathered from three cohorts followed from adolescence into late life:

- The *College Study* (Grant study): This ongoing study consists of 268 men selected as Harvard sophomores circa 1938 and followed prospectively for the next 70 years. (The name Grant derived from the William T. Grant Foundation, which provided early financial support for the study.) Selected for psychological, physical, and academic "soundness," these college men have now passed age 85 with only minimal attrition of the study population. Privileged socioeconomically, chosen for mental and physical health, the College Study men are perhaps better positioned to do well than any other cohort of adults currently being followed.
- The *Core City Study* (Glueck study): This ongoing study consists of 456 inner-city schoolboys selected for study during junior high school circa 1940 and followed prospectively to the present. The Core City men originally made up the nondelinquent (control) arm of Sheldon and Eleanor Glueck's study of juvenile delinquency. At the time of selection, these youth typically had endured multiple forms of social disadvantage, including poverty, modest to low IQs, and family dysfunction, yet did not become delinquent. The Core City men are now approximately age 75.
- The *Study of Gifted Women* (Terman women sample): The Study of Adult Development researchers interviewed 40 women chosen from Lewis Terman's study of 672 women who had exceptionally high measured intelligence (an IQ of >140) (Terman 1925). Originally selected from the California public schools in 1920, women in this sample were interviewed at age 78.

Together, these cohorts constitute arguably the longest-running study of adult development in existence. Although admittedly each of these cohorts is composed of white subjects, they contain much socioeconomic diversity and have the rare virtue of providing nearly lifelong longitudinal follow-up. The College Study, Core City, and Gifted Women subjects are among the best means we are likely to have available for studying the protective value of healthy coping over extended periods of time.

A Hierarchy of Coping Styles

In the section that follows, our goal is to help the busy mental health clinician learn to do what Stuart Hauser calls "seeing in the dark" (Hauser et al. 2006)—discerning strengths that bode well for the future, even in the midst of difficult psychopathology. The task is daunting, for in the moment of stress, adaptive coping styles can seem like the colors in a rainbow: evanescent, if very real. With time and practice, however, clinicians can begin to recognize and name the component colors more reliably, as if using a prism to refract light.

We present below a differentiated hierarchy of coping styles (defenses) that has been empirically validated (Vaillant 1976). Of note, this hierarchy builds on the work of Elvin Semrad (1967), professor of psychiatry at Harvard Medical School and clinical director at the Massachusetts Mental Health Center in Boston circa 1960–1976, as well as on the contributions of Norma Haan (1963) and Anna Freud (1937). Although we focus here on the mature defenses, detailed discussion of the intermediate and immature defenses can be found elsewhere (Vaillant 1992a, 1993).

In broad outline, *immature defenses* are characteristic not only of children but of individuals with psychiatric illnesses, in the form of either acute Axis I disorders or long-term maladaptive personality styles (Axis II disorders) (see Vaillant and Drake 1985). For example, after the death of a loved one, a school-age child may complain of a stomachache, but not of sadness or grief. After a similar loss, an adult who suffers from major depression may be convinced that she has an undiagnosed cancer. Both are examples of *hypochondriasis,* the unconscious use of somatic preoccupation to ward off intolerable psychic pain. Who wishes to acknowledge overwhelming grief? But while protecting the user, immature defenses also tend to drive away support—in part by inducing feelings of helplessness and frustration in others. A primary care physician who tries to reassure a hypochondriacal patient by telling her that nothing is wrong is likely to fare badly in the clinic. He may do far better if, rather than endless workups, he offers an empathic acknowledgment of his patient's psychic pain (Brown and Vaillant 1981).

In contrast, users of *intermediate (neurotic) defenses* spare the feelings of others but are often unsparing to themselves. A habitual user of intellectualization, for example, can see problems accurately. She may be able to describe the impact of career triumph or a loss with impressive clinical detachment. But she cannot feel joy or sadness spontaneously. Conversely, a user of repression can feel intensely, but he cannot hold onto the context or reasons for his feelings, and thus loses the power to harness the feelings and use them productively. In adaptive value, intermediate defenses are located somewhere between the immature and mature coping styles. They are not strongly associated with severe psychopathology, but in general they are not good predictors of mental health or psychosocial outcome (Vaillant 1976).

Mature (Adaptive) Coping Styles

T.S. Eliot famously said that humans cannot bear very much reality, but the mature (adaptive) coping styles creatively increase the range of what humans can bear. We all need our illusions. But unlike the coping styles used by individuals with personality disorders, mature coping styles help their users deal constructively with stress and conflict while introducing only minimal distortion of reality and minimizing the cost to others. They allow painful conflicts to be experienced in advance, converted into play, or held temporarily in abeyance. In that way the mature coping styles help users achieve in life what Semrad defined as the task of psychotherapy: to help the patient acknowledge, bear, and put into perspective difficult feelings (Razo and Mazur 1980, p. 30).

The adaptive coping styles, listed in Table 19–1, function as protective factors that make resilience more likely. They are defined and illustrated below.

Suppression

Suppression is the deliberate directing of attention away from painful feelings toward what can be controlled and toward tasks that need to be done. Suppression may take the form of a stiff upper lip, the ability to delay gratification, or a stoic resignation to what cannot be altered. Winston Churchill's speech of 1940—"I have nothing to offer but blood, toil, tears, and sweat"—is a famous example. So is the remarkably durable Serenity Prayer of Alcoholics Anonymous. Stoics may appear uninterested in discussing feelings, and for this reason suppression is often mistrusted by clinicians, who tend to regard it as pathology rather than as strength. In fact, however, this coping style has one of the strongest correlations with adult adjustment (see Vaillant 1976; Vaillant et al. 1986).

TABLE 19–1.   Hierarchy of coping styles

Mature (adaptive) coping styles

Suppression

Anticipation

Sublimation

Humor

Altruism

Intermediate (neurotic) coping styles

Intellectualization

Reaction formation

Displacement

Repression

Immature (maladaptive) coping styles

Projection

Dissociation

Passive aggression

Fantasy

Hypochondriasis

Acting out

Source.   Adapted from Vaillant 1976, 1993.

At age 80, a college man who scored highly on suppression was forced to move when his lower Manhattan home was covered by debris during the attacks of September 11. Notably, he did not deny the pain or elaborate on his feelings—he described being close to Ground Zero as "a severe inconvenience"—but said simply, "We have weathered it well." In suppression, difficult reality (inner or outer) is not denied but takes its place alongside realistic positive thinking (accepting what one cannot control). A Core City man exemplified suppression in midlife when he described his job on the subway as "grueling" but said, "It means a good living." Suppression is seldom dramatic, but it pays off handsomely in stability and resilience.

Anticipation

Anticipation is the affective experiencing of anxiety about the future. Under ordinary circumstances, this coping style may be almost invisible. But the College and Core City studies bear out the truth of the observation attributed to Benjamin Franklin: "Look before, or you'll find yourself behind."

Whether it was studied in the socially privileged or the socially disadvantaged, anticipation correlated positively with adult adjustment in midlife (Vaillant 1976; Vaillant et al. 1986).

One way to study anticipation is to contrast it with its absence. When asked about his plans for the future, one Core City man at 50 replied simply, "No idea." When he was asked about retirement plans, his answer was a similar "I couldn't say." (In the absence of dementia, these examples also illustrate the intermediate defense of *repression*.) In contrast, when asked the same question, another Core City man replied that in 10 years he expected to be working at his same job. But unlike the first man, this man acknowledged worries about having enough money to retire. To address his worries, he had taken on a second job. Similarly, after recovering from a drinking problem, he warded off relapse by reminding himself of the likely consequences.

Sublimation

Sublimation includes expressing conflict through creative activities such as art, music, writing, and scientific study. These activities put something into the world that was not there before. Sublimation also has the fringe benefits of providing the unique experience of "flow," or losing oneself in one's creative work (Csikszentmihalyi 1990), and of summoning the admiration of others. For example, one subject in the Study for Gifted Women had been deprived of career opportunities early in life but coped with her divorce by taking violin lessons at age 60. She focused intently on her music and eventually played solo concerts in Los Angeles to great acclaim (Vaillant 1993).

Douglas O'Keefe, a Core City man, had been deserted by his father and placed in foster care during childhood. By the time he was 16 years old, he had lived at 21 different addresses, most of them in congested slum neighborhoods. O'Keefe dropped out of school in the tenth grade. But he showed early competence in drafting and photography, and he stayed with both, eventually attending art school and supporting himself and his young family by doing commercial drawing and photography—"the only work I've ever liked." The admiring Study of Adult Development interviewer agreed: "He loved his work and it helped him to manage his feelings." At 68, O'Keefe was happily working at his studio at home, surrounded by his family and by his stunning photographs of nature. His wife was working at a desk nearby, and the interview was punctuated by warm interruptions from his children. O'Keefe illustrates the way adaptive coping can bring joy while keeping loved ones close.

It is frequently suggested that there is an association between creativity and mental illness. Yet longitudinal study suggests that the causation may be in the opposite (protective) direction. A Parisian psychoanalyst who conducted multiyear analyses of creative artists and their inhibitions concluded that in cases where psychopathology was present the "part of the personality which allowed them to create, and to keep on creating, must be considered as the healthy part!" (McDougall 1997, p.79). Her conclusion is buttressed by empirical study of creativity in our cohorts. In our early studies the correlation of sublimation with adult adjustment was positive albeit weak. In Core City men the use of this coping style correlated strongly with overall mental health in middle age (Vaillant et al. 1986).

Humor

At age 85, Bernard Baruch observed, "To me, old age is always 15 years older than I am." Perhaps because of its dependence on timing and context, humor is elusive and difficult to document in somber psychological investigations and interview transcripts. Few writers have tried harder than Freud, who produced a remarkably humorless book on the subject; yet in old age, when the Nazis demanded a letter certifying that they had not mistreated him, he had the defiant wit to write: "I can most highly recommend the Gestapo to everyone" (Gay 1988, p. 628).

As Freud's example shows, adaptive coping runs the risk of miscalculating. As Freud's admirers we may laugh along with him from the safety of our armchairs, but even his biographer wondered whether the sarcastic comment, made on the brink of his release, didn't amount to a death wish. With defiant rage (acting out) a risk on one hand, and self-destructive clowning (passive aggression) a risk on the other, the wonder of contagious humor is that it manages to be so finely calibrated.

In our study of Core City men, the correlation of humor with global mental health was robust (Vaillant et al. 1986).

Altruism

Helping others is an additional way to turn lemons into lemonade. Adam Carson, a physician in the College Study, turned from the research career his father wanted for him to a satisfying career seeing patients and promoting medical ethics. Similarly, Ben Aguilar, the Core City man with hypochondriasis at age 45, transformed his conflict into a satisfying retirement, which he spent visiting the sick and helping them overcome their pain. Triangulation helped the interviewer see that the change was real and not imagined. During Aguilar's interview at age 67, his 95-year-old neighbor called to ask his advice on dealing with arthritis.

In our early studies, the correlation between altruism and adult adjustment was positive, though weaker than for the other mature defenses (Vaillant 1976; Vaillant et al. 1986). However, in Core City men, its correlation with overall mental health in midlife was robust (Vaillant et al. 1986).

Coping Style and Successful Aging

In summary, as deprived and fortunate children grow into middle age, the adaptive (mature) coping styles have empirically demonstrable value to adult mental health. By using the hierarchy of coping styles as a prism, clinicians can reliably identify the spectrum of mature coping styles that promote healthy adjustment.

But does mature coping style also have protective value over longer periods of time? Table 19–2 shows our effort to test the power of coping style to guide adults (in this case, men) through the second half of the life span (Vaillant and Mukamal 2001). We contrasted six predictor variables that were uncontrollable with seven variables that were at least partially controllable, all measured before age 50. Uncontrollable variables were major depression, parental social class, warmth of childhood, ancestral longevity, childhood temperament, and physical health (objective disability). Relatively controllable variables were coping style (maturity of defenses), smoking, alcohol abuse, exercise (for men in the College Study only), and education (for men in the Core City Study only)—all assessed independently. Subjects were 237 College Study men and 332 Core City men who were still participating in the study at age 50. Outcomes assessed at ages 70–80 included overall quality of aging, physical health, death and disability before age 80, social supports, subjective life satisfaction, and objective mental health.

In summary, the controllable factors made a powerful contribution to successful aging, while the contribution of the uncontrollable factors was surprisingly weak. As predictors of poor outcome, alcohol and smoking remained impressive. But maturity of coping style proved more potent than a stable marriage, exercise, or body mass index in predicting a positive outcome in late life. Men who used mature defenses before age 50 were two to three times more likely to be both happy and well in late life, rather than sad and sick (odds ratio=2.65 for 162 College Study men at ages 75–80; odd ratio=2.98 for 217 Core City Study men at ages 65–70; P<0.05):

It is important to note that coping style did not correlate with every aspect of successful aging. In particular, mature coping did *not* predict objective physical disability in late life. Yet mature coping did predict subjective physical disability, or the men's perception of how disabled they were. In other words, men who coped adaptively were able to make the most of their real disabilities. (In contrast, ancestral longevity is an excellent predictor of objective physical disability but has little ability to predict subjective physical disability; see Vaillant 1991). Thus, the mature defenses appear to have spe-

TABLE 19–2.   Predictors of successful aging

Predictor variables	Quality of aging[a]	
	College men	Core City men
Controllable factors assessed before age 50		
Maturity of defenses	0.32**	0.23**
Pack-years of smoking	0.35**	0.31**
Alcohol abuse	0.42**	0.19**
Exercise or education[b]	0.22**	0.20**
Body mass index	0.14*	0.11*
Stable marriage	0.27**	0.22**
Uncontrollable factors assessed before age 50		
Major depression	0.22**	0.12*
Parental social class	NS	NS
Warmth of childhood[c]	0.18*	NS
Ancestral longevity	−0.15*	NS
Childhood temperament	NS	NS
Objective physical disability at age 50	0.39**	0.40**

Note.   NS=not significant.
*$P<0.05$; **$P<0.001$.
[a]Quality of aging was assessed at approximately ages 75–80 for 237 College Study men and at ages 65–70 for 332 Core City Study men. This global measure made use of independent ratings of disability and psychosocial adjustment based on interview, questionnaire, and medical data, and of the subject's own rating of his subjective life satisfaction to categorize overall quality of aging: 1=*happy-well:* survival to age 75 (College Study men) or age 65 (Core City Study men), no objective or subjective physical disability, objective psychosocial adjustment in top three-quarters, subjective life satisfaction in top two-third, and (College Study men only) social supports in top three quarters; 2=*intermediate:* survival with either physical disability or psychosocial disability, but not both; 3=*sad-sick:* survival with 5 or more years of objective or subjective disability and psychosocial adjustment in bottom quarter or life satisfaction in bottom third, or (College Study men only) or social supports in bottom quartile; 4=*prematurely dead* (before age 75 for College Study men or before 65 for Core City Study men).
[b]Exercise was measured for College Study men only; education was measured for Core City Study men only.
[c]Warmth of childhood was rated by research assistants blind to all later data. This score was a composite of ratings of family cohesion; relations with mother, father, and siblings; and the rater's global impression of the subject's childhood.
Source.   Adapted from Vaillant and Mukamal 2001.

cial relevance to the ability to play the hand that fate deals us—something akin to the Serenity Prayer.

When we studied satisfaction during retirement in Core City men, poor health and income proved less important than the presence of other strengths, such as marital satisfaction and sanguine personality style. For men with these strengths, retirement offered a "third chance at a contented life" (Vaillant et al. 2006, p. 688), regardless of what childhood and midlife had held for them. Notably, the happily retired were more likely than others to report finding meaning in activities that reflect sublimation and altruism, such as the following:

- "Writing my memoirs"
- "Playing piano"
- "Watching grandchildren"
- Helping others (One man remarked, "I know what it is like to be poor so I try to help others.")

As Ben Aguilar said, it's not what happens to you that matters, it's what you do with it.

Can Coping Style Mature With Age?

The Berkeley Longitudinal Study has recently shown that overall psychological health improves from age 30 to age 62 (Jones and Meredith 2000). Although our prior work has documented a shift toward more adaptive coping in college men from age 19 to age 30 (Vaillant 1976), the potential for coping style to mature in later life remains relatively unexplored.

One of the few studies to document changes in coping in the elderly is the Berlin Aging Study, which carefully followed six 5-year age cohorts of urban elderly individuals between ages 70 and 100. In the younger of these cohorts, the strategies of information seeking and "giving up" were commonly used, while in the older cohorts it was more common to perceive life as being without meaning. The study documented increases in spirituality and serenity—the latter probably paralleling suppression—from age 70 to 95 (Baltes and Mayer 1999).

Clinical Implications

In closing, as Table 19–2 suggests, there is solid empirical evidence to show that as we age, our fate is not in our stars but in our selves. Clinicians may not be able to block the aging process, but they can strive to promote what is controllable and to help their patients accept what is not. The following suggestions, grounded in the empirical studies described in this chapter, offer ways for clinicians to begin strength-based work with older adults.

1. *Adapt to slowness.* Of all the cognitive changes associated with aging, reduced processing speed is the most consistent and the most widely discussed. The decrease in processing speed is observed both cross-sectionally and longitudinally and may help explain other cognitive changes that occur with advancing age, such as declining performance on visuoconstructive tasks and modest decreases in the ability to learn new information (Dunkin and Amano 2005). But in the clinic, the more important issue may be to combat the busy clinician's impatience with slowness. Be aware of the temptation to rush, to use a first name, to omit a formal title, or to patronize in other ways. It may help to remind yourself that your patient is not a child but a vastly experienced adult moving in slow motion.

2. *Get out of the way of strengths.* Become familiar with the adaptive coping styles presented in Table 19–1, and then inquire how your patient dealt with the latest challenge at home. What does the patient do to feel better when he or she is feeling down? If the answer is "I don't think of it that way. I just go ahead and do what I have to do," as it was for one man from the College Study, consider applauding. Deployed at the right moment, suppression may have more adaptive value than the therapist's reflexive wish to explore and formulate. If your patient is able to laugh contagiously about his erectile dysfunction, laugh along with him. At age 80, shared laughter may be the best medicine. Finally, ask about volunteer activities and involvement with others (altruism). Charting symptoms is important, but DSM-IV's Global Assessment of Functioning Scale also awards points for the presence of strengths, such as "is sought out by others because of his or her many positive qualities" (American Psychiatric Association 1994). If you're curious only about your patient's suffering, you may never know that he or she is volunteering at a soup kitchen—or, like Ben Aguilar at age 67, tending to even older neighbors.

3. *It's not all about death.* In our experience many clinicians erroneously name the approach of death as the overwhelming issue facing 80-year-olds. But in fact, late life is a diverse and interesting place. Most seniors have other concerns. Advance planning for the future (anticipation) is obviously prudent. But if an 80-year-old spends most of his or her time thinking about death, the person is probably depressed. Ask about sleep, appetite, energy, and regrets. Otherwise, ask about relationships, grand-

children, friendships, bridge games, and books. In therapy, fostering new goals is at least as important as traditional late-life psychotherapy tasks such as grieving losses, saying good-bye, or completing a life review. Develop the capacity for play. Exciting new choices may represent the beginning of a new chapter in life, not merely a manic defense against loss or a denial of death.

4. *Sometimes it's all about sex.* When the Study of Adult Development began its pilot study of late-life marriage, men and their wives reported that we were not asking enough about sex (R.J. Waldinger, personal communication, 2008). Our experience turns out to be typical. Studies consistently reveal that large numbers of older adults are sexually active, yet in the clinic physicians ask about sex far less often than their older patients would like (Lindau et al. 2007; Smith et al. 2007). Again, busy clinicians run the risk of overlooking a great source of joy in the lives of their elderly patients.

More generally, taking a competent social and relational history remains important in working with older adults, yet is easily overlooked. Take 5 minutes in an initial diagnostic interview to establish your patient's longest relationship and most satisfying job. A patient may be described responsibly as "a 72-year-old white female with a history of progressive dementia, hypertension, and elevated transaminase levels who presents with severe anxiety." But the experience becomes more powerful if you present that patient as "a popular, long-married high school math teacher who was forced to retire early as her memory failed and who began dipping into the sherry at home." If a patient's romantic life is in decline, a clinician should ask not only "When did the sex stop?" but "What made it good?" and "What was going right?" And although "How has your memory loss affected your marriage?" is a perfectly responsible question, your patient may come to life (or be moved to tears) if you ask, "Who has most touched your heart?" or "In your life, who has understood you best of all?"

In making use of this or any such list of recommendations, a few caveats are in order:

- First, clinicians interested in working with a patient's strengths need to be sensitive to context, timing, and mutuality. For example, as Leston Havens (1986, p. 115) reminds us, the self-recriminating patient may enter therapy "looking to find something bad about himself." Such a patient may feel the need to be "seen" and validated in his or her pathology; poorly timed praise may be experienced as an abandonment, or even as a value judgment, what Havens calls "a turning over of power and judgment to the therapist" (Havens 1986, p. 116). One's admiration for the patient should perhaps be used tentatively—not pronounced as a final verdict, but offered as the first step in an ongoing dance of mutuality.

- Similarly, if a clinician directs her or his attention exclusively to a patient's strengths, the clinician may well be perceived as a Pollyanna and may lose credibility with the patient. Hope needs to be realistic if it is to be helpful.

- Finally, in working with older adults, it is always wise to remember that individual differences in the aging process can be considerable. As Schaie (1990) notes, by age 85 almost all adults show a decline in at least one cognitive function, but few show declines in all. Recognize areas of specific competence for each individual, and tailor an approach that includes those areas.

Conclusion

Empirical study over the adult life span suggests that the adaptive coping styles or mature defenses—suppression, anticipation, sublimation, humor, and altruism—function as promoters of successful aging. By focusing on how their older patients deal with stress and change, including the aging process itself, clinicians can learn to recognize adaptive coping styles in the consulting room and on the hospital ward. Without minimizing pathology, clinicians interested in how a patient is coping can gracefully inquire about the patient's relationships and joys, thereby replacing a sterile DSM-IV checklist with a portrait of a three-dimensional human being. Such a collaborative effort, albeit undertaken late in the journey of life, can produce an inventory of strengths for the clinician and older patient to use together in the service of promoting resilience.

KEY POINTS

❚ *Adaptive coping style* (i.e., mature choice of ego mechanism of defense) is a key facet of mental health in midlife and predicts successful aging 25 years later.

❚ With practice, clinicians can begin to recognize examples of adaptive coping styles. These include *suppression* (stoicism), *sublimation* (channeling conflict into creative outlets), *humor, altruism*, and *anticipation*.

❚ *Adapt to slowness.* Older adults process information slowly, but the more important issue may be our own impatience with slowness. Be aware of any temptation to rush or to patronize.

■ *Recognize healthy coping.* Become familiar with the adaptive coping styles presented in Table 19–1, and then inquire how your patient dealt with his or her latest challenge at home. At times, your patient's use of suppression and humor may be more valuable than your own need to explore pathology.

■ *Ask about sex—and about relationships.* Many older adults are sexually active, but often we fail to ask about this source of joy. Take 5 minutes to establish your patient's current level of sexual activity, ask about his or her longest relationship, and also ask about the patient's most satisfying job.

■ *It's not all about death.* Most seniors have other concerns; exciting new choices need not be merely a manic defense against loss or a denial of death.

■ In summary, a gracefully conducted inquiry into coping, relationships, and joy can help replace a sterile DSM-IV checklist with a portrait of a unique, three-dimensional human being.

References

American Psychiatric Association: Diagnostic and Statistical Manual of Mental Disorders, 4th Edition. Washington, DC, American Psychiatric Association, 1994

Baltes PB, Mayer KV (eds): The Berlin Aging Study. Cambridge, UK, Cambridge University Press, 1999

Brown HN, Vaillant GE: Hypochondriasis. Arch Intern Med 141:723–726, 1981

Csikszentmihalyi M: Flow: The Psychology of Optimal Experience. New York, Harper & Row, 1990

Dunkin JJ, Amano SS: Psychological changes with normal aging, in Kaplan and Sadock's Comprehensive Textbook of Psychiatry, 8th Edition. Edited by Sadock BJ, Sadock VA. Philadelphia, PA, Lippincott Williams & Wilkins, 2005, pp 3624–3631

Erikson EH: Childhood and Society (1950), 2nd Edition. New York, WW Norton, 1963

Erikson EH: The human life cycle, in A Way of Looking at Things: Selected Papers From 1930 to 1980. Edited by Schlein S. New York, WW Norton, 1968, pp 595–610

Freud A: The Ego and the Mechanisms of Defence. London, Hogarth Press, 1937

Freud S: Fragment of an analysis of a case of hysteria (1905), in The Standard Edition of the Complete Psychological Works of Sigmund Freud, Vol. 7. Translated and edited by Strachey J. London, Hogarth Press, 1953, pp 1–122

Freud S: The ego and the id (1923), in The Standard Edition of the Complete Psychological Works of Sigmund Freud, Vol 19. Translated and edited by Strachey J. London, Hogarth Press, 1961, pp 1–66

Gay P: Freud: A Life for Our Time. New York, WW Norton, 1988

Haan N: Proposed model of ego functioning. Psychol Monogr 77:1–23, 1963

Hauser ST, Allen JP, Golden E: Out of the Woods: Tales of Resilient Teens. Cambridge, MA, Harvard University Press, 2006

Havens LH: Making Contact: Uses of Language in Psychotherapy. Cambridge, MA, Harvard University Press, 1986

Jones C, Meredith W: Developmental paths of psychological health from early adolescence to later adulthood. Psychol Aging 15:351–360, 2000

Lindau ST, Schumm LP, Laumann EO, et al: A study of sexuality and health among older adults in the United States. N Engl J Med 357:762–774, 2007

McDougall J: The artist and the outer world, in The Inner World in the Outer World. Edited by Shapiro ER. New Haven, CT, Yale University Press, 1997, pp 77–96

Roston D, Lee KA, Vaillant GE: A Q-sort approach to identifying defenses, in Ego Mechanisms of Defense: A Guide for Clinicians and Researchers. Edited by Vaillant GE. Washington, DC, American Psychiatric Press, 1992, pp 217–233

Razo S, Mazur H (eds): Semrad: The Heart of a Therapist. New York, Jason Aronson, 1980

Rutter M: Psychosocial resilience and protective mechanisms. Am J Orthopsychiatry 57:316–331, 1987

Schaie KW: The optimization of cognitive functioning in old age, in Successful Aging. Edited by Baltes PB, Baltes MM. Cambridge, UK, Cambridge University Press, 1990, pp 94–117

Seligman ME: Authentic Happiness: Using the New Positive Psychology to Realize Your Potential for Lasting Fulfillment. New York, Free Press, 2002

Semrad E: The organization of ego defenses and object loss, in The Loss of Loved Ones: The Effects of a Death in the Family on Personality Development. Edited by Moriarity DM. Springfield, IL, Charles C Thomas, 1967, pp 126–134

Smith JL, Mulhall JP, Deveci S, et al: Sex after seventy: a pilot study of sexual function in older persons. J Sex Med 4:1247–1253, 2007

Terman LR: Genetic Studies of Genius, Vol 1: Mental and Physical Traits of a Thousand Gifted Children. Palo Alto, CA, Stanford University Press, 1925

Vaillant GE: Natural history of male psychological health, V: the relation of choice of ego mechanisms of defense to adult adjustment. Arch Gen Psychiatry 33:535–545, 1976

Vaillant GE: The association of ancestral longevity with successful aging. J Gerontol 46:292–298, 1991

Vaillant GE: The beginning of wisdom is never calling a patient a borderline; or, the clinical management of immature defenses in the treatment of individuals with personality disorders. J Psychother Pract Res 1:117–134, 1992a

Vaillant GE (ed): Ego Mechanisms of Defense: A Guide for Clinicians and Researchers. Washington, DC, American Psychiatric Press, 1992b

Vaillant GE: The Wisdom of the Ego. Cambridge, MA, Harvard University Press, 1993

Vaillant GE, Drake RE: Maturity of ego defenses in relation to DSM-III Axis II personality disorder. Arch Gen Psychiatry 42:597–601, 1985

Vaillant GE, Mukamal K: Successful aging. Am J Psychiatry 158:839–847, 2001

Vaillant GE, Bond M, Vaillant CO: An empirically validated hierarchy of defense mechanisms. Arch Gen Psychiatry 43:786–794, 1986

Vaillant GE, DiRago AC, Mukamal K: Natural history of male psychological health, XV: retirement satisfaction. Am J Psychiatry 163:682–688, 2006

Recommended Readings

Vaillant GE: Natural history of male psychological health, V: the relation of choice of ego mechanisms of defense to adult adjustment. Arch Gen Psychiatry 33:535–545, 1976

Vaillant GE: The Wisdom of the Ego. Cambridge, MA, Harvard University Press, 1993

Vaillant GE, Mukamal K: Successful aging. Am J Psychiatry 158:839–847, 2001

20 Gaining Wisdom Through Multiage Learning

The Story of The Intergenerational School

Peter J. Whitehouse, M.D., Ph.D.
Danny R. George, A.B.D., M.Sc.
Catherine C. Whitehouse, Ph.D.

Aging successfully means various things to different individuals across different cultures. Success is relative to expectations and goals defined both idiosyncratically by members of society and by the conventions of a society itself. Alternative concepts encapsulating the notion of successful aging are profuse: *productive aging, positive aging,* and *conscious aging* have all been used to develop a sense of what the appropriate aspirations and behaviors of older individuals should entail.

Each concept, however, creates limits just as it attempts to liberate. Aging is of relevance throughout the life span and is not just something that people do as they near life's end stages. Aging takes place between birth and death (arguably even in utero), and thus there is no universal threshold at which someone is confronted with the opportunity to age successfully. In a country such as the United States, our successful aging discourse is socially constructed and mirrors our cultural obsession with material well-being, lifelong productivity, fear of death, and unbridled optimism in human possibility. In this chapter, we critique the limitations of the successful aging discourse and draw on the lessons we have learned at The Intergenerational School (TIS), an 8-year-old community charter school in Cleveland, Ohio, to develop a more integrative, life span–oriented conception of aging in the twenty-first century.

Caveats to the Concept of Successful Aging

There is some concern in the field that successful aging discourse has created a narrative that ignores the diverse ways in which people age and the range of limitations faced by many aging individuals (Martinson and Minkler 2006; Moody 2001). The multitude of successful aging models that have been created with the good intention of countering negative stereotypes and guiding individuals toward more salutary health outcomes has actually served to promote homogenized and proscriptive models of aging that emphasize individual responsibility; ignore the structural inequities that affect life course experiences, expectations, and late-life opportunities; and tend to frame "success" in terms of economic usefulness (Estes et al. 2003).

By creating proscriptive models for successful aging, we risk imposing negative value or even deviant status onto those who do not fit the mold. Because some may not possess sufficient amounts of personal resources (time, money, personal skills, knowledge, transportation, health, mobility, stamina) to allow them to participate at normative levels of social engagement , such a narrative is unfair. We must honor and support other experiences of aging without making absolute value judgments that productivity and community participation necessarily equate with successful aging. So, too, must we foster a sense that there are infinite pathways for self- and social development—we must not fall into the trap of assuming that everyone in our diverse society has the same personal and social priorities (Martinson and Minkler 2006). With these caveats in place, we present our vision for successful aging as it has emerged at TIS.

Aging and Wisdom

Perhaps one of the essential goals of aging enumerated in Western culture is the possibility of gaining wisdom or, as expressed in Eastern traditions, enlightenment. *Wisdom* is an elusive concept that involves the integration of knowledge and positive values through life experience (see also Chapter 6, "Wisdom: Definition, Assessment, and Relation to Successful Cognitive and Emotional Aging"). Wisdom itself has taken on a multitude of meanings over time; the Greeks, progenitors of the concept, believed that wisdom came in many forms—philosophical, practical, and even feminine (*sophia*). As part of the successful aging discourse, wisdom has come to include attributes such as the capacity for solving problems and making complex judgments, and possessing moral imagination and self-knowledge. But in its broadest sense, wisdom encompasses the notion that being able to assimilate life experience and apply it wisely in the world makes possible a larger contribution to the lives of others. Thus, although wisdom is often conventionally viewed as a rare property of a few, the more democratic concept of *collective wisdom* incorporates the idea that each of us is wise to a degree and that we gain wisdom primarily through relationships with others.

Most people know that wisdom is gained in many individualized ways—perhaps through formal education, or through conquering adversity—but there is also a sense that the creation of collective wisdom—for instance, the knowledge that humans have compiled about medicine, nature, technology, or ethics—is its most powerful emanation. Because we are never extricated from our communities, the opportunities to gain wisdom through experiential learning and to contribute to a larger wisdom over the course of our lives are always present. One essential aspect of wisdom that must not be forgotten is the recognition that there is a limit to our knowledge of the world and to knowledge in our own lives. Wisdom comes from knowing what we do not know (and perhaps cannot know) as well as what we do know. Personal morality provides both a limit to our biological existence and a source of inspiration for the value of our life and the lives of all living creatures.

A Collective Wisdom: Sustainability in the Twenty-First Century

With this larger, more integrative understanding of collective wisdom in mind, we would urge that there is an impetus to define *successful aging* in the context of larger global issues. The number of older people is rising dramatically around the world in both developed and developing countries. At the same time, the entire species is threatened by global warming and related health and environmental challenges. Our vulnerable populations—both the elderly and our children—will be subject to these challenges much more so than middle-aged adults. And so, in the twenty-first century, with questions of ecological sustainability taking on crucial importance, contributions to a collective wisdom are coveted now more than ever. Built into the basic notion of sustainability is an intergenerational ethic that asks older citizens, the current stewards of our earth, to leave behind ecosystems and societies that can meet the needs of the next generation and create opportunities for successful aging for them as well.

In order to realize a more holistic model of successful aging in this complex and increasingly troubled world, a variety of approaches can be adopted. According to mainstream medicine, especially as represented by molecular-oriented researchers and clinicians and multinational pharmaceutical companies, successful aging can be accomplished by managing disease, particularly through the use of multiple medications. Health is maintained by polypharmacy—the usage of multiple drugs. We are inundated with marketing pitches about successful aging that imply that with the right pills we can lead a near-perfect physical, emotional, and sexual life. Yet these claims are being made at a time when the numbers of actual new, effective chemical entities being developed are diminishing, and direct-to-consumer advertising expenditures are increasing. Moreover, we are coming to realize that our systems of monitoring the long-term safety of drugs are abysmal.

Information technology, perhaps more than biotechnology, provides many opportunities for both individuals and communities to thrive. Computers can connect us through social networking sites such as Facebook and YouTube. Symbiotic information processing between people and computers can assist our planning about the future through, for example, modeling ecosystems. Computers can teach us about the beauty of the world through distributed and shared music and photography. Interventions to improve cognitive abilities are focusing on use of computer learning programs (Smith et al. 2009). For instance, claims are being made by software vendors that if one sits in front of a computer and listens to and processes various sounds and sights, one can age more successfully, at least in a cognitive sense. Despite claims that such programs have been proven scientifically, the generalizability of benefits of such programs is uncertain. Certainly we can improve skills, but can we create practical incremental improvements in cognitive performance in daily life? The potential damage lies in people spending too much time trying to develop focused cognitive skills and ignoring holistic approaches to learning, especially of a social nature. Pseudoscience and exaggerated scientific claims are being used to foist products of uncertain value on an ill-informed public itching to "age successfully" through their consumer choices.

Quality of Life and Successful Aging

It is essential to underscore a basic truth: that the broadest, richest, and deepest concepts of successful aging relate to the individual in the larger context of society. Ample research has demonstrated that older people who have a sense of purpose associated with meaning in life and who interact to keep themselves cognitively and physically active with groups of other individuals are most likely to enjoy a higher quality of life (Morrow-Howell et al. 2003, 2005). Quality of life is a concept that is intimately related to and perhaps equally elusive as wisdom. From our perspective, attaining and enjoying a good quality of life would seem to depend on practical problem solving, having enduring values, relating well to others, and having expectations congruent with the likelihood of attaining one's goals. This goes far beyond pills or "successful aging" computer products.

Our approach to successful aging is integrative, ecological, and focused not only on individual life spans, but on the collective aging of humanity. Therefore, in this chapter we consider only in passing the individual biological or psychological approaches elaborated on elsewhere in this book. Whereas we do believe that appropriate attention to biological health and psychological abilities is reasonable, we also believe that these are overhyped in society at present, and that some of the richest approaches to successful aging involve lifelong learning across the generations with children. When so many children are living in poverty, do not have health insurance, and are dying around the world from preventable causes (such as a lack of clean water), it is a time for older adults to recognize the opportunities to age successfully by building relationships with, and with regard to, young people. Such an intergenerational perspective helps us view successful aging as a lifelong process undertaken by individuals in both local and shared ecological communities rather than as an end-of-life issue endured in the solitude of one's living room.

The Intergenerational School

TIS is the only known public intergenerational school in the world. The school's vision is to serve as a model to encourage and invigorate communities to create new environments that empower learners of all ages as they become lifelong contributors to a democratic society. Since its inception, TIS has broken new ground in innovative public education, and it continues to further its mission of fostering an educational community of excellence for learners of all ages. TIS began in 1998 as the brainchild of its three founders: Catherine C. Whitehouse, Ph.D., educator and developmental psychologist; Peter J. Whitehouse, M.D., Ph.D., a geriatrics authority from Case Western Reserve University; and Stephanie FallCreek, D.S.W., executive director of the Fairhill Center and an expert on successful aging. TIS is a free public charter school where families in the Cleveland area benefit from a unique, high-quality educational option. The desire of the school's founders to offer a school that challenges traditional concepts of age segregation and creates a community of learning where individuals, regardless of age, race, and socioeconomic factors, thrive and excel together remains the driving force of the organization.

TIS opened its doors to its first 32 young learners in August 2000 and has grown to serve 145 children in kindergarten through eighth grade, with continued expansion planned. TIS has grown from having three elder reading mentors and one long-term-care facility partner in its first year, to having more than 200 adult and older adult volunteers from numerous organizations who participate as an integral part of the school. (Adults include undergraduate and professional students from Case Western Reserve University and other educational institutions. Older adults, roughly defined as those over 65, come from the community and area residential facilities, such as Judson Park.) TIS is committed to providing a high-quality, developmentally appropriate education in a community of diverse participants. Its ultimate mission is to foster an educational community of excellence that provides experiences and skills for lifelong learning and spirited citizenship for learners of all ages.

TIS Model and Philosophy

TIS's unique developmental curriculum organizes instruction by learning stages (Emerging, Beginning, Developing, Refining, Applying, and Leadership) rather than traditional grade levels. The progressive curriculum was designed with an emphasis on student decision making, self-assessment, and fostering a lifelong love of learning by Catherine Whitehouse, who is the principal and chief educator. Students thrive in small (16 students per classroom), multiage classrooms based on individual learning needs. Students are able to learn in their own way and at their own pace, creating an individually tailored experience. This is in sharp contrast to arbitrary (in terms of learning levels), age-segregated grade levels. After each academic year, learning starts up again where it left off, precluding the need to repeat a grade or accelerate to a level for which a student may not be fully prepared. Students move progressively through the stages, meeting objectives and benchmarks based on mastery. This ensures that a solid foundation is being built as the student moves ahead. Extensive individual assessments are given frequently throughout the year to show clear evidence of progress, and as a public charter school, TIS also administers Ohio Achievement Tests yearly.

The educational philosophy behind the curriculum is held up by two pillars. The first is that learning is a lifelong developmental process. All members of the TIS family, regardless of age or background, are considered learners.

The second pillar is that knowledge is constructed in the context of culture, experience, and community. Differences are valued and respected and are often the impetus for further exploration and study. Teaching is holistic in that the whole student is considered, taking into account his or her existing knowledge, talents, culture, interests, attitudes, and experiences. Learning is also meaning based and constructivist. The emphasis is on process and problem solving as opposed to rote memorization. Each learner is actively engaged and proactively creates his or her own understandings, and TIS educators strive to meet each child where he or she is in his or her learning. Visitors to TIS classrooms often see students busy working on various tasks or projects either independently or in small groups, as opposed to the traditional teacher-led lessons where students are passive participants.

Another core feature is the values-driven culture of the school. TIS adopted a set of values that is woven into the fabric of the organization, from students in the classroom to the board of directors. These values include personal integrity, a work ethic, choice and accountability, celebration of diversity, interpersonal skills, shared and responsible use of resources, and honoring the interconnected web of life and time. Students are assessed on exhibiting these values throughout the year, and this assessment is communicated in each trimester's progress report along with the academic assessments. The schoolwide discipline plan holds students accountable for demonstrating these values daily. The presence of older adult volunteers throughout the school also helps to create an atmosphere of respect. Adults serve as reading mentors, computer learning partners, intergenerational gardeners, field trip participants, career development models, and examples of spirited citizens. Younger adultsm such as undergraduate honors students, nurses, and medical students, work on projects with TIS students that focus on learning through providing service to the community, such as in public health initiatives. For example, an interprofessional project involving nursing and medical students developed ways of raising the visibility of lead poisoning prevention programs. A strong emphasis on character development and service learning leads to an environment that is conducive to learning and achievement.

This new model of education has produced outstanding results for the children who attend, most of whom are poor and African American. Although one may question the merits of achievement test scores as an important measure of success, those scores have earned TIS a state ranking of "excellent" for the past 4 consecutive years. Indeed, TIS is the only charter school in Ohio with this record. As a result of this success in "closing the achievement gap," TIS has been recognized by the U.S. Department of Education and included as one of only seven charter schools highlighted in a recent publication (Center for Education Reform 2007). TIS was also recently featured in *The Achiever,* the U.S. Department of Education's newsletter, in an article entitled "Bridging the Gap, Ohio Charter School Surmounts Age, Achievement Barriers" (Ashby 2007). TIS is a member of Schools That Can, a selective national organization whose member schools provide excellence in urban education.

Multiage Learning in the TIS Community

It is not only the developmental model and progressive pedagogy that have led to these successes. The intergenerational learning model incorporates an atmosphere where learning takes place through relationships with the community. On a daily basis, a corps of regular volunteers, including retired seniors and other community members, share their time and wisdom with TIS students through intergenerational learning programs that include reading mentors, computer classes, museum exploration, gardening, and creating narrative histories. Each classroom also partners with a long-term-care facility for a yearlong schedule of visits, during which the children and residents interact through art, song, literature, and storytelling. The curriculum regularly integrates the exchange of older adult wisdom, the active involvement of the children's family members, and daily life connections to people of diverse backgrounds, often through service-oriented learning. All students are considered *mentors in training* as they learn and grow, and the oldest (Leadership stage) students work very closely with the youngest (Emerging stage) students during the school year.

Along with the TIS administration and teaching staff, Dr. Whitehouse has been instrumental in the development of many of the programs for adults. He has directed undergraduate honors and service learning programs and other projects with professional students (in medicine, nursing, law, and management) at TIS. Moreover, as a geriatric neurologist, he has encouraged the participation of his own patients and other elders as reading mentors and in other opportunities at TIS. Just as TIS has helped children learn in better ways, so too, we believe, has TIS offered adults not only opportunities for lifelong learning but a place to find purpose and meaning.

TIS is also an essential aspect of the authors' attempts to reframe the concept of *Alzheimer disease* (Whitehouse and George 2008; Whitehouse et al. 2000). The mainstream myth of Alzheimer disease is that it is a single condition unrelated to normal aging. In fact, very few experts believe that Alzheimer disease is one condition (Whitehouse and George 2008). At all levels of description, from genetic to neuropathological to clinical, Alzheimer disease represents a heterogeneous collection of processes. Moreover, these processes overlap and are probably coextensive with the processes of aging. Hence, those who are unfortunate enough to have their brains age particularly severely are said to have Alzheimer disease. The world is not divided into two groups of people—those with Alzheimer disease and those afraid of getting the disease. Rather, we all exist on a continuum of brain aging, a view that should inspire solidarity and hope rather than segregation and fear.

Evaluation of Intergenerational Programs in Relation to Successful Aging

Outcomes on standardized tests and other quantifiable measures have validated the range of benefits TIS confers on its young students (for more information on outcome measures, see www.tisonline.org). However, because the school extends the definition of *learner* to persons of all ages who participate in the pedagogical community—even older volunteers with age-related dementia—research has been undertaken to determine the benefits TIS may provide for its older mentors.

The Protective Pathways of Volunteering

For decades, the benefits of social activity have been inferred by social scientists. In his writings on suicide, Émile Durkheim (1897) observed that involvement in the community confers mental, physical, and spiritual benefits. Durkheim's linkage of suicide rates with the loss of social cohesion has been challenged (Kunitz 2004), but over the past several decades, a growing body of evidence in the gerontological literature has suggested that social participation has a positive correlative effect with mental and physical health outcomes, lower mortality rates, less morbidity, and a lower risk of cognitive decline (Bassuk et al. 1999; Bennett et al. 2003; Berkman and Breslow 1993; Fratiglioni et al. 2000; Menec 2003; Musick et al. 1999; Rowe and Kahn 1987, 1998; Seeman and Crimmins 2001; Stuck et al. 1999; Verghese et al. 2003, 2006; Zunzunegui et al. 2003).

Of the social activities found to be most protective, researchers have accumulated a solid evidence base to support the claim that volunteering promotes biopsychosocial well-being for older adults (Morrow-Howell et al. 2005). From a psychological standpoint, it has been suggested that volunteering may act to influence health by reducing depressive symptoms, anxiety, and stress, which are common in patients with dementia, and elevate levels of endogenous stress hormones that may be toxic to neurons at prolonged exposures (Hunter and Linn 1980–1981; Krause et al. 1992; Lyketsos et al. 1997; Morrow-Howell et al. 2003b). There is also evidence that volunteering provides social pathways that give the volunteer feelings of usefulness, growth, fulfillment, and self-respect (Monk 1995; Okun 1994) and protect the individual against role loss (Chambre 1987, 1993) and social isolation (Moen et al. 1992). By providing a strong and diverse social network, volunteering may render an individual more likely to seek professional care and other sources of information, guidance, and advice during times of mental or physical duress than individuals who do not engage in volunteer activities.

At the biological level, some have proposed that the basic human-to-human interaction engendered by volunteering may help preserve cognition throughout the course of brain aging by fortifying an individual's *cognitive reserve*—the capacity of neuronal connections to tolerate a greater amount of brain pathology such as the amyloid-β plaques and neurofibrillary tangles commonly held as the two hallmarks of so-called Alzheimer disease (but also found in normal aging) (Katzman et al. 1988; Scarmeas and Stern 2003, 2004; Unger et al. 1997; Welin et al. 1992). There is also evidence that acting altruistically may activate the body's cellular immune response, lower blood pressure and heart rate (Berkman 1995), and delay mortality (Harris and Thoresen 2005).

Existing knowledge is largely derived from longitudinal, nonexperimental research, which limits the ability to make causal inferences about volunteerism and biopsychosocial benefits. In other words, clarity is lacking as to whether social engagement causes wellness or whether persons with better health are more likely to be engaged. Randomized, controlled studies are desirable, but employing such rigorous research designs is challenging, time-consuming, and expensive. Over the course of the 2007–2008 school year, one of the authors (George) received grant funding from the University of Oxford and from the Shigeo and Megumi Takayama Foundation in Japan (through Whitehouse) that supported a yearlong randomized, controlled study to assess how five biopsychosocial variables that the World Health Organization (1993) declares relevant to quality of life—cognitive functioning, stress, depression, sense of purpose, and sense of usefulness—are influenced by intergenerational volunteering at TIS among individuals with mild to moderate dementia.

Engaging Local Partnerships to Measure the Benefits of Intergenerational Volunteering

Successful aging is a community undertaking. Thus, in conducting the research described in the previous subsection, a partnership has been forged with Judson Park, a local assisted-living facility in Cleveland. Sixteen Judson Park residents, all of whom have been diagnosed with clinical dementia, and two of whom reside in the locked unit for residents diagnosed with Alzheimer disease, were recruited and randomly assigned to one of two groups: an intervention group of eight persons who volunteered at TIS for 1 hour per week, and a control group of eight persons who participated in a biweekly educational seminar at Judson Park. To address the complexities of this study, a variety of mixed methods—spanning psychometric data (the Mini-Mental State Examination, the Beck Depression Inventory, and the Beck Anxiety Inventory), narrative data from one-on-one interviews and focus groups, and ethnographic data from participant-observation fieldwork—have been employed. There are early signals that suggest intergenerational volunteering may indeed promote quality of life, especially through the mechanism of decreased stress. The population size in our pilot study is small, and future studies must include more participants—nevertheless, research is beginning to evince the range of benefits conferred by intergenerational volunteering.

Discussion: The Future of Intergenerational Learning

Intergenerational learning is hardly a novel concept. It is embodied in all families, particularly extended families, which have existed as kinship patterns for countless centuries across all societies. However, international trends toward urbanization are creating situations in which parents and children may move to urban centers seeking better employment, leaving older adults in rural settings. Hence, developing new community-based opportunities for intergenerational learning has appeal in many countries. For example, Japanese society is reorienting toward different conceptions of aging (e.g., focusing on the development of children- and elder-friendly communities), motivated particularly by the reduction in Japan's population due to the low birth rate and extended longevity. TIS is currently collaborating with an afterschool program in Tokyo, St. Luke's College of Nursing Afterschool Program, which involves middle school students and elders of various sages. Even in Finland, which has excellent public schools, the concept of intergenerational learning has prompted interest as a possible response to what they call the loss of *silent knowledge,* the knowledge of elders that may not be passed on to young children, which might also be referred to as *wisdom.*

Intergenerational learning will also create new opportunities for resituating schools at the epicenter of vibrant communities. Schools can become the heart of intergenerational neighborhoods, in which civic life is viewed as a more explicitly lifelong process and where sharing across generations and building collective knowledge are sought after rather than learning in isolation. Such environments can actively create collective wisdom that will help our species face the mounting challenges of the twenty-first century. The future of our world will depend on many factors that are being dramatically affected by global warming. Health, viewed as psychosocial well-being rather than just a biological state, requires not only a health care system, but the entire society to focus on the well-being of all its citizens. Intergenerational schools could play a central role in improving public health. For example, in Cleveland, TIS students and volunteers worked on a project teaching them about lead abatement strategies. Lead poisoning is a threat not only to children, but to older adults as well. Toxins, including lead, likely contribute to late-life dementia; for example, early exposure to lead kills nerve cells, which diminishes cognitive reserve in later years. There is evidence in animal models that lead exposure early in life leads to the overexpression of amyloid-β protein in adult brains, which may play a role in the neuronal death observed in the dementia of so-called Alzheimer disease (Basha et al. 2005; Wu et al. 2008).

Intergenerational learning communities could also contribute to making the world of commerce healthier. Business is rapidly developing opportunities for creating sustainable enterprises that make profits by providing products and services that save energy and improve lives and communities. Schools can actively encourage students to understand the world of business. Students can learn to appreciate as both consumers and potential entrepreneurs how businesses can better attend to their environmental impact, avoid greenwashing (marketing false images of a company's ecological consciousness), and contribute to true sustainability.

Any form of education in the future needs to address the role of information technology. Such technology can support the development of relationships between schools and communities, between current students and alumni, and even between students on different continents. Multimedia narrative can be used as a form of education not only within a school but also on the Internet through the emerging social networking tools of the Web 2.0 world. Thus intergenerational learning communities can provide opportunities for positive aging in many different settings with different age groups using different technologies. At the heart will be the creation of collective wisdom to facilitate lifelong learning and community solidarity.

Conclusion

The future of intergenerational learning will be built around deeper intergenerational ethics. By bringing people together to learn how to address community challenges—of both the social and the natural variety—intergenerational schools can create a sense of historical perspective in young people, while concurrently giving older adults an important sense of contributing to a legacy for the future. If we are to survive as a species, we must learn to think more broadly and deeply across longer ecological life spans. In aspiring to new heights for our cognitive and emotional lives, we must learn to tell richer stories in which successful aging is viewed from a lifelong perspective and as a process that is based on meaningful relationships among individuals and with our natural surroundings.

KEY POINTS

- There are infinite pathways for successful aging—we must not fall into the trap of assuming that everyone in our diverse society has the same personal and social priorities.

- Opportunities to gain wisdom through experiential learning and to contribute to a larger wisdom over the course of our lives are always present.

- An intergenerational ethic asks older citizens, the current stewards of our earth, to leave behind ecosystems and societies that can meet the needs of, and create opportunities for successful aging for, the next generation.

- The broadest, richest, and deepest concepts of successful aging relate to the individual in the larger context of society.

- The world is not divided into two groups of people—those with Alzheimer disease and those afraid of getting the disease. Rather, we all exist on a continuum of brain aging, a view that should inspire solidarity and hope rather than segregation and fear.

- Intergenerational learning can create new opportunities for making our communities more vibrant and sustainable. The future of our society will be built around deeper intergenerational ethics.

- Research conducted at TIS in Cleveland, Ohio, and elsewhere is beginning to evince the range of benefits conferred by intergenerational volunteering, both for older individuals and for communities at large.

References

Ashby N: Bridging the gap: Ohio charter school surmounts age, acheivement barriers. The Achiever 6(7), 2007. Available at: http://www.ed.gov/news/newsletters/achiever/2007/0907.html#2. Accessed June 29, 2009.

Basha MR, Wei W, Bakheet SA, et al: The fetal basis of amyloidogenesis: exposure to lead and latent overexpression of amyloid precursor protein and beta-amyloid in the aging brain. J Neurosci 25:823–829, 2005

Bassuk SS, Glass TA, Berkman LF: Social disengagement and incident cognitive decline in community-dwelling elderly persons. Ann Intern Med 131:165–173, 1999

Bennett DA, Wilson RS, Schneider JA, et al: Education modifies the relation of AD pathology to level of cognitive function in older persons. Neurology 60:1909–1915, 2003

Berkman LF: The role of social relations in health promotion. Psychosom Med 57:245–254, 1995

Berkman LF, Breslow L: Health and Ways of Living: The Alameda County Study. New York, Oxford University Press, 1983, pp 83-85

Center for Education Reform: Stories of Inspiration, Struggle, and Success. Washington, DC, U.S. Department of Education, 2007

Chambre SM: Good Deeds in Old Age: Volunteering by the New Leisure Class. Lexington, MA, Lexington Books, 1987

Chambre SM: Volunteerism by elders: past trends and future prospects. Gerontologist 33:221–228, 1993

Durkheim É: Le suicide: étude de sociologie [Suicide: Study in Sociology]. Paris, Alcan, 1897

Estes C, Biggs S, Phillipson C: Social Theory, Social Policy and Ageing: A Critical Introduction. London, Open University Press, 2003

Fratiglioni L, Wang HX, Ericsson K, et al: Influence of social network on occurrence of dementia: a community-based longitudinal study. Lancet 355:1315–1319, 2000

Harris AH, Thoresen CE: Volunteering is associated with delayed mortality in older people: analysis of the Longitudinal Study of Aging. J Health Psychol 10:739–752, 2005

Hunter KI, Linn MW: Psychosocial differences between elderly volunteers and non-volunteers. Int J Aging Hum Dev 12:205–213, 1980–1981

Katzman R, Terry R, DeTeresa R, et al: Clinical, pathological, and neurochemical changes in dementia: a subgroup with preserved mental status and numerous neocortical plaques. Ann Neurol 23:138–144, 1988

Krause N, Herzog AR, Baker E: Providing support to others and well-being in later life. J Gerontol 47:P300–P311, 1992

Kunitz SJ: Social capital and health. Br Med Bull 69:61–73, 2004

Lyketsos CG, Steele C, Baker L, et al: Major and minor depression in Alzheimer's disease: prevalence and impact. J Neuropsychiatry Clin Neurosci 9:556–561, 1997

Martinson M, Minkler M: Civic engagement and older adults: a critical perspective. Gerontologist 46:318–324, 2006

Menec V: The relation between everyday activities and successful aging: a 6-year longitudinal study. J Gerontol B Psychol Sci Soc Sci 58:S74–S82, 2003

Moen P, Dempster-McClain DD, Williams RM: Successful aging: a life-course perspective on women's multiple roles and health. American Journal of Sociology 97:1612-1638, 1992

Monk A: Volunteerism, in The Encyclopedia of Aging. Edited by Maddox GL. New York, Springer, 1995, pp 958–960

Moody HR: Productive aging and the ideology of old age, in Productive Aging: Concepts and Challenges. Edited by Morrow-Howell N, Hinterlong J, Sherraden M. Baltimore, MD, Johns Hopkins University Press, 2001, pp 175–197

Morrow-Howell N, Hinterlong J, Rozario PA, et al: Effects of volunteering on the well-being of older adults. J Gerontol B Psychol Sci Soc Sci 58(3):S137-S145, 2003

Morrow-Howell N, Carden M, Sherraden M: Volunteerism, philanthropy, and service, in Perspectives on Productive Aging: Social Work With the New Aged. Edited by Kaye LW. Washington DC, NASW Press, 2005, pp 245–259

Musick MA, Herzog AR, House JS: Volunteering and mortality among older adults: findings from a national sample. J Gerontol B Psychol Sci Soc Sci 54:S173–S180, 1999

Okun M: The relation between motives for organizational volunteering and frequency of volunteering by elders. J Appl Gerontol 13:115–126, 1994

Rowe JW, Kahn RL: Human aging: usual and successful. Science 237:143–149, 1987

Rowe JW, Kahn RL: Successful aging. Aging (Milano) 10:142–144, 1998

Scarmeas N, Stern Y: Cognitive reserve and lifestyle. J Clin Exp Neuropsychol 25:625-633, 2003

Scarmeas N, Stern Y: Cognitive reserve: implications for diagnosis and prevention of Alzheimer's disease. Curr Neurol Neurosci Rep 4:374–380, 2004

Seeman TE, Crimmins E: Social environment effects on health and aging: integrating epidemiologic and demographic approaches and perspectives. Ann NY Acad Sci 954:88–117, 2001

Smith GE, Housen P, Yaffe K, et al: A cognitive training program based on principles of brain plasticity: results from the Improvement in Memory with Plasticity-based Adaptive Cognitive Training (IMPACT) study. J Am Geriatr Soc 57:594–603, 2009

Stuck AE, Walthert JM, Nikolaus T, et al: Risk factors for functional status decline in community-living elderly people: a systematic literature review. Soc Sci Med 48:445–469, 1999

Unger JB, Johnson CA, Marks G: Functional decline in the elderly: evidence for direct and stress-buffering protective effects of social interactions and physical activity. Ann Behav Med 19:152–160, 1997

Verghese J, Lipton RB, Katz MJ, et al: Leisure activities and the risk of dementia in the elderly. N Engl J Med 348:2508–2516, 2003

Verghese J, LeValley A, Derby C, et al: Leisure activities and the risk of amnestic cognitive impairment in the elderly. Neurology 66:821–827, 2006

Welin L, Larsson B, Svärdsudd K, et al: Social network and activities in relation to mortality from cardiovascular diseases, cancer and other causes—a 12 year follow up of the study of men born in 1913 and 1923. J Epidemiol Community Health 46:127–132, 1992

Whitehouse PJ, George DR: The Myth of Alzheimer's: What You Aren't Being Told About Today's Most Dreaded Diagnosis. New York, St Martin's Press, 2008

Whitehouse PJ, Maurer K, Ballenger JF (eds): Concepts of Alzheimer Disease: Biological, Clinical and Cultural Perspectives. Baltimore, MD, Johns Hopkins University Press, 2000

World Health Organization: Measuring quality of life: the development of the World Health Organization Quality of Life Instrument (WHOQOL). Geneva, World Health Organization, 1993

Wu J, Basha MR, Brock B, et al: Alzheimer's disease (AD)–like pathology in aged monkeys after infantile exposure to environmental metal lead (Pb): evidence for a developmental origin and environmental link for AD. J Neurosci 28:3–9, 2008

Zunzunegui MV, Alvarado BE, Del Ser T, et al: Social networks, social integration, and social engagement determine cognitive decline in community-dwelling Spanish older adults. J Gerontol B Psychol Sci Soc Sci 58:S93–S100, 2003

Recommended Readings and Web Sites

Whitehouse PJ, George DR: The Myth of Alzheimer's: What You Aren't Being Told About Today's Most Dreaded Diagnosis. New York, St Martin's Press, 2008

Whitehouse PJ, George DR: The Myth of Alzheimer's: What You Aren't Being Told About Today's Most Dreaded Diagnosis. New York, St Martin's Press, 2008; http://www.themythofalzheimers.com

The Intergenerational School: http://www.tisonline.org

21 Epilogue

Dilip V. Jeste, M.D.
Colin A. Depp, Ph.D.

For the busy practitioner who may or may not yet be an older adult, we hope that this volume has yielded some useful insights as to how the science of successful aging can be applied in his or her own daily life, as well using these insights to counsel patients. These chapters remind us that we are only in the early stages of understanding how to maintain and thrive as an aging person in the twenty-first century, and although there are many promising leads, much remains to be done in terms of translating basic science to empirically based treatments. In many ways, we still do not have satisfactory answers to the fundamental questions of why we age and what we can do about it. Furthermore, exact definitions of successful cognitive and emotional aging are not agreed on by researchers and laypeople. How processes such as compensation and resilience can lead to successful aging remains uncertain, along with the multiple other paths to attaining success described in this text.

Nevertheless, the chapters in this book do indicate that there are some compelling pieces of evidence that can be used to promote successful cognitive and emotional aging. Just as basic scientists are beginning to uncover fundamental roots of the aging process that cut across diseases and syndromes, there appear to be some common recommendations that can enhance the probability of aging well (at any age). Even if we cannot, and perhaps should not, define who among older adults can be described as having aged successfully, there are risk factors and protective factors, along with interventions derived from randomized, controlled trials, that guide us toward the ways to modify cognitive and emotional aging. We have compiled below a list of some of these strategies, applicable to a large majority of the population. As Cutler and Mattson (2006) point out, many human faculties, such as muscle strength and respiratory volume, peak at ages younger than 20 years. Therefore, it is never too early nor too late to try following some of the recommendations below.

Strategies for Successful Aging

Physical Activity

1. Engage in regular aerobic physical exercise—moderate exercise for 30 minutes five times per week or 25 minutes of vigorous exercise three times a week.
2. Stretch every day.
3. Do strength-building activities two to three times per week.
4. Attend to (and address) barriers to physical activity in the built environment (e.g., steps without handrails).

Nutrition

5. Follow the food pyramid.
6. Eat colorful vegetables and fruit (e.g., broccoli, kale, blueberries).
7. Take multivitamins.
8. Follow the research on dietary supplements and be mindful of upper limits.
9. Stay hydrated and know that perception of thirst may change with age.
10. Consider caloric restriction or at least limit dietary intake to recommended levels.

Health Hygiene

11. Don't smoke or use tobacco products.
12. If you choose to drink alcoholic beverages, drink to a moderate degree but no more than what is recommended or allowed by your physician.
13. Practice good sleep hygiene.
14. Treat sleep apnea.
15. Keep a healthy skepticism about claims regarding antiaging supplements, products, and procedures.
16. Follow recommendations for screening for cancers and other chronic illnesses to catch problems early.

Cognitive Stimulation

17. Engage in cognitively stimulating work.
18. Attain as high a level of education as possible.

19. Consider yourself a lifelong learner and utilize community resources for continuing education.
20. Work or volunteer in something meaningful to you and your community.
21. Take part in intergenerational programs.
22. Keep in mind that not all cognitive abilities decline with age.
23. Recall that the brain retains a remarkable level of plasticity in older age.
24. Engage in cognitively stimulating leisure activities that are novel and challenging.
25. Remember that cognitive changes can sometimes be mitigated by taking one's time, using memory aids, and having a healthy lifestyle.
26. Be aware of signs such as difficulty driving, getting lost, and impairment in day-to-day functioning, and seek a medical evaluation.
27. Try a "brain training" program but don't spend too much money on it, and don't let it get in the way of other meaningful activities.

Social/Pleasant Activity

28. Be a part of a social organization, such as a club, sports league, spiritual/religious organization, or class.
29. Spend some time with other people every day.
30. Try to maintain a ratio of three pleasant activities to one negative activity.
31. If an activity that used to be enjoyed can no longer be performed at the same level (e.g., bridge, strenuous sports), adapt or adopt a new activity.
32. Seek help for depressive symptoms and be sure depression is treated aggressively.
33. Consider, and, if appropriate, enhance, the role of spirituality in your life.

Coping

34. Consider your strengths, including those that have developed out of hardships you have experienced.
35. Maintain a positive attitude toward aging and be mindful of negative aging-related stereotypes that exist.
36. Study developments in the evidence for the safety and efficacy of cognition-enhancing and mood-enhancing medications before initiating such treatments.
37. Remember that optimistic people tend to live longer.
38. Employ the coping strategies of humor, sublimation, and sometimes even suppression.

Stress Management

39. Avoid prolonged exposure to stress if possible.
40. If stress is unavoidable, such as in caregiving, structure respite periods, engage in support groups, and learn to handle problem behaviors.

Beyond these 40 suggestions, we hope that readers of this book have found many more opportunities to enhance their own and their loved ones' likelihood of healthy aging. Although there are many legitimate economic and other societal concerns about the aging of the population, it is important to recognize that the rapid increase in the human life span that we are seeing represents a remarkable achievement. Scientific and cultural revolutions will teach us much in the coming years about how one can live a long, healthy, happy, and socially and intellectually engaging life—we hope that this book, even if in a very small way, contributes to these efforts. In doing so, we expect that the foretold "gray tsunami" that some people are concerned about can instead be turned into a "golden revolution."

References

Cutler RG, Mattson MP: The adversities of aging. Ageing Res Rev 5:221–238, 2006

Index

*Page numbers printed in **boldface** type refer to tables or figures.*